Whittingham's text is a rich, accessible, and creative synthesis of the evidence base that guides the expert practice of focused brief group therapy (FBGT). FBGT is tailored to real-world, time-sensitive, clinical environments. The FBGT model comes to life through Whittingham's illuminating the central importance of interpersonal communication and connectedness, and the powerful ways group therapy fosters that connectedness. This book will be of great value to both beginners and experienced group therapists, students, and teachers.

—**Molyn Leszcz, MD, FRCPC, CGP, AGPA-DF,** Professor of Psychiatry, University of Toronto, Toronto, Ontario, Canada, and Past-President, American Group Psychotherapy Association

This book is an incredible resource for group therapists of all levels of experience—from graduate students to advanced group therapists. Whittingham seamlessly integrates evidence-based theories and assessment into a new model of focused brief group psychotherapy that offers short-term group treatment to people with diverse needs, including interpersonal struggles and loneliness. His model can be applied to groups in private practice, counseling centers, and hospital settings. He focuses on research-based assessment, thoughtful screening strategies, and important interventions for before and after group therapy begins. Readers will be able to quickly apply his model as he has provided many interesting and useful clinical examples throughout his book. I will definitely recommend this book to my students learning group therapy and to colleagues who are looking to strengthen their group practice.

—**Cheri L. Marmarosh, PhD,** licensed psychologist in private practice and associate professor, George Washington University, Washington, DC, United States

Whittingham takes an empirically sound model of interpersonal interactions and applies it skillfully to create an innovative brief focused group therapy. This book is a must-read for anyone who wants to do brief group therapy that goes beyond simply educating patients and that harnesses the power of groups to create lasting change. Whittingham blends the best research evidence and clinical wisdom in his focused brief group therapy model.

—**Giorgio A. Tasca, PhD,** Professor, University of Ottawa, Ottawa, Ontario, Canada

W0193387

FOCUSED BRIEF GROUP THERAPY

FOCUSED BRIEF GROUP THERAPY

An Integrative Approach to Reducing Interpersonal Distress

MARTYN WHITTINGHAM

 AMERICAN PSYCHOLOGICAL ASSOCIATION

Published by
American Psychological Association
750 First Street, NE
Washington, DC 20002
https://www.apa.org

Order Department
https://www.apa.org/pubs/books
order@apa.org

Typeset in Charter and Interstate by Circle Graphics, Inc., Reisterstown, MD

Printer: Lake Book Manufacturing, Melrose Park, IL
Cover Designer: Beth Schlenoff, Beth Schlenoff Design, Bethesda, MD

Library of Congress Cataloging-in-Publication Data

Names: Whittingham, Martyn, author.
Title: Focused brief group therapy : an integrative approach to reducing
  interpersonal distress / Martyn Whittingham.
Description: Washington, DC : American Psychological Association, [2024] |
  Includes bibliographical references and index.
Identifiers: LCCN 2023017213 (print) | LCCN 2023017214 (ebook) |
  ISBN 9781433836510 (paperback) | ISBN 9781433841040 (epub)
Subjects: LCSH: Group psychotherapy. | Brief psychotherapy. |
  BISAC: PSYCHOLOGY / Psychotherapy / Group | PSYCHOLOGY / Psychotherapy /
  Counseling
Classification: LCC RC488 .W474 2023 (print) | LCC RC488 (ebook) |
  DDC 616.89/152--dc23/eng/20230710
LC record available at https://lccn.loc.gov/2023017213
LC ebook record available at https://lccn.loc.gov/2023017214

https://doi.org/10.1037/0000389-000

Printed in the United States of America

10 9 8 7 6 5 4 3 2 1

For Felisa and Felisa Iris

Contents

Preface

In 2006, the group program at Wright State University (WSU) Counseling and Wellness Services had not been running well, so I was tasked—as a new faculty member—to help inject new life into it. My initial responsibility was to ensure groups began, ran well, and could take clients with a wide variety of presenting problems and diagnoses. I looked to Yalom and Leszcz's (2020) work for inspiration. Students loved to learn Yalom and Leszcz's method of group therapy within an interpersonal framework, and clients enjoyed the vitality and energy of interacting with each other in real time using the group process as a force for change. The method held students' interest and gave them a deep dive into the art of therapy that was beyond the didactic teaching that comprises many manualized approaches.

The WSU campus is diverse, having significant numbers of students from minoritized backgrounds who attend the counseling center. WSU also has a larger percentage of students with disabilities than is found on most campuses. Major restrictions on the setting at the time, though, were that WSU ran on the quarter system, which was only 10 weeks long, and it was a commuter campus, meaning students were seldom able to continue groups from one quarter to the next. So, groups had to begin, run, and finish within those 10 weeks.

The challenge was whether anything meaningful could actually happen in a dynamic model in such a short time. Yalom's (Yalom & Leszcz, 2020) one-session agenda model suggests that a brief, inpatient, interpersonal process could be meaningful, and the literature on brief groups (Piper & Ogrodniczuk,

2004) also offers guidelines for best practices. Moreover, my own dissertation work (Whittingham, 2007) had left me fascinated by the interpersonal circumplex, which I had always thought might have clinical value if it were applied within a person-centered framework. It also needed to be multiculturally responsive.

So, I developed the focused brief group therapy (FBGT) model and researched it using a client group comprising around 30% of clients identifying as people of color. The largest group identified as African American, and smaller percentages of clients identified as Latinx and Asian American. However, race and ethnicity were only a part of the picture; important issues related to marginalized intersectional identities also informed how to deliver treatment.

To ensure the model was effective, I researched every group from multiple different perspectives: conducting clinical observations via live supervision; looking at screening, process, and outcome data; obtaining client feedback during debriefing; seeking group leader input (many of whom were practicum students or interns); reviewing multiple student dissertations that explored effectiveness; and using something I ended up labeling as "failure analysis." *Failure analysis* is the examination of every problematic outcome from multiple perspectives to prevent self-serving bias from being used to explain away any treatment failures, an issue that can sometimes occur when therapists are seeking closure (Dandachi-FitzGerald et al., 2021). Exercising care to avoid any self-serving bias that "the client wasn't ready for change" or that "they got what they needed," I was able to treat every problematic outcome with a rigorous analysis that led to many of the techniques and refinements in FBGT, such as inoculation, habituation, and other model-specific innovations found in this text.

From the beginning, I designed FBGT to work in real-world practice settings. Many of the techniques and innovations in the approach came not from asking how to treat a specific condition but, rather, how to ensure that effective treatment starts, reduces dropout, and finishes with evidence of outcomes at the local level for people with a broad range of presenting problems and diagnoses. Therefore, issues such as ensuring client retention and individualized success took primacy.

Acknowledgments

Many people have influenced this model—focused brief group therapy (FBGT)—and its development. Going back to the very start, mentor and guide Rex Stockton stoked my passion for group therapy, and his research on feedback impacted how this is delivered in FBGT. The intellectual progenitors of FBGT—Don Kiesler, Dennis Kivlighan, Len Horowitz, Aaron Pincus, Rex Stockton, Bill Piper, Gary Burlingame, Irv Yalom, and Molyn Leszcz—have been an inspiration.

So, FBGT began. Erin Frick, my colleague at Wright State University, was the initial sounding board for the ideas and helped run some of the first groups. A skillful group therapist who was a major part of the initial implementation, she was endlessly supportive as well. Her input and skills were invaluable. Several of my trainees, notably, Jennifer Lotz and later Jordan Allison, also contributed to the development of FBGT. Jennifer created the first beta version of the manual under my guidance, an effort that became an important milestone and was vital in training new leaders. She also coined the term "Going for Goldilocks," which refers to the search for the optimal level of anxiety (see Chapter 6). Jordan practiced, researched, and presented with me for several years and showed considerable clinical skill in doing so. Jordan as well as multiple other students, including Sarah Rotsinger-Stemen, Kacey Greening, David Yutrezenka, and Michelle Sobon, contributed important insights from research dissertations they undertook; the resulting insights added important information and data that helped me refine the model.

Myriad colleagues at WSU, in American Psychological Association (APA) Division 49 (Society of Group Psychology and Group Psychotherapy), and in the American Group Psychotherapy Association offered encouragement, commentary, and constructive criticism, all of which are important in ensuring a model is well thought out. The input of Dennis Kivlighan, Gary Burlingame, Phil Flores, George Tasca, Daniela Burnworth, and others has never failed to make me think. Cheri Marmarosh also provided considerable inspiration with her writing on attachment theory as well as her feedback and thoughts on FBGT. She remains a wonderfully supportive colleague and friend.

Ming "Grace" Zhou and Shi Min Liew, with whom I worked with in China and Singapore, respectively, have proven invaluable partners in helping me understand cross-cultural differences as they apply to FBGT. They also have helped me to continually appreciate the ongoing need for cultural humility. Thanks also go to Jian Xing and Changzhi "Ben" Li from the China Institute of Psychology; both have been wonderful partners in promoting and training FBGT therapists in China.

Len Horowitz also gave generously of his time by consulting on the nuances of the interpersonal circumplex and consistently offering his encouragement. His passing in 2019 was a great loss to the field. Most recently, Molyn Leszcz and Irv Yalom have generously provided their support and encouragement of this work, and I have found their wisdom and counsel invaluable.

I also thank all the workshop participants in the United States, China, and Singapore for sharing your thoughts not only about the nuances of the FBGT model, but also about cultural adaptations. I never fail to learn something new from participants, and I look forward to doing so for many years to come.

Over the years, many others have provided feedback, or their work has served as an inspiration. Thanks to all of you for your work, your dedication to the field, and your contributions.

I thank friends who have continued to offer me encouragement and support as a person and professional throughout this process of developing the model. In particular, Rick Browne, Amy Nitza, and Cheri Marmarosh have been wonderful friends and supporters during both the celebrations and challenges that have come my way during this process. Your friendship has been invaluable.

Thanks go to the APA staff for their ongoing belief in this project. For their patience, support, and guidance in completing this project, I thank Susan Reynolds, acquisitions editor; Ida Audeh, development editor; Elizabeth Brace, production editor; and Laurel Vincenty, copyeditor.

Finally, thanks to my family for all their support throughout the process of developing and growing the model. To my parents and brother: Thank you. Your support of me through my journey has made everything possible. Most of all, thanks to Felisa, my always encouraging wife, and to Felisa Iris, my wonderful daughter. You both are the inspiration for so much of what I do.

FOCUSED BRIEF GROUP THERAPY

INTRODUCTION
Overview and Rationale

Relationships provide the fuel for our happiness. Longitudinal data from Harvard's study of adult development (Waldinger & Schulz, 2023) showed that the most significant factor in lifelong happiness is the quality of social relationships. The authors described the concept of *social fitness*—of being able to navigate relationships successfully—as an essential component of that journey. Thus, our lifelong happiness is significantly determined by how successful we are in establishing and maintaining high-quality relationships. However, problems in relationships can also prove problematic to people's well-being. Such problems have been particularly pronounced in recent years: Loneliness, for example, has been described as an epidemic (Weissbourd et al., n.d.).

INTERPERSONAL RELATIONSHIPS AND MENTAL HEALTH

The importance of interpersonal relationships has catapulted into the public consciousness in the past decade. In a summary of loneliness research, Heu et al. (2019) reported that loneliness increased in the United States from

11% to 17% in the 1970s to more than 40% for those middle-aged and older in the 2010s. They also pointed out similar increases internationally. COVID-19 lockdowns brought a heightened focus on the role of loneliness in mental health. People locked down in their homes were unable to establish or maintain the social relationships necessary for their sense of well-being; as a result, mental health problems worsened across the world (Ernst et al., 2022; T. Wu et al., 2021). Concerns emerged that loneliness would cause significant increases in mental health problems (Killgore et al., 2020). This focus on the connection between relationship quality and mental health honed in on how interpersonal relationships contribute to one's mental health.

Loneliness

Mental health problems are closely tied to poor relationships and loneliness, and research has shown that loneliness is linked to everything from depression, suicidality, and social anxiety disorders to personality disorders (Beutel et al., 2017; Lutz et al., 2020). As Marmarosh et al. (2009) pointed out in their review of the literature, attachment style—the corollary of interpersonal style—has shown that insecure attachment impacts how people cope with stress (Mikulincer, 1998), regulate affect (Fonagy, 1999; Fonagy & Target, 1997; Fonagy et al., 2002, F. G. Lopez & Brennan, 2000; Schore, 2000), how they relate to romantic partners (Collins, 1996; Collins & Read, 1990; Mikulincer, 1995, 1998), how people deal with conflict in close relationships (Simpson et al., 1996), and how they deal with the transition to adulthood (Rholes et al., 2001). Further, depression, substance abuse, eating disorders, and suicidal ideation all have links to problems with attachment (Dozier et al., 1999; Flores, 2006).

The link to suicidal ideation is particularly notable. Studies have shown that increased levels of suicidal ideation relate to thwarted belonging and loneliness (Ogrodniczuk et al., 2023); that is, people's inability to meet their needs in terms of desire for relational connection was strongly related to thoughts of suicide. As Klonsky et al. (2021) described in their three-step model of suicide, now one of the most cited models in suicide research and treatment, "Whereas pain provides the push away from life (Step 1), connectedness provides the pull toward life (Step 2). Thus, connectedness can make life worth living (despite the presence of pain that is not expected to abate)" (p. 2). They found that pain *plus* loneliness and then lack of connections to others were responsible for two of the three steps toward suicide (with the third step being capability). Thus, connectedness and belonging form important mediating and protective factors against an increase in suicidal ideation. Satisfying relationships make us more resilient.

Rejection and Pain

Social connection is also something that can be broken, and the consequences can be equally deleterious. Research has shown that social pain, such as rejection, ostracism, and betrayal, lasts far longer in the memory than physical pain (Meyer et al., 2015). Social pain leaves an indelible mark that people can relive throughout their lifespan. The pain of exclusion, according to research, mirrors that of physical pain in our brains (Eisenberger et al., 2003; Kross et al., 2011).

Relationship Quality

Whether loneliness affects mental or physical health, the scientific literature is clear about loneliness as a definition. It is not always just social isolation. Rather, loneliness is a dissatisfaction with either the quantity or quality, or both, of one's relationships. Therefore, loneliness depends on many factors, ranging from personality and attachment style to cultural expectation or contextual factors (Ernst et al., 2022). It is not just the absence of relationships but can also result from the presence of unsatisfying relationships. As Albert Schweitzer reportedly once remarked, "We are all so much together, but we are all dying of loneliness" (Leavitt, 2022, para. 4).

While other humans have the capacity to be our greatest source of joy, they also can cause us the most pain. A large-scale international research study found that the leading cause of nightmares across the world is interpersonal aggression and the top-rated cause of bad dreams is to be in conflict with others (Robert & Zadra, 2014). Feeling misunderstood, taken for granted, dominated, betrayed, ridiculed, ignored, overlooked, and attacked are feelings that lead to sleepless nights and angst and can sometimes cause life-changing reactions. If love, joy, passion, closeness, connection, belonging, and moments of intimacy are what make life living, then the worst human interactions can provide the pain and suffering that lead to misery.

Conversely, the presence of positive relationships provides broad-based effects and impacts on mental and physical health. Pietromonaco and Collins (2017) in an overview of the field pointed out three main benefits of positive relationships: (a) support to moderate against stressful life events (i.e., safe haven support); (b) support when striving to meet goals and trying new things (i.e., secure base support) and cheerleading during positive life events; and (c) love, intimacy, and belonging. These and other factors not only provide protective factors against mental health episodes, but they also promote movement toward physical health and existential goals.

RELATIONSHIPS AND PHYSICAL HEALTH

The link to physical pain extends beyond just experiencing it as equally acute. Relationship quality and quantity have also been found to affect not just happiness and mental health but also physical health. The absence of or poor quality of relationships has been shown to shorten lifespans and increase the risk of physical diseases, such as cancer, heart disease, and even joint pain (Mushtaq et al., 2014; Quadt et al., 2020). This action occurs through the mechanism of *cortisol*, a hormone released when the body is under stress (Cole et al., 2015). The persistent presence of cortisol resulting from loneliness acts as an inflammatory agent in the body, creating a negative impact on organs, musculature, and physiological functions.

Further research has pointed out that loneliness also has downstream effects. It can lead to unhealthy coping behaviors, such as overeating, excessive drinking, and smoking (Kassel et al., 2003), all of which have health consequences. Research has suggested that loneliness may have as much impact on mortality as smoking seven cigarettes a day (D'Ippolito et al., 2017), leading to a life expectancy that is shortened by 15 years.

However, much as we would wish for a utopian life in which everyone treats everyone else with dignity and respect, a more realistic stance is to be able to move toward responding as effectively as possible to the meet the challenges of connecting to others. People can seldom control how others respond to them, but they can be at play in determining how they approach and respond to others. Although this stance will not magically solve every situation and will not result in permanent blissful happiness, it will allow people to be more agile in pursuit of what they want from relationships and to ultimately find ways to make relationships more satisfying and meaningful. So, how can psychotherapy help?

TREATMENT FOR INTERPERSONAL PROBLEMS: FOCUSED BRIEF GROUP THERAPY

With constant innovations in mental health ranging from use of genetic testing and brain mapping to psychedelic-assisted therapy, it is easy to forget the practice of mental health is based around the *biopsychosocial model*, which posits that social aspects of functioning are one of the primary factors in mental health. The endurance of this model as a premise is based on decades of supporting research. It all points to one major thing: Humans are social animals (Aronson, 2018), and treatment should address social relationships. People are hardwired to live and function in groups, and although societies and individuals within them find different ways to coexist, the need for human contact is universal (Feldman, 2017). As Stack Sullivan (1947) first pointed out, a great deal of human distress and symptomatology emerge from problems with relationships. Therefore, carefully evaluating and treating the cause—difficulties in relationships—should be a central part of any treatment.

Establishing treatment pathways requires an understanding of the core constructs underlying interpersonal problems. Sheffield et al. (1995) found a clear correlation between mental health problems and interpersonal distress (see also Hardy et al., 2011), and a recent study even showed links between interpersonal cognitive inflexibility to greater problems related to individuals with psychosis (García-Mieres et al., 2020).

Focused brief group therapy (FBGT) is a model that addresses the underlying causes of interpersonal distress. It is a semistructured, integrative, interpersonal process group approach designed to reduce interpersonal distress in fewer than eight sessions. FBGT offers a greater application to a wider range of clients and engenders improved client flow in an agency or practice. It is also transdiagnostic: FBGT addresses etiology, not symptomatology. It is a strengths-based approach that tailors treatment transparently and collaboratively around the client's strengths as well as their self-identified highest level of interpersonal distress. This model is designed to address loneliness and belonging by helping the client either develop new relationships or improve existing ones. The approach allows the therapist to blend the science and art of therapy, strengthening the working alliance so that treatment goals are both achievable and measurable. By marrying process-based therapy with individualized treatment goals, FBGT provides a means of providing focused treatment in a way that accelerates change (S. C. Hayes et al., 2019).

FBGT also blends principles and techniques from Yalom and Leszcz's (2020) interpersonal process model, interpersonal circumplex theory (Horowitz & Strack, 2011; Kiesler, 1996), and measurement-based care (MBC; Lewis et al., 2019) into a multiculturally responsive (Owen et al., 2011) model of therapy. FBGT is based on the idea of mobilizing evidence-based processes and evidence-based relationships (Burlingame & Strauss, 2021; Norcross & Wampold, 2011), that is, how to use all that is known about the evidence-based processes in therapy at every stage of treatment. It relies on the fact that evidence-based relationship variables between the therapist and the client (and also between the group and the therapist) offer considerable explanatory value for the size of treatment effects. Wampold and Imel (2015) showed that effect sizes for relationship variables, such as the alliance, unconditional positive regard, and multicultural competence of the therapist, accounted for stronger outcomes than specific techniques in therapy.

More recent evidence is now also showing that the use of MBC has a statistically significant impact on treatment (Lewis et al., 2019). This set of learnings infuses FBGT throughout. Evidence-based relationships inform every aspect of treatment, including serving to enhance outcomes and reduce premature dropout. These relationships work within the idea that being multiculturally sensitive and responsive is an essential part of being evidence based (E. C. Chen et al., 2008). Further, FBGT involves developing methods to help therapists work better with clients who typically are considered "difficult to treat." FBGT is part of a new wave of therapies that are process based and led by evidence-based, relational mechanisms of change that have been proven to work (Hofmann & Hayes, 2019).

Interpersonal Flexibility and Mental Health

Reducing interpersonal distress in ways that feel meaningful to a client can have an impact on their overall distress (Allison & Whittingham, 2017). *Interpersonal flexibility*, the ability to adapt to various interpersonal responses and situations—and the main mechanism of change in FBGT—has been linked to improved mental health (Wei et al., 2021), and working on becoming more proficient in meeting needs of the self involves expanding skills in being able to manage the needs of others.

FBGT work focuses on reducing a client's highest interpersonal distress score by adding interpersonal behavioral options. A greater range of behavioral choices allows for the client to have a broader range of possibilities for adaptively responding to situations (Wright et al., 2022). This is an important concept. Sometimes people's interests are served by getting along with others or sometimes by standing up for themselves, even at the cost of a relationship or a wide range of responses in between. People's value systems, sense of identity, cultural and religious beliefs, career goals, dreams, and aspirations are all lived out in the social sphere. Without the skills to navigate that sphere, the choices that might lead people to their goals and having their needs met become more elusive. For one person, this might mean finding ways to ease back on pleasing others at the expense of themselves. For another, it might mean finding ways to let go of the need to excessively protect themselves in situations in which they are seeking intimacy.

Each person has their own set of life goals, from achieving career success to establishing relationships, managing a romantic relationship, or just living their own truth. Whatever a person's raison d'être, they also bring a different set of social strengths *and* inflexibilities to the table. People are capable of considerable interpersonal skills, but it is not uncommon for them to develop along narrow corridors of functioning. One person might be a highly skilled arguer, who lays waste to courtrooms with precise language, skilled oratory, and ruthless confrontation of inconsistencies. However, at home, this same person may not always find it as easy to meet the emotional needs of their partner or to offer softness and warmth to their child. Everyone has blind spots in their interpersonal functioning: Sometimes they are highly skilled in one or more areas but may have large deficits in functioning in others.

That lack of skill may be difficult for others to identify because it is easy to be blinded by high levels of functioning in areas of strength, such as a CEO of a billion-dollar company who is conflict avoidant, an actor who is painfully introverted, or a child care worker who prefers considerable interpersonal distance. All are examples of people who might still thrive in their chosen professions, who may rise to the challenge of flexibly adapting to a situation they value. The type of interpersonal problems people deal with are both generalizable in form but also unique to them in terms of situations and contexts. How one person's social inhibition will play out is different for them based on their respective life choices, cultural contexts, and life circumstances.

Brief Treatment

Providing the work of FBGT is manageable and well defined; clients will fit work into the available time (e.g., Corpas et al., 2021). Once clients understand the parameters and are in agreement that the tasks and outcomes are achievable and realistic, then work takes place more rapidly. In groups, this process can be sped up by tailoring therapy before the group even starts, an essential task in brief groups in which quickly finding a focus is vital (Piper & Ogrodniczuk, 2004).

In personalizing therapy (Fisher & Boswell, 2016), the therapist uses assessment to tailor treatment to each client's unique distress patterns and identities (Norcross & Wampold, 2011). This use of MBC (Lewis et al., 2019) involves a collaborative assessment with the client. FBGT uses both personalized therapy and MBC to propel clients toward change. This approach provides an opportunity to craft individual goals ahead of time and use the group to act these goals out. Participating in an individual session once group sessions have concluded helps clients to cement their interpersonal learning and consider how to continue their growth in their natural environments outside of group.

FBGT does not provide a one-size-fits-all solution but, rather, collaboratively generates new strategies for growth for each client. It also provides a psychologically safe space to practice behaviors that are new for them.

So, if there is only a brief treatment period to address this duality—that people bring considerable strengths but also significant deficits in social relationships—how does treatment begin? Therapy must treat people as individuals with specific life circumstances, identities, and goals while also finding ways to connect people around common solutions. That's no easy task. Longer term therapy groups have the luxury of allowing people to both come together and establish their own identities among one another. Short-term groups seeking to mobilize those same mechanisms of change need to organize them very differently. As top chefs will tell you, good food can take a long time to make but can also emerge from a more rapid process, providing there has been enough thoughtful preparation and planning. With the right preparation and organization of contents and good processes, the same outcome can take place in far less time.

PURPOSE OF THE BOOK

This book aims to help psychotherapists understand the premises behind FBGT and offers strategies and techniques for implementing the approach. As a semistructured process, FBGT provides enough guidance so the therapist has a clear rationale for every intervention, understands the mechanisms of change, and knows what they are working toward. However, the therapist must understand themselves, be mindfully centered, and be aware of the techniques at their disposal that permit the art of this therapy to take place. The therapist uses key elements from science in the art of the here-and-now of therapy. They also use measurement, not to replace clinical judgment but to inform it. Therefore, the art and science of therapy are intended to mesh in ways that allow the therapist to find the right balance between having structure and allowing an organic process to develop.

Although the approach integrates assessment into every stage of therapy, the book is not a technical manual for every instrument. It does not have chapters that show how to score instruments in minute detail. Rather, the practitioner using the instruments in FBGT should avail themselves of the instruction manuals and available trainings (see https://www.focusedbriefgrouptherapy.com). However, the book does explain how to think about the assessment tools and how to integrate multiple data points to enhance the therapeutic process. Where there are more concrete examples of instrument use, the clinician should always consider how the client in front of them can benefit from that case example—and also how the client may differ from that example.

The book is also a guide to, but not a substitute for, reflective, deliberate practice. Use of consultation and supervision is essential for this approach. Group therapy is a specialty, designated as such in 2018 by the Commission for the Recognition of Specialties and Subspecialties in Professional Psychology (Whittingham et al., 2021); this recognition acknowledges that group therapy is not just individual therapy in a group. This book can give considerable guidance on how to implement the model as intended, but it would be well supported by an attitude of continuous movement toward expertise in group therapy in general and FBGT specifically.

SECONDARY PURPOSE OF THE BOOK

Readers will find applications of this book useful. Practitioners are now reporting using the 32-item Inventory of Interpersonal Problems (IIP-32; Horowitz et al., 2000)[1] for a variety of purposes in clinical and training work, including in training physicians in interpersonal skills, working with clients on interpersonal problems in individual therapy, and working on understanding group dynamics. Others may find the book useful for understanding more general principles of the practical application of interpersonal theory or as an aid to running brief groups. The theory behind FBGT has innovative approaches to deconstructing group dynamics, conceptualizing transference and countertransference, predicting into and preventing premature termination, and understanding coleader dynamics. Each of these theoretical and practical applications has potential value.

Equally, FBGT may be of interest to those who find it difficult to get groups started and to prevent premature dropout. Because this model was developed in a real-world setting, it was designed from the beginning to consider how to form a strong enough alliance to ensure that therapies "stick." FBGT, which focuses on what is needed for a brief therapy to work in a practice setting, is instructive for anyone attempting this kind of work. Both the underlying theory and the specific techniques (e.g., inoculation, which is outlined in Chapters 2 and 6) shed light on the reasons why groups fail and how to prevent the causes of those failures.

FBGT is an example of how to enact MBC and to tailor group therapy (MacNair-Semands & Whittingham, 2023). This book offers an exemplar of how to tailor treatment using assessment collaboratively with the client. MBC is becoming more widespread around the world (Lewis et al., 2019) and is now required as a part of clinical practice in countries such as the United Kingdom and Australia (Whittingham et al., 2023) because of its proven

---

[1]Inventory of Interpersonal Problems (IIP) items reproduced by special permission of the Publisher, Mind Garden, Inc. Further reproduction requires the Publisher's written consent. Copyright © 2000 by Leonard M. Horowitz, Lynn E. Alden, Jerry S. Wiggins, & Aaron L. Pincus. All rights reserved in all media. Published by Mind Garden, Inc., www.mindgarden.com

impact on a variety of client outcomes. Models that have thoughtfully integrated MBC have a strategic advantage in this endeavor because they are not adding a measure onto an existing intervention; rather, those models have woven measurement into the therapy from the beginning, resulting in a proliferation of uses for each measure.

FBGT provides guidance on group leadership and coleadership supervision and training. Its use of the circumplex to inform coleadership dyads and to help leaders understand themselves, their coleadership issues, and their place in the overall dynamic can provide guidance for the supervisory or consultation process. FBGT also has implications for groups and teams in general, with applications to sports, to the military, and in educational settings (e.g., Whittingham, 2021). Applications of interpersonal theory have the potential to shed light on a variety of conditions, such as the prediction of how people with different interpersonal styles might react when encountering a trauma (Whittingham, 2022). Further, FBGT's use of Kiesler's quarter turn (described in Chapter 2) to understand the pathways to interpersonal change has implications for groups and individual therapies that deal with everything from assertiveness training to substance and alcohol abuse.

STRUCTURE OF THE BOOK

This book explores how FBGT provides the personalization of group therapy to match clients' individual needs by offering guidance on how to create a safe space where members can work interdependently. It does so by providing phenotypic examples from which therapists can personalize and individualize treatment. It explores how to use the common factors of therapy (Wampold & Imel, 2015), how to integrate assessment with multicultural concerns and contextual variables, and how to manage groups according to principles of evidence-based relationships.

This Introduction gives the background and rationale for FBGT. The rest of the book is structured into two major sections: Part I consists of four chapters that offer an overview of the underlying constructs, integrated theory, and overall structure of the approach. In Part II, Chapters 5 through 10 focus on implementation of the model. The final chapter offers future directions for FBGT.

Chapter 1 explores the theoretical underpinnings of the model, paying particular attention to the key role of interpersonal theory in informing the model. This chapter focuses on understanding key constructs and principles that underlie the thinking behind FBGT. However, each of these principles is woven into the model at different stages. For example, polyvagal theory, although important throughout, has particular significance during the therapy, pregroup preparation, and screening (TPS) session. Equally, homeostasis and habituation are particularly salient during debriefing. Therefore, this chapter represents the Rosetta stone for many of the other chapters.

Chapter 2 explains the structure of FBGT and its main mechanisms of change. It also outlines inclusion and exclusion criteria. In terms of implementation, the chapter offers concrete steps that guide the practitioner in how to both plan and execute the model.

Chapters 3 and 4 represent a shift in the book to more concrete details about clients and therapists. Chapter 3 outlines the eight subscales used in the approach that are based on the main instrument, the IIP-32. The chapter explores the strengths, challenges, and implications of each phenotypic client and therapist style, serving as a foundation for a more thoughtful clinical integration later.

Chapter 4 explores core leadership attitudes and techniques that inform the model as a whole. It serves as the foundation for Chapters 6 through 13, which explore the model step by step.

In Part II, Chapter 5 discusses the all-important process of intake referral process and inclusion/exclusion procedures. It explains how to set up a successful referral process to ensure thoughtful referrals take place. It also provides the first look at how to use and interpret the assessment tools that are so vital to the implementation of FBGT. The chapter also covers assessment administration and interpretation and gives case examples demonstrating how to begin to form the tentative hypotheses that drive the TPS session.

Chapter 6 explains the TPS session, which is the foundation of the approach. A successful TPS is essential to the success of FBGT. The TPS session is complex and requires much of the therapist, but successful completion of the task sets the rest of the group up for success. This chapter outlines tasks that need accomplishing and includes key innovations coming from the model, such as inoculation, that can promote good outcomes and prevent premature dropout.

Chapter 7 covers Sessions 1 and 2 because each has specific tasks to accomplish that are different than those of the middle to later sessions. These two sessions set the stage for the middle sessions and therefore require slightly different techniques and levels of activity of the therapists.

Chapter 8 outlines the middle and later sessions, explaining leadership techniques ranging from here-and-now activation to working the axes and managing alliance ruptures. It also offers suggestions on how to maintain fidelity to the treatment while allowing clinical flexibility. The chapter covers termination and outlines how to close the group. It also reintroduces structure from the group leader and illustrates how to manage the competing forces and agendas in the group as members struggle with the idea of ending.

Chapter 9 explains the process of triangulation of data. This process involves combining multiple data points: outcomes prepost, leader observation of behavior, a count of the number of times a goal was attained, and other relevant clinical data as determined by the therapist.

Chapter 10 covers the all-important debriefing session. This involves taking the hypothesis from data triangulation and working with the client to determine for them the success or otherwise of the group. Debriefing also entails managing the process of generalization and transfer: where to implement change and where not to as well as preparation of the client for any homeostatic pushback from contexts.

Chapter 11 covers directions for the future. It describes possible applications of the model and research projects emanating from the approach.

All clients and therapy sessions described in this volume are amalgams used to illustrate certain dynamics in group therapy and are not based on specific clients. Three appendices for this book are available at https://www. apa.org/pubs/books/focused-brief-group-therapy and require a password to access. Appendix A is the Group Therapy Questionnaire–S (the short form of the questionnaire). Appendix B is a diagram of the interpersonal circumplex model; you might find it helpful to print it and refer to it when reading this book and in clinical practice. You can also use this diagram to map out a score for a client. Because the original circumplex uses labels that are more pejorative and less person centered, this tool is better for working collaboratively with clients than the ones supplied with the instruments itself. It can be helpful in reminding those seeking to learn the approach where the different subscales are in relation to each other. Appendix C is a sample referral sheet.

For this approach to be implemented successfully, clinicians should purchase the IIP-32 from Mind Garden (https://www.mindgarden.com).

PART **I** **THE MODEL**

1 THEORETICAL UNDERPINNINGS

Focused brief group therapy (FBGT) is an integrative, process-based model of psychotherapy. However, to understand how the model fits together, it is first necessary to outline its theoretical underpinnings. The model is theoretically integrative—a tightly woven set of interrelated techniques with a unifying structure and a clear progression toward change. This chapter explores the relevance of the main theoretical strands to FBGT and outlines their central premises. Chapter 2 then outlines how these theories connect, describes the structure, and explains how mechanisms of change evolve throughout the model. This chapter begins by explaining FBGT's stance on human development and functioning, which provides an overarching background for the theories, structure, and change processes used.

THE GENESIS OF INTERPERSONAL BEHAVIOR

FBGT takes the position that interpersonal behavior begins with trait-level genetic dispositions that evolve across the lifespan (Costa & McCrae, 2011; Horowitz, 2004). Those dispositions are influenced by parental reactions

https://doi.org/10.1037/0000389-002
Focused Brief Group Therapy: An Integrative Approach to Reducing Interpersonal Distress, by M. Whittingham

and life events (e.g., trauma, friendships) and become an attachment style (Marmarosh, 2015). This attachment style carries with it a set of interpersonal behaviors that can then be broken down into smaller units of measurement that allow for a finer grain analysis (and that form the basis for FBGT) of interpersonal strengths and areas of inflexibility. These styles are embedded as schemas, which act as cognitive maps for behavior (Shaver & Mikulincer, 2011). Interpersonal behaviors emerging from these processes are then either flexible or inflexible and can lead to a person's either becoming skillful at getting their needs met or becoming increasingly distressed and developing symptoms that eventually cluster into diagnoses. These interpersonal behaviors are also reciprocally shaped by wider developmental-ecological forces (Bronfenbrenner, 1992) operating at different levels of society, ranging from local neighborhoods to wider societal structures that dictate power and affiliation relations. Thus, local and larger cultural forces also impact developmental progression of interpersonal behaviors (see Figure 1.1).

People also have role demands (e.g., parent, worker, romantic partner, friend) that demand certain proscribed behaviors, albeit ones that can flex and change over time. For example, a romantic relationship may begin with warmth and mutual enjoyment of leisure activities, but over time, it requires that each partner negotiate boundaries more carefully as their lives become more complicated and demanding. Equally, some of these roles require skills that overlap with other roles. For example, being a warm, sociable person may engender positive results as a romantic partner and also as a friend. However, skills deficits may not show up in one environment (e.g., a friendship group keeps appropriate boundaries and does not need to be confronted about overstepping) but may be particularly germane to another (e.g., the same person becomes distressed at work, and they feel unable to say no to unreasonable expectations).

Thus, in this model, both interpersonal strengths and deficits are important to consider, as are the settings in which they take place. Because those settings may demand very different things from a person, some contexts have good fit between a person's strengths and the demands of the situation, whereas others expose difficulties that person may have in certain areas of interpersonal functioning. Thus, *interpersonal flexibility*—the ability to successfully draw on different interpersonal skills to meet the needs of different situations—is at the heart of FBGT's sought outcomes for each client.

People's choices are, of course, also constrained to varying degrees by the power and status structures that allow people access to the resources that enable them to have choices or to severely limit choices. Contextual and cultural factors operating in the macrosystem filter down into the mesosystem

FIGURE 1.1. The Focused Brief Group Therapy Model of Interpersonal Functioning in a Multicultural Context

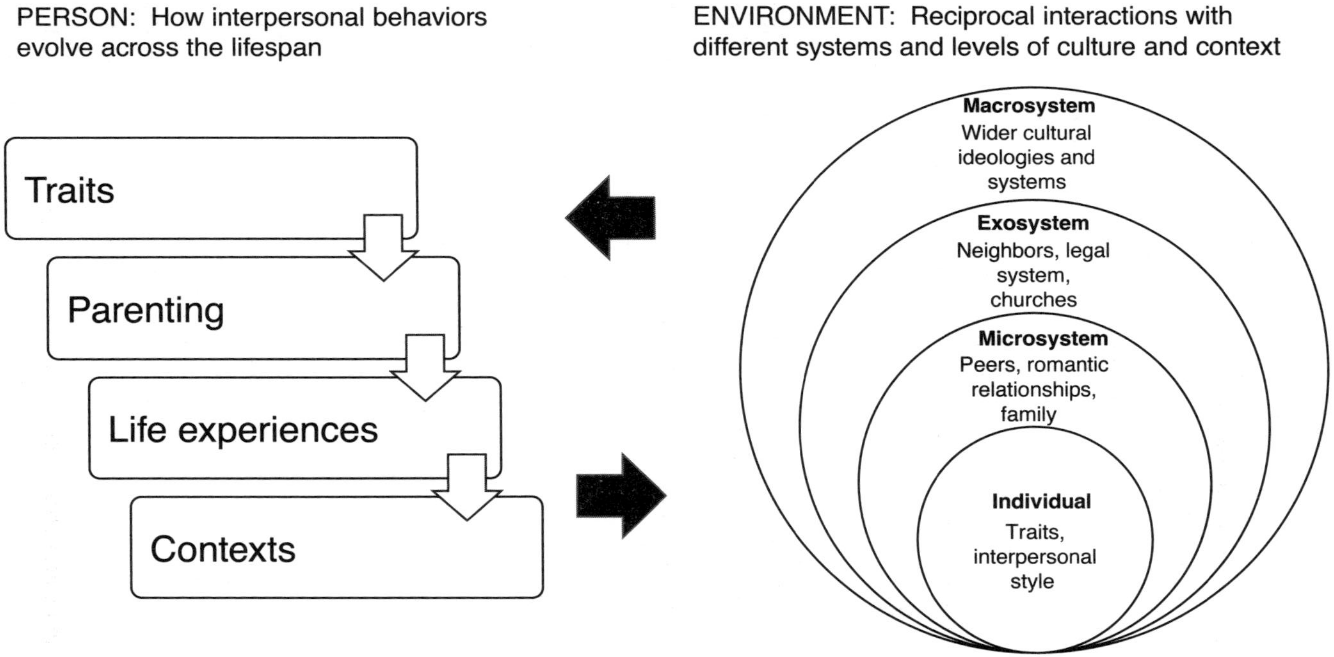
PERSON: How interpersonal behaviors evolve across the lifespan
ENVIRONMENT: Reciprocal interactions with different systems and levels of culture and context
Traits
Parenting
Life experiences
Contexts
Macrosystem
Wider cultural ideologies and systems
Exosystem
Neighbors, legal system, churches
Microsystem
Peers, romantic relationships, family
Individual
Traits, interpersonal style

Note. Data from Bronfenbrenner (1979).

and microsystems (see Figure 1.1) and have a significant impact on choice. The roles of privilege, oppression, and systematic power structures and their influence on relationships and life course thus play an important part in understanding this process (Kliman, 2010).

Interpersonal flexibility is therefore the core tenet of FBGT, but it is seen within multiple contexts, roles, and systems of power and privilege. FBGT works on increasing options to navigate those multiple interpersonal spaces. In cases in which this involves considerable interaction with systemic inequity, FBGT can also facilitate clients' acquisition of skills that allow them greater choices in how to respond to each interpersonal situation so they may maximize the possibility of positive outcomes or mitigate the possibility of negative ones.

Loneliness, Connectedness, and Belonging

FBGT allows clients to work on issues related to agency and autonomy. It also focuses on issues related to loneliness, connectedness, and belonging, such as forming or improving the quality of relationships (e.g., romantic, platonic, collegial), the two main components of that construct (S. Hayes et al., 2022). Initiating and forming relationships are important to interpersonal belonging, but so is ensuring quality in relationships: Interpersonal skills can significantly impact quality by allowing clients to select from previously unused behavioral options. For one person, this might mean becoming better able to assert reasonable boundaries; for another, it could mean learning to listen empathically and be supportive; and for yet another person, it might mean learning to express the importance of their cultural identity to others. While initiating relationships typically involves use of more warmth, improving the quality of relationships can also sometimes involve usage of techniques such as knowing how to self-disclose more, offer encouragement, set boundaries, and how to manage conflict.

As is explored in Chapters 2 and 3, people with distress on different interpersonal scales often have different reasons for either the absence of relationships or the presence of dissatisfying ones. For example, the absence of relationships could be caused by someone's being too socially inhibited to initiate relationships; by somebody who is so aggressive that they frighten others away; or by a person who begins relationships too intensely, leaving potential friends seeking an exit. Being able to understand the interpersonal strengths and deficits clients bring for each scale not only helps clarify what the issues are, but also helps the client better understand what is occurring and to begin to work on solutions. Improving interpersonal flexibility means adding behavioral options for the client to choose from that might allow them to better meet their needs and goals in life related to connectedness.

Frustration of Needs and Goals

The model rests on the interpersonal theory assumption that interpersonal distress is caused by an individual's feeling frustrated in their interpersonal goals and motivations (Wright et al., 2023). These goals are specific to that person and could involve motives that are either agentic (i.e., that raise self-esteem and a sense of personal power or control) or communal (i.e., that increase feelings of belonging and connection), or some combination of both. These goals and motives can also be related to different contexts. For example, someone may be successful in meeting their needs and goals in one context (e.g., in their romantic life, friendships) but be frustrated that their skills are not proving successful in meeting goals in other contexts (e.g., at work). As is discussed later in this chapter, the therapist is looking for areas of rigidity or extremeness in interpersonal behavior that might be causing the client difficulty.

FBGT also looks for areas of strength. It is therefore important to understand both an individual's specific interpersonal strengths and challenges as well as the arenas in which they feel successful or unsuccessful. People may be frustrated in all their relationships (e.g., romantic, friendship, family) and contexts (e.g., work, recreation, family), or some but not others. Therefore, it is important within the approach to collaboratively understand how pervasive and cross-situational the problem is. This is done during by combining the 32-item Inventory of Interpersonal Problems (IIP-32; Horowitz et al., 2000) with the interpersonal interview, as described in Chapter 6.

COLLABORATIVE EXPLORATION OF CHOICES

With respect to the working alliance between client and therapist, FBGT, working from a person-centered and multiculturally responsive framework, takes the stance of collaboratively exploring issues, such as the meaning of interpersonal distress, the role of identity in that distress, and the shaping of goals. As is discussed throughout the book, the process involves using measurement-based care (MBC; Lewis et al., 2019) in combination with exploring a client's identity variables and the interpersonal spaces in which they operate. This is done in a way that is nonshaming and nonblaming with the intent of helping clients understand and build on strengths while allowing for the possibility that small changes can make a big difference.

Collaboration also takes place with the group, which becomes both a place to practice new behaviors and to collaborate with others who are working on their goals. Learning from and about others while working on one's own goals allows for opportunities to benefit from the power of group processes. This collaboration continues through the life of the group and, most importantly, continues during the individualized debriefing session. Discussions take place based on what changes may be helpful to the client but also help them to assess the relative likelihood of success, including the possible risks and rewards of attempting changes in different contexts.

Client autonomy is therefore tightly interwoven with informed consent as to the risks and benefits of change. FBGT assumes that systems will push back against change—a homeostatic response from people and systems that prefer interactions to remain stable and predictable (Seshadri, 2019). The model therefore encourages spending substantial time and thought during individualized debriefing sessions considering both that people are embedded within systems and the possible consequences of interpersonal change. The model therefore works on the idea of promotion of client choice—based on the client's preferences, needs, and goals. These choices are important because the approach is also based on the idea that the client's goals are paramount to establishing a treatment focus and that understanding what client needs or goals are being frustrated is key to forming treatment goals and generating the working alliance.

FBGT also inquires about clients' identity variables and seeks to understand to what degree they are salient to treatment. This involves thoughtful discussion and listening carefully to how the client describes their diversity variables, how these variables impact them interpersonally, and whether and how they wish to make them a focus of treatment. Understanding the different spheres and environments in which a person feels comfortable or distressed can help form goals appropriate to each context and cultural space in which a person is experiencing distress. The therapist and client also note preexisting strengths and work to ensure that clients do not overgeneralize change to places where it is not needed (e.g., where they are already feeling interpersonally competent in how they manage situations). This is all done within the context of understanding an individual's traits and preferred interpersonal style. Therefore, blending data about interpersonal challenges with contextual information is key to forming goals that are meaningful to the client. Chapter 3 explores in more detail how goals relate to each phenotypic scale, and Chapter 6 further describes integrating data.

Underpinning FBGT are multiple theory bases, each of which informs the model at different times. Some processes represent the deep structure and drumbeat of FBGT; these processes need to be continuous within the therapy. Other theories, though, inform the model at key moments but are less pervasive throughout the model. Each is now addressed in turn.

THEORETICAL APPROACHES

The FBGT model is based on Yalom's interpersonal process approach (Yalom & Leszcz, 2020) combined with Kiesler (1996) and others' interpersonal theories that integrate the interpersonal circumplex (as can be seen in Horowitz & Strack, 2011). After exploring Kiesler and Yalom's approaches, this section explains the premises of brief group therapy to demonstrate how they resulted in modifications to Yalom's approach and now inform the treatment (Piper & Ogrodniczuk, 2004; Yalom & Leszcz, 2020). The section then explores the principles of polyvagal theory (Porges & Dana, 2018) to show how they are used to help clients and therapists manage the change process. To enhance screening, pregroup preparation, process, and therapy, FBGT also uses the following approaches: multicultural orientation (MCO) theory (Owen et al., 2011) to integrate identity and context into treatment, behavioral activation (Stein et al., 2021), a common factors/evidence-based relationships approach (Wampold & Imel, 2015), and measurement-based care (MBC; Burlingame et al., 2006; Scott & Lewis, 2015). Each of these approaches is outlined in turn.

Exploring interpersonal approaches first, distinctions need to be made between seemingly identical terms that are similar and yet very different: Interpersonal "theory" is distinct from interpersonal "therapy." Although both originated from the work of Harry Stack Sullivan (1947), who first considered the idea that relationship issues could be etiological to diagnoses, over time, they split into two distinct camps. Interpersonal *theory* was rigorously scientifically studied under the auspices of personality and social-psychological basic and applied science using psychometrically sound measures (e.g., Horowitz & Strack, 2011). Interpersonal group process *therapies* became more aligned with psychodynamic approaches and the art of therapy (e.g., Yalom & Leszcz, 2020). FBGT integrates both these strands and basic and applied science with the art of psychotherapy. Let us first consider interpersonal theory.

Interpersonal Theory

Derived from Sullivan's (1947) work, the interpersonal circumplex was invented in the 1950s by Leary (1957) and, over the years, has become recognized as the gold standard in interpersonal research; studies using the model number in the thousands (Gurtman, 2009; Horowitz & Strack, 2011). It is well correlated with the five-factor model of personality (Costa & McCrae, 2011) and has also been suggested in the fifth edition of the *Diagnostic and Statistical Manual of Mental Disorders* (American Psychiatric Association, 2013) as an alternative underpinning models of personality disorder (Wright et al., 2022). In addition, interpersonal circumplex measures used within the model have been validated across multiple cultures, including China (L. Z. Wu et al., 2015); South Africa (Clifton, 2018) and Iran (Chelmardi et al., 2018). Over time, the theory has evolved and has been expanded into a model to describe human social functioning (Pincus & Hopwood, 2012; Wright et al., 2022).

Interpersonal theory has two main tenets that are particularly important for FBGT: (a) the use of the interpersonal circumplex and (b) the notion of complementarity (Sadler et al., 2011). Let us first explore the interpersonal circumplex.

The Interpersonal Circumplex

The *interpersonal circumplex* maps interpersonal behavior onto a circular plot with scales that are similar to each other when close together and scales that are opposite when farthest apart (see Figure 1.2; Horowitz & Strack, 2011). For example, Socially Inhibited (Scale 4) is close to Distant (Scale 3) but

FIGURE 1.2. The Interpersonal Circumplex

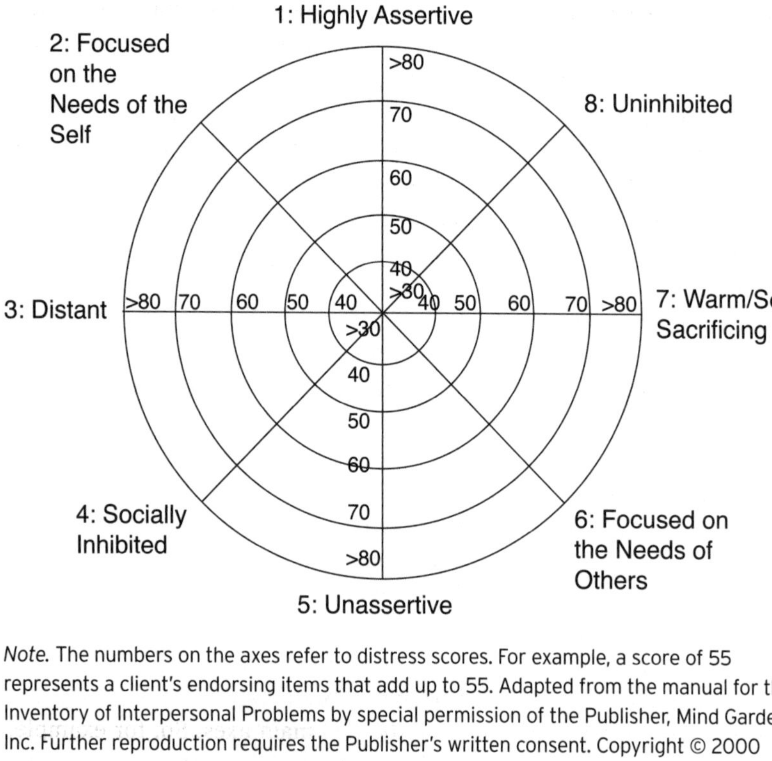

Note. The numbers on the axes refer to distress scores. For example, a score of 55 represents a client's endorsing items that add up to 55. Adapted from the manual for the Inventory of Interpersonal Problems by special permission of the Publisher, Mind Garden, Inc. Further reproduction requires the Publisher's written consent. Copyright © 2000 by Leonard M. Horowitz, Lynn E. Alden, Jerry S. Wiggins, & Aaron L. Pincus. All rights reserved in all media. Published by Mind Garden, Inc., www.mindgarden.com

furthest from Uninhibited (Scale 8), which represents the conceptual opposite of this construct. The two main axes are "agency," which runs vertically north to south (ranging from Highly Assertive at the top to Unassertive at the bottom), and "affiliation," which runs horizontally east to west (ranging from Warm/Self-Sacrificing on the far right to Distant on the far left).

These axes represent two major dimensions: (a) *agency*, the way in which people form hierarchies and organize themselves with respect to feeling a sense of personal power or control and being able to influence others; and (b) *affiliation*, the way in which people manage belonging, social connections, and boundaries. These two constructs can also be found in psychoanalytic literature. There, they have been described as the two fundamental tasks of life: (a) balancing the need for autonomy, individuation, status, power, and control against (b) needing to connect, belong, and maintain social ties (e.g., Bakan, 1966). Or, put more simply, how people manage their own needs in relation to the needs of others. As Fournier et al. (2011) pointed out, these constructs can also be found in literature ranging from evolutionary psychology's discussions on status hierarchy versus alliance formation (Buss, 1991) to cross-cultural literature on individualism versus collectivism (e.g., Kitayama et al., 2022). This balance between the needs of the self and the needs of others is constantly being negotiated at every level of every system, ranging from the wider culture and its power structures and hegemonic practices to individuals' negotiating within their microsystems—with reciprocal influence taking place between all levels. Balancing the needs of self against the needs of others is a major organizing thread of humanity's existence. Both these constructs have also been found to be connected to emotional states (Watanabe & Yamamoto, 2015), suggesting that they are hardwired into our systems.

The tension between these two sometimes well aligned but occasionally deeply conflicting motivations has been posited to create considerable stress that can lead to distress if the needs emanating from those motivations (to belong or to feel one's individual needs are met) are unfulfilled (Beck, 2007). People struggle significantly with their emotions when they do not achieve the balance between influence/autonomy and the connection that they want.

Reflecting these two main constructs—affiliation and agency—an interpersonal circumplex was developed. It allows different interpersonal preferences and styles to be conceptualized around these two main axes.

Interpersonal Scales

Those two main scales are then further subdivided into eight scales that represent weighted combinations of the two main axes. So, for example, as seen in Figure 1.2, Scale 4: Socially Inhibited is a weighted combination of Scale 3: Distant and Scale 5: Unassertive. Higher scores on each scale represent a tendency toward that particular scale. Midpoints between the two axes—for example, Scale 8: Uninhibited—represent a weighted combination of the two main axes. So, in this example, Scale 8 is a combination of Scale 1: Highly Assertive and Scale 7: Warm/Self-Sacrificing—for instance, someone who prefers to be dominant who is also high in Warmth. Similarly, Scale 2: Focused on the Needs of the Self represents someone Highly Assertive and more Distant. Scale 4: Socially Inhibited represents aspects of Unassertive and Distant, whereas Scale 6: Focused on the Needs of Others represents a combination of Warm/Self-Sacrificing and Unassertive.

Interpersonal circumplex label changes for the IIP-32. Given that the interpersonal circumplex was going to be used therapeutically and transparently, rather than for scientific studies and more opaquely, it was important to change the labels as originally written because of their pejorative nature (e.g., Scale 8 was originally labeled "Intrusive/Needy" on the IIP-32; Horowitz et al., 2000). As is discussed throughout this book, the IIP-32 measures interpersonal distress and not interpersonal style, allowing it to be used as a means for further exploration of what might be causing that distress, which might be a client's interpersonal inflexibility, problems in the environment, or interactions between the two.

The original labels were adapted using student feedback from clients at a nearby university counseling center. Those students described what would represent the distress around the construct without leaving clients feeling negatively labeled. These labels were then cross-validated with an author of the original instrument; that author concurred that the labels still represented the original constructs. See Table 1.1 for the label changes.

TABLE 1.1. Comparison of Original IIP-32 Labels With FBGT Modifications

Scale	IIP-32 original labels	IIP-32 FBGT modified labels
1	Domineering	Highly Assertive
2	Self-Centered/Vindictive	Focused on the Needs of the Self
3	Cold/Distant	Distant
4	Socially Inhibited	Socially Inhibited
5	Non-assertive	Unassertive
6	Overly Accommodating	Focused on the Needs of Others
7	Self-Sacrificing	Warm/Self-Sacrificing
8	Needy/Intrusive	Uninhibited

Note. IIP-32 = 32-item Inventory of Interpersonal Problems (Horowitz et al., 2000); FBGT = focused brief group therapy.

Items on the IIP-32 ask how a person feels about certain aspects of their own interpersonal behavior and what kind of reactions they get from others that cause them distress, as in the following example:

It is hard for me to:
- Understand another person's point of view
- Be firm when I need to be

The following are things that you do too much:
- I try to control other people too much.
- I tell personal things to other people too much.[1]

Person-centered scales. Changes to the labels of these scales were important because no one scale behavior or style should be considered "wrong"; every behavioral stance has a moment or situation in which it is applicable and helpful. Most interpersonal behaviors can be adaptive depending on the context. For example, being distant and aloof would be extremely helpful in a situation in which strong and clear boundaries are needed, such as in a setting where concealment of emotions, composure, and role-based professionalism are preferred. Equally, being focused on the needs of others would be highly effective in a role as a caregiver, friend, or parent. The scales therefore formed important conceptualizations of how people with different interpersonal styles might interact and behave while allowing for study of how those interactions take place.

The therapeutic value of mapping out scales and discussing them with clients is considerable. As is discussed throughout the book, scales can shed light on both interpersonal strengths and potential areas for improvement. They can also be used to map out group dynamics, anticipate transference and counter-transference, and improve the working alliance; however, for these factors to be operationalized, the idea of complementarity must also be added to the conceptual mix.

Complementarity

Complementarity is an important concept in interpersonal theory and FBGT (particularly with respect to the client–therapist relationship and group dynamics) and has been well tested in the scientific literature (see Sadler et al., 2011). Underlying this concept is the idea that people want to both maintain a sense of internal stability and a clear sense of self (Carson, 1969;

---

[1] Inventory of Interpersonal Problems (IIP) items reproduced by special permission of the Publisher, Mind Garden, Inc. Further reproduction requires the Publisher's written consent. Copyright © 2000 by Leonard M. Horowitz, Lynn E. Alden, Jerry S. Wiggins, & Aaron L. Pincus. All rights reserved in all media. Published by Mind Garden, Inc., www.mindgarden.com

Kim & Rose, 2014) while also accomplishing interpersonal goals (e.g., to have more or less autonomy or more or less warmth; Horowitz et al., 2006).

People seek a stable sense of self, a stable sense of others, and a predictable sense of how interactions will play out. For example, someone seeking to be in control (an agentic motivation) will act in ways that promote that agenda, perhaps by demanding someone to adhere to their wishes. If that demand is met with a complementary response—the other person acquiesces—then the motivation is satisfied.

Therefore, this seeking of stability can also be linked to motives (Horowitz et al., 2006), which, if frustrated, can lead to tension and anxiety. For example, if someone is seeking friendship or communality with a warm invitation and receives a cold or distant reply, then that motivation is frustrated. When relationships become unpredictable, people often become anxious and then act in ways to reduce that anxiety (e.g., by leaving the situation or changing their interpersonal behavior) to restore a sense of homeostasis. This drive to get motivational needs met (whether that need is to increase or reduce distance from others or to be in control or let someone else be in control) to reduce anxiety and maintain consistency is what underpins the idea of complementarity in interpersonal theory (K. D. Locke, 2015): that people are constantly sending out invitations to others that they hope will result in others' responding in predictable and expected ways.

Complementarity is also linked to emotional states. For example, Halberstadt et al. (2023) found that complementary interactions resulted in an overall more positive affect for people. Consider the emotional impact of when someone behaves rudely in response to a polite request. The resulting emotional upset can often parlay into later discussions with support systems to emote about that rude person's behavior or even into difficulty sleeping. Therefore, the links between interpersonal motives, interactions, and emotional states are important for overall well-being and affect regulation.

Complementary and Noncomplementary Invitations and Responses

Interpersonal theory posits that every interpersonal act contains within it an invitation to the other person to respond within a proscribed way. For example, an outstretched hand and a smile send an invitation for reciprocation in the form of a smile and a handshake. However, if that smile and outstretched hand is met with a disdainful look and a refusal to offer a hand in return, immediate tension is created. These interactions are called "complementary" and "noncomplementary" interactions, respectively.

Complementary responses. Complementary responses involve a matching of invitation to the desired response. They are correspondent (the opposite) on the agency axis and reciprocal (the same) on the affiliation axis. So, on the agency axis, dominance invites submission, and submission invites dominance. For example, dominant behavior (e.g., "Bring me my phone!") invites an opposite (called "reciprocal"), submissive response (e.g., "I will get that right away"). The reverse is also true: A submissive invitation (e.g., "Tell me what shirt to wear") is complementary when met with a dominant response (e.g., "You should wear the blue one").

On the affiliation dimension, complementary responses are called *correspondent* and involve the response being the same as the invitation. Warmth (Warm/Self-Sacrificing) invites the return of warmth, and distance (Distant) invites a response of distance. For example, a warm smile when met with a warm smile in response is complementary because it is correspondent (it matches). Equally, a distant invitation from a manager at work (e.g., "Let's not waste time on small talk, we have a lot to do") is complementary if met with the correspondent reply (e.g., "Agreed. Let's get on with it and get this done"; Sadler et al., 2011).

Noncomplementary responses. However, in instances in which the invitation is not met with the hoped for response, tension arises; these are called *noncomplementary* interactions. For example, in the previous example of a distant invitation, if the employee responds aggressively (e.g., "What is the matter with you? Why are you so rude? Can't you at least say hello first?"), tension and anxiety increase, and the situation is now noncomplementary. The manager could further escalate and invite an unassertive response (e.g., "We don't have time for niceties. If you don't get to work, you are fired!")— an escalation of Highly Assertive distance [Distant], repeating the same invitation—or choose to change their invitation to a different stance, such as warm dominance (e.g., "Ha! Good for you for standing up for yourself. Let's connect for a minute, then get to work"). Whatever sequence occurs, the situation is not resolved until the tension is dissipated with complementarity. In the example, the roles of each person also mediate the situation. If manager to employee were replaced with parent to child or friend to friend, sequences can look very different and have different meanings. That is why understanding in which roles a client is distressed is critical to understanding interpersonal distress. It is also important to be aware of two different types of noncomplementary responses: acomplementary and anticomplementary.

Responses that meet one part of the invitation but not the other are called *acomplementary*, such as when a warm and dominant invitation is met with a distant (does not match the invitation) and submissive (does match the invitation) response. An example is the following exchange: If "I am so happy to meet you. I am looking forward to leading this team and am glad you are going to be a part of it" is responded to with "I heard you were going to be the new boss. We will certainly listen to what you have to say." The response would have been complementary if the employee had replied with enthusiasm, "I can't wait to start this next phase of work now you are here!" Instead, the coldness of the reply created a sense of tension and doubt in the employer as to how the relationship would progress.

If the invitation is met with both parts of the invitation not being matched, then it is called *anticomplementary*. Anticomplementary responses create greater tension than acomplementary ones because both invitations are rebutted. For example, using the earlier example of the new boss, say the employee responds instead with "I gather you think you are going to tell us all what to do. Good luck with that!" This response rejects both premises—warmth and dominance—in that it is one expressing more dominance with the implication that the employee and the team will not acquiesce to any demands and will respond with coldness. Because such a response creates the greatest tension, it makes situations anxious and difficult. This kind of response is often considered so improper in work situations that it is labeled insubordination and may be considered a cause for termination.

FBGT encourages group leaders to meet clients with acomplementary (meeting an invitation on one axis but not the other) responses at times during treatment but to avoid anticomplementary (not meeting invitations on either axis) responses, particularly during alliance formation. Later chapters cover this concept in greater detail.

Complementarity has major implications for FBGT. Understanding how it operates prepares the client for a range of technical issues, including having transference–countertransference reactions, predicting into group dynamics, and creating the working alliance and repairing alliance ruptures. All are discussed in later chapters.

These two topics—the interpersonal circumplex and the idea of complementarity—show how interpersonal behaviors and motivations can lead to distress. However, if we are to work on reducing this distress, then a model is needed to identify key mechanisms of change that can be the focus for clinical work. FBGT drew on the work of Kiesler (1996) to determine the main foci for treatment.

Problematic Behaviors

Interpersonal distress emerges from people's struggles to meet their own needs, goals, and motivations (Wright et al., 2023). Given that people are required to constantly adapt to different situations and to achieve their own goals (e.g., get a promotion at work, form or maintain a loving romantic relationship), the need for a range of interpersonal skills that will enhance their likelihood of doing so is paramount. Within FBGT, recognizing the strengths of people's interpersonal traits, but also prizing interpersonal flexibility, is an important premise. In other words, people should be proud of their strengths and seek out situations that play to those strengths. However, they should also be willing, at times, to be flexible to adapt to situations so they can meet their needs or the needs of others.

The FBGT approach also targets what can limit people's abilities to meet their own needs: the presence of behavioral problems that can frustrate those motivations—rigid and extreme behaviors, two interpersonal problems identified by Kiesler (1996). Whether problems arise from a client's own behavioral inflexibility, emanate from interactions with dysfunctional people and systems, or are one of many different combinations of those, giving clients more coping tools that can help them navigate successfully toward goals they value are going to help them thrive. Rigidity and extremeness first need to be understood from a definitional point of view.

Rigid behavior. *Rigid behavior* is a lack of flexibility in being able to meet the needs of different situations. Life demands a great deal from people in terms of interpersonal flexibility. Consider this example: If a child is about to run into a busy street, it requires the person to use a commanding voice to shout, "Stop!" As a romantic partner arrives for dinner, the same person requires an ability to listen and respond with emotional resonance. Their sister later calls to say that they are feeling depressed and suicidal and asks for help. At work, the next day, that same person realizes that their regional manager is arriving the next day to interview employees about readiness for an overhaul of the workplace procedures and personnel, and the manager wants to talk to that person. Each situation demands flexibility in interpersonal responses. Failure to use the appropriate interpersonal skills in each situation can have deleterious consequences for the individual or for others.

A behavior might be seen as rigid when it is the only interpersonal scale behavior a person can exhibit. In the preceding example, imagine if the person had only one interpersonal strategy to draw on: a singular strategy of meeting every situation with high assertiveness and no empathy or understanding of other people. This would likely result in a mixture of success and disaster, depending on each prior situation that was mentioned. Tasks, such stopping the child running into the street, may be successful, but the other scenarios would have much more uncertain outcomes. As can be seen from that example, a rigid, restricted range of interpersonal behaviors can sometimes lead people to be unable to achieve their goals.

This rigidity is not just for this style. Other examples include the college student high in warmth (Warm/Self-Sacrificing) who is constantly taken advantage of by acquaintances and does not know how to set boundaries (a Distant strategy). Another example might be someone who is rigidly stuck on Scale 6: Focused on the Needs of Others. They become a carer and receive considerable praise for helping other people and being giving of themselves. However, they struggle with asking for help for themselves, setting boundaries with others, and ensuring their own needs are being met. Over time, they become angry, resentful, and burned out. Lacking the flexibility to set limits and establish two-way mutually beneficial relationships, and being conflict-avoidant, they become increasingly depressed. This last example illustrates how other people may also miss the consequences of that rigidity. Friends, family, and work colleagues sometimes find it easier to notice externalizing behaviors in others (e.g., angry outbursts) than they do internalizing behaviors (e.g., resentment that is internalized and becomes depression). However, rigidity is not the only problematic interpersonal issue.

Extreme behavior. *Extreme behavior* is when an interpersonal strategy occurs too often and/or in ways that are inappropriate to the situation such that the person who exhibits the extreme behaviors is also not getting their needs met. An example is the person high in uninhibition (Uninhibited) who is perceived by others as someone who excessively self-discloses too quickly, who is overly intrusive, and who ignores other's boundaries. This same behavior—being able to express concern for others and to self-disclose—is useful when at less intense levels, but in excess, it can become aversive and counter-productive to that person's having their needs met or meeting the needs of others. Their intent—to develop deep and meaningful relationships—is frustrated by their extreme interpersonal strategies for doing so. The same could be said for shyness (introversion is a positive unless it is preventing that person from achieving their goals), assertiveness (being able to defend oneself or to stand up for loved ones is a positive, but loudly and aggressively berating people at every opportunity often results in negative consequences), or any of the other scales.

FBGT and Interpersonal Flexibility

FBGT primarily seeks to work on those two main areas, rigidity and extremeness. It focuses on areas in the client's life in which those two approaches leave the client frustrated that they cannot seem to meet their goals or get their needs met. If an extreme behavior is working in a setting and achieves the desired goal and end state for a client, then it is left alone or, in some cases, is reinforced. For example, if a client keeps extreme distance at work because this suits their work style, they are more productive and have little need for interaction. Providing that they are satisfied with this, then there is not a problem, and it might be considered a wise choice. However, if they identify that they wish for more closeness in a romantic relationship and do not have the skills to do that, then this becomes the focus for treatment. Goals are not just person specific in FBGT; they are also setting specific and are based on clients' accomplishing goals in contexts in which their goals are currently being frustrated. Goals in FBGT (see Chapter 3) can sometimes work on reducing rigidity; in other cases, goals can seek to reduce extremeness or can be compound goals that work on both.

Interpersonal theory's ideas involving the interpersonal circumplex and complementarity form important structural components of understanding processes in FBGT that range from understanding interpersonal subtypes and forming a working alliance to understanding transference, countertransference, and group dynamics. Yalom and Leszcz's (2020) interpersonal theory draws on similar strands of theory but without embedding the deep structure of the interpersonal circumplex and ideas about invitations directly into groups. However, it has significant overlap with interpersonal theory and provides significant therapeutic direction to the model by suggesting the therapeutic milieu for the approach.

Interpersonal Process Group Therapy

FBGT shares many premises with Yalom and Leszcz's (2020) interpersonal process group therapy. Central to both approaches are the importance of early attachment experiences that lead to inaccurate and maladaptive cognitions, something that Sullivan (1947) called *parataxic distortions*. These cognitions or schemas create cyclical maladaptive patterns (Levenson, 2010) in people's relationships because they are based on inaccurate perceptions resulting from schemas about people that were helpful in childhood but do not generalize well to adaptive functioning in the world beyond the family home. For example, faced with domineering parents who refuse to let a child exercise any personal choice or power, the child learns passive-aggressive techniques to gain covert power. These strategies are repeated into adulthood, resulting in difficult relationships and resentment as others react angrily to these same covert power strategies. What was once adaptive is no longer helpful and can be self-defeating. However, the schemas have become so ossified that they are resistant to change. People therefore tend to move through life seeking predictability, even if it makes them unhappy.

In particular, the role of self-fulfilling prophecy ensures the continuation of these behaviors. For example, a person learns as a child that their parents will not give them any time, love, or attention regardless of how they behave. They come to see people as unlikely to ever give them love and as fundamentally untrustworthy, an interpersonal schema that forms a template for behavior. Seeing people as untrustworthy and having learned to rely only on themselves, they act in ways that greet people with distance and suspicion. People respond to this seeming disdain with rejection. Once rejected, the schema that people are untrustworthy and rejection is reinforced, creating a self-fulfilling prophecy that reinforces the schema. Thus, a dismissive attachment style becomes reinforced and solidified. As can be seen, this approach is linked to the idea of attachment style (e.g., Marmarosh, 2017). The central idea is that an initial problem in parental response to a child can lead to a secure attachment style or to an insecure attachment style (e.g., preoccupied, dismissive, fearful), which results in difficulties attaching to others as an adult.

Interpersonal styles, which are used in FBGT, represent two sides of the same coin with respect to attachment style (Whittingham, 2017). If attachment style represents the underlying motivation with respect to behaviors (to confirm negative or positive views of the self and others), then interpersonal style is the behavior that accomplishes that goal. Interpersonal circumplex scales map onto attachment styles with good statistical fit: Preoccupied and dismissive attachment styles map onto Scales 8 (Uninhibited) and 2 (Focused on the Needs of the Self), secure attachment maps onto Scale 7 (Warm/Self-Sacrificing), and anxious/avoidant attachment maps onto several interpersonal styles at the base of the interpersonal circumplex (Alden et al., 1990; Bailey et al., 2018). Therefore, when considering the research on attachment style and group (e.g., Marmarosh et al., 2013; Tasca & Maxwell, 2021), it is important to note that the overlaps between the two are significant.

However, when developing FBGT, a conscious decision was made to root the approach in interpersonal behavior because it was observable by client and therapist and was not directed at the client's core sense of self. Equally, the eight octants of the interpersonal circumplex offered a more nuanced and fine-grained analysis of how people's distress manifests and can be changed than the far broader categories (ranging from two to four dimensions) seen in attachment-based approaches (Slade & Holmes, 2019). The literature on attachment theory in psychotherapy, when paired with the literature on interpersonal theory, has considerable additive value. Each informs the other.

Yalom and Leszcz's (2020) solution to these attachment-based, cyclical maladaptive patterns is group therapy using an interpersonal process model based on the idea of the *social microcosm*, which means, when placed into a group, members will eventually display the attachment problems and associated interpersonal behaviors that are causing them problems in their outside lives (Kivlighan, Gullo, et al., 2021; Yalom & Leszcz, 2020). The model posits that people seldom have awareness about their interpersonal processes and patterns. The premise is that other people rarely communicate accurate feedback to others regarding how they come across. So, someone who is behaving in ways that are overwhelming to others will seldom experience someone else's taking the time to explain how that behavior is causing problems and what they can do to change it. Instead, others typically just depart the situation, leaving the person confused and upset or feeling that their assumptions about people were correct. A Yalom group provides a safe space for people to explore how their behaviors come across to others and to develop new ways of relating. As other group members witness and experience those maladaptive behavioral patterns, they share how they are impacted by them, so the person receiving feedback gains insight into how they are both acting and impacting others.

The interpersonal process group leader sets up the group by setting facilitative conditions of placing the group into the here and now and encouraging process illumination. The *here and now* means that group members are invited to share their perceptions of each other in real time. For example, clients are encouraged to share how they feel about each other interpersonally in the present moment, using the concept of immediacy to share observations about the impact they have on each other. *Immediacy* involves real-time feedback on how a person is coming across and feedback from the group on each other's behaviors. This use of the group and the act of giving each other feedback on their reactions to each other in the present moment are key to the process of change.

Another stage of change is *process illumination* (Yalom & Leszcz, 2020), which involves the therapist's or clients' sharing how the process of interaction is impacting individuals and the group. Therefore, the content of a discussion (e.g., a person's discussing feeling upset with a relative) is less important than the process (that the person has been upset for months with the relative but has kept denying this to the other group members, thereby blocking any potential that the group may have had to help).

The power of the group is primarily seen as being how group members help each other by offering feedback, by modeling, and through a range of other therapeutic factors that promote change. A central mechanism of change in a Yalom group is acquisition of insight into the maladaptive pattern followed by a process of behavior change within the group. However, this insight is emergent and organic. That is, Yalom's (Yalom & Leszcz, 2020) idea of the social microcosm suggests that, over time, people will eventually bring the same problematic interpersonal patterns into the group that they follow in their life (Kivlighan, Gullo, et al., 2021). The group leader's job and the group's job are to help illuminate those patterns as they become apparent.

It is a model that typically lasts several months and sometimes runs for years. FBGT takes these ideas and implements some of them in a slightly different sequence; it is more driven by semistructured and collaboratively established expectations of goal achievement, as discussed in the next chapter. However, it uses the here and now, immediacy, and process illumination as key drivers of the group itself.

Brief Group Therapy

Unlike the prior Yalom groups, which run for the medium to long term, FBGT is a brief group that runs eight or more sessions (although many groups run for eight sessions, as originally conducted, in other settings, groups run for 12–15 sessions). Brief therapy groups change a great many assumptions about the organization of mechanisms of change and what must be added to accommodate for the increased pace of change.

Brief therapy groups have certain conditions that make them different than longer groups. They are seen as needing to meet the following conditions (Piper & Ogrodniczuk, 2004; Yalom & Leszcz, 2020):

• Not everyone will get all their goals achieved within the life of the group.
• Group is a jumping-off place, not a final destination.
• Leaders must keep the group time focused.
• Goals must be clear and achievable within prescribed time limits.
• Members must have realistic expectations.
• Groups must be built around rapid cohesion.
• Group members must have a strong working alliance with the therapist.

FBGT made these alterations to the Yalom model to enhance best practices. Instead of allowing the interpersonal behaviors to emerge organically, which may take weeks and months (time FBGT does not have), it predicts into them in the individualized therapy, pregroup preparation, and screening (TPS) session (see Chapter 6) using assessment tools. This accelerates the process of insight with the help of the interpersonal circumplex to preidentify the problem (see Chapters 5 and 6). This *rapid movement to insight* using assessment provides a preview of the expected behavior of the client in the social microcosm of the group.

FBGT also anticipates that, for some clients, enactment of interpersonal patterns can result in self-sabotage early in the life of the group that can be hard for both the client and the group to recover from. *Inoculation* (Whittingham 2015), a key technique developed for FBGT, is used to anticipate this self-sabotage and to prophylactically prevent it, simultaneously including it as a treatment goal (see Chapter 6). The here and now and process illumination are also important parts of FBGT, except that instead of being used to promote insight, they are used as a space in which to activate new behaviors and to receive feedback. Each FBGT goal must be able to be enacted in the here and now of the group.

One of the differentiators between a medium-term interpersonal process group and an FBGT group is its relationship to anxiety and conflict. Given that FBGT greatly accelerates the process of change, some emotional guardrails need to contain the process so it does not cognitively and emotionally flood the client and reduce the opportunity for learning. FBGT also works on maintaining realistic expectations, keeps a time focus, and prioritizes a strong working alliance and group cohesion as foundations. These processes also require an understanding of how to manage group and client stress levels to promote optimal levels of anxiety that are required for brief group members to be successful. Because, given their accelerated nature, brief groups are particularly stressful for clients, the need to manage anxiety is paramount. Understanding polyvagal theory (Porges & Dana, 2018), therefore, becomes an important strand within FBGT.

Polyvagal Theory

Polyvagal theory is the study of how the brain and body interact via the central nervous system. The two main systems are (a) the *sympathetic nervous system*, which prepares people to defend themselves against threats via fight, flight, or freeze mechanisms; and (b) the *parasympathetic nervous system*, which operates to facilitate calmness, learning, and relaxation via what are described as rest and digest mechanisms (Porges, 2007; Porges & Dana, 2018).

As Flores and Porges (2017) pointed out, process groups that focus on relationships have inherent potential gains in helping people self-regulate. They enable people to securely attach and to develop relationships that allow them to effectively coregulate emotions. However, the key component of this potential is that the group must be experienced as safe, and the therapist must set the conditions early in the group for that safety. This then allows members to increase their ability to self-regulate and to improve their neuroception. As the authors pointed out, *neuroception* involves the person's ability to notice the cues (e.g., facial expressions, posture) and intentions of others to determine whether they are a threat. For the person, the group then becomes a secure base to explore and improve their ability to acquire a safe base in their real world contexts. The authors also recommended that group leaders help group members manage themselves and help members apply a *vagal brake*, the ability to move between moments of calmness and activation so that they can manage, tolerate, and learn from difficult moments.

FBGT group leaders provide the safety and predictability at the beginning of the group by using inoculation and titrating both conflict and other extremes of behavior (e.g., unboundaried warmth or uninhibited and extreme self-disclosure), thereby providing a sense of safety and stability in the initial stages. As the group progresses and those behaviors inevitably reappear, the group's cohesion can then act as a safety net that allows the more extreme behavior to be integrated into social learning.

The sympathetic and parasympathetic nervous systems are inextricably interlinked to social learning. When the body is in fight, flight, or freeze mode, the sympathetic nervous system is engaged. The body prepares for action by releasing hormones, such as adrenalin, into the system and begins to prepare people for immediate physical action requiring fast thoughts. The responses become automatic and based on a sense of self-protection. To experience social learning, the parasympathetic system needs to be engaged (Flores & Porges, 2017). Therefore, when social threat is perceived as too great, social learning is difficult, and people instead retreat into familiar, automatic, and unthinking responses to that threat.

Social threat and social support do not look the same for everyone (Collins & Feeney, 2004; Kivlighan & Angelone, 1992), however. For someone comfortable with aggressive confrontation (e.g., with a style high on Scale 2: Focused on the Needs of the Self), conflict and argument are actually relatively safe spaces. What is vastly more terrifying for them is the possibility of vulnerability—a part of themselves they have split off from themselves, often early in childhood, and that they associate with victimhood. By contrast, someone with an unassertive style will perceive that same conflict as highly activating and will quickly move into a position in which they may become immobilized or frozen as the feelings of threat become overwhelming. It is important in FBGT to understand what "comfort" looks like for each person. The same conflict can be energizing for one participant and immobilizing for another.

Therefore, careful calibration of stress to ensure the client is kept at a level of optimal anxiety to facilitate social learning is another key precept of FBGT.

Too little anxiety and social learning will fail to take place because the goals are seen as irrelevant or too easy and therefore are boring. Too much anxiety (e.g., with an intense conflict in the first 5 minutes of the group or goals that are too challenging) and some clients are catapulted into fight, flight, or freeze mode, and little learning takes place. Therefore, polyvagal theory is important throughout the life of FBGT at various points, including the idea of "Going for Goldilocks" described in Chapter 6 that explains how to establish goals that are optimally anxiety provoking. Polyvagal theory is critical to goal setting (see Chapter 6), the bond to the therapist (see Chapters 3, 5, and 6), cohesion with the group (see Chapters 7 and 8), inoculation techniques (see Chapter 6), and titration of conflict (see Chapters 7 and 8).

This concept is also important to understand in relation to the concept of how much interpersonal change is realistic to expect before a client decompensates or leaves because of the strain. The construct of the quarter turn, noted by Kiesler (1996) and discussed in Chapter 2, became a key principle in FBGT.

Diversity variables are also an important factor in helping clients be successful in group. FBGT looks to help the client feel connected, understood, and aligned with the therapist and the group by working on understanding what diversity variables are important to the client.

MULTICULTURAL THEORY

FBGT looks at both within-group differences (interpersonal styles based on different traits and developmental factors) as well as the different contexts and cultural spaces that can also impact interpersonal distress. FBGT prioritizes valuing and respecting cultural identity and values as strengths. It seeks out information about how the client defines themselves, using assessment tools as a way to broach the subject followed by an interpersonal interview that seeks out more information about the interface between interpersonal distress and culture. From this discussion, the therapist and client work together to understand the connections (if any) between interpersonal distress and cultural identity.

At one end of the scale, a client may identify that their interpersonal problems straddle all their cultural spaces and contexts. For example, they identify considerable distress around being socially inhibited across all cultural groups and settings, including those with which they most identify. In other cases, a client may report that their distress only arises when encountering cultural forces, such as discrimination and prejudice from specific contexts that they are in.

Remember that contexts can also be maladaptive and send incorrect signals about someone's behavior, identity, and worth. For example, acts of interpersonal racism can lead to significant interpersonal distress and worsening mental health for the target of that discrimination (Chao et al., 2012). Equally, microaggressions can impact people of color and other minoritized people in negative ways, when at work (King et al., 2023), online (Awad & Connors, 2023), and in other settings (Nadal, 2023). Research has found that microaggressions can have a significant impact on mental health via the concept of thwarted belongingness, resulting in depression and anxiety (Wike et al., 2023). Therefore, the links between societal discrimination, feelings of exclusion and rejection, and negative mental health outcomes are important to understand and treat. Equally, because loneliness is also linked to social identity and emotional regulation (S. Hayes et al., 2022), it is important to elicit from clients how they define themselves and what diversity variables are most important to them. Asking a client to share how they define what identity or identities are important to them opens the door to understanding how these factors impact them in more complex ways and promotes a stronger alliance.

The nuances of how clients' identities interact become important to explore because how they explain what is causing the clients the most distress then helps to guide treatment. For each client, it is important to understand the possible attributions for interpersonal distress and to then determine what goals make sense. In some cases, this may mean exploring the opportunity to build skills that help them assert their identity, an interpersonal skill that is not easy for some clients, depending on their interpersonal style. In other cases, it may mean exploring the other connections between identity and interpersonal goals to uncover what the client would define as a helpful change. For example, a person who identifies as lesbian, gay, bisexual, transgender, questioning or queer, and others (LGBTQ+) states that they feel able to assert themselves around their identity. They also state that they are thriving as an advocate for LGBTQ+ rights and their skills in assertive public speaking are proving successful. However, they report that they struggle to keep friends or romantic partners, leaving them feeling lonely and unsupported as well as more stressed and depressed because they feel like they are helping everyone else without being able to meet their own needs. The therapist supports this client's successes in public speaking while exploring with the client how they can better meet their personal need for intimacy. With such careful thought and collaboration with the client, FBGT can help clients find ways to improve their interpersonal flexibility with the intent of meeting their interpersonal goals.

FBGT explores all areas of a client's life to determine how the client identifies themselves and how that identity combines with their interpersonal strengths and distress. Within the approach, helping clients find more adaptive behaviors to meet their goals is always the sought out outcome. Whether the client is learning new interpersonal skills to counter interpersonal acts of discrimination, is learning to ask for help and support, or is working on other interpersonal goals, listening to what the client finds distressing and working on the areas of their life that are important to them is the sought end goal. Clients may also find benefit from other mechanisms of change common with therapy groups, such as universality (e.g., "I am not alone"), altruism (e.g., "I can help other people in the group, helping me realize I have something to give people"), and other therapeutic factors (Yalom & Leszcz, 2020).

Important issues related to leadership behaviors and multicultural skills also need to be considered. Studies of psychotherapy have found that therapists are not equally effective with clients based on their racial–ethnic minority background (J. A. Hayes et al., 2015, 2016). FBGT is an approach that requires therapists to be multiculturally sensitive and to adopt the attitudes associated with the MCO framework (Owen et al., 2011): maintaining cultural humility and looking for opportunities to elicit cultural material and develop cultural comfort, which entails self-awareness on the part of the therapist in becoming more comfortable discussing multicultural issues over time. Therapists should adopt a position of learning about other cultures while also listening for how culture impacts each client individually: the nomothetic (what people within cultural groups share in common) and the ideographic (how culture plays a part in an individual person's life; Ridley, 2005). Group leaders must be prepared to broach the topic of diversity both in the TPS session and also in the group.

Cultural missed opportunities are a key factor in group member improvement. Grimes and Kivlighan (2022) found that when the group missed cultural opportunities for discussion, but the group leader addressed them, or when the group leader missed them but the group addressed them, client outcomes improved. In other words, when one compensated for the other, clients achieved better therapeutic change. However, although group members can feel supported and can grow from discussions emanating from either leaders or groups, the group leader must always be ready to broach the topics and be ready to discuss culture, diversity, and issues related to identity.

Therapists must make careful decisions on when to adopt and when to adapt FBGT. Over the past 15 years, FBGT has been used across the United

States (in dozens of agencies from the East Coast to the West Coast) as well as in Singapore, China, and elsewhere (Jia, 2021; Whittingham & Liew, 2020). As Hewitt and Liew (2023) described via an example in which FBGT was successfully run at a psychiatric hospital in Singapore, careful consideration needs to be made regarding evaluating the norms for each instrument, using item analysis, and seeking out areas in which the approach may need to be adapted. Engaging in clinical interviewing, seeking out local cultural experts, and using triangulation of data for each client and group also form an important part of making the process both clinically and culturally responsive. With the use of FBGT in China, careful attention has been paid to the need to consider when to adopt and where to adapt. While leading workshops in China it became clear through clinical observations and consultation with cultural experts that corrective feedback was received very differently than in the United States. Some Chinese workshop participants actively sought out corrective feedback and indicated being honored by it being given, while showing some suspicion of positive feedback. Thus, at times, adjustments were made to account for those cultural norms. Thus, adjustments were made to account for those cultural norms by sometimes allowing for more corrective feedback (per the request of the clients) than might be given in the United States.

Consistently and carefully listening to each client, broaching discussions about culture, checking assumptions, and being willing to show humility with respect to cultural learning are keystones of FBGT practice. Promoting discussion of identity also contains within it not just the healing processes that occur internally and cognitively, but also provides opportunities for clients to practice new behaviors.

Behavioral Activation

Research is now showing the importance of behavioral activation as a unifying mechanism of change that is fundamental to treatment for a range of emotional disorders (e.g., Santos et al., 2021). The role of approach and avoidance in theories of behavioral activation is a basic principle in behavioral theory. The theory is that underlying depression and anxiety are avoidance of feared stimuli, including interpersonal situations that the person perceives as potentially threatening (Boswell et al., 2017).

A precept of FBGT, therefore, is the idea that insight is necessary but insufficient for interpersonal change. A person must move that insight into action. To change the fixed, maladaptive schemas that promise disaster when attempting new behaviors, behavior change must also occur. The resultant emotional and cognitive flooding that then takes place must be managed by the client via group processes facilitated by the group leader.

This focus on making these interpersonal goals behavioral and then activating them during the group became a defining foundation of the approach. As Gold and Kivlighan (2011) noted, the sequence of experiencing in a group is an important one for interpersonal change. They also noted that when group members were actively involved in the group process, including both emotional responses and behavioral activations, and were then able to reflect on what had happened, positive interpersonal outcomes occurred. The two conditions that this same study found to be unhelpful were either (a) clients were passive or (b) members had experiences with the group's having a more unpredictable and chaotic climate. FBGT works on overt activation of behavior that also involves an emotional response (that may be overtly or covertly experienced) followed by an integration of that material cognitively. It also relies on a strong basis of group cohesion, which provides the secure base for behavioral activation to take place.

Common Factors/Evidence-Based Relationships

The need for a strong working alliance and group cohesion to help clients manage the anxiety surrounding new interpersonal behavioral changes is also essential. Common factors are becoming more understood in the field as being the transtheoretical building blocks of any good therapy (Lo Coco et al., 2015; Wampold & Imel, 2015). Research has shown that they account for more change than any one specific technique in individual therapies (Imel & Wampold, 2008; Wampold et al., 2017). Research in group therapy has found similar effects: Group cohesion and the working alliance have proven to be particularly important to client change and retention (Arnold, 2021; Clough et al., 2022) in group therapy. As Chapter 2 demonstrates, FBGT mechanisms of change are built around a particular emphasis on a strong working alliance and group cohesion; the working alliance is a prerequisite for group cohesion (Arnold, 2021). Each represents the "glue" that helps promote attendance and reduces premature dropout by acting as the container for the challenging work. These two constructs represent the metaphorical drumbeat of and baseline to the work of FBGT.

A key common factor is also the need for unconditional positive regard and the ability to maintain a strengths focus. The anxiety of possible ostracism is pronounced in groups. Establishing and maintaining a bond with the client is key to success, even when their behavior is sometimes designed to test the therapist or even, as is common, invites rejection. Keeping unconditional positive regard at the forefront is therefore imperative. Wampold and Imel's (2015) common factors research showed that unconditional positive regard represented a stronger effect size than differences between treatment theories. It represents the underlying thread that must be maintained to keep the client–therapist bond.

Unconditional positive regard in FBGT involves the process of understanding the deeper feelings and motives driving clients' behavior and finding a way to care about them. No matter what the overt behavior and how off-putting and emotionally activating for the therapist the cyclical maladaptive pattern is, the group leader must maintain a focus on the client's underlying strengths, the operating principle being that they are always trying their best, and have empathy for the pain that repeated interpersonal frustrations and distress causes the client. Chapter 6 discusses this idea in more detail. Notably, despite assessment sometimes being seen as antithetical to a strong therapeutic relationship, when used in the right way, the working alliance can be strengthened by thoughtful and collaborative use of measurement to inform treatment.

Measurement-Based Care

MBC (Lewis et al., 2019) is a method in FBGT that allows many of the prior threads—interpersonal functioning; common factors, such as the working alliance; and MCO theory—to be optimized. By approaching the process collaboratively and transparently, what could have been a process that labels and distances instead becomes a shared journey of understanding and meaning.

The use of MBC has been shown to add considerable value to psychotherapy. It prevents client worsening and premature dropout, two factors that therapists tend to miss (Lambert & Harmon, 2018). As Fortney et al. (2017) pointed out, a significant amount of the difference between randomized clinical trials and routine, real-world care is accounted for by using routine monitoring in real time to make adjustments to treatment. Research has shown that treatment outcomes were improved for more than two thirds of therapists and that deterioration reduced while outcomes improved for those most at risk of poor outcomes (Lambert et al., 2018). Research has also found that use of MBC reduces the differences in effectiveness between more and less effective therapists (Delgadillo et al., 2022).

New studies are also showing the impact of using MBC with racial and ethnic minoritized youths. E. H. Connors et al. (2023) suggested that it can be used to improve the working alliance and to track progress while enhancing shared decision making and improving client satisfaction.

Several components of MBC differentiate it from using assessment to simply measure outcome: (a) the therapist reviews measures in real time, rather than later; (b) the client reviews the assessments too; and (c) the therapist and client collaboratively review the measures and decide together on how to make adjustments to improve treatment (Lewis et al., 2019). FBGT shares a similar premise in that all assessment tools are used as part of the therapeutic relationship. They are used transparently with every client. They are used to inform but not supplant clinical judgment during screening and pregroup preparation; to inform group process; to understand the group dynamic; to inform therapist analysis of transference and countertransference, thereby aiding the working alliance; and to help understand outcomes and translate them into the outside world. Assessment in FBGT is comprehensive and client centered and is designed to help the client and therapist at every stage of the group. As is discussed in later chapters, any preassessment of clients is used to develop hypotheses that are held lightly. On meeting the client, listening to their story, experiencing their interpersonal invitations, and discussing the results, the therapist can validate those hypotheses or consider which need refining or changing. Thus, assessment is responsive to client input, and clinical judgment remains key (Whittingham et al., 2023).

MBC was woven deeply into FBGT from the very beginning because it enhanced clinical decision making, improved outcomes, allowed the therapist to anticipate and prevent deterioration, and was seen as helpful by clients. Therapists also found the assessment helpful in understanding transference and countertransference, goal setting, establishing a bond, working with a coleader, and analyzing group dynamics, all of which are explored throughout this book in later chapters. Measurement in FBGT is always collaborative and nonshaming and is designed to be conducted using unconditional positive regard, as the next chapter shows. The attitude toward the client in FBGT is to walk together with caring curiosity.

SUMMARY

Together, these theories form key underpinnings of FBGT. Interpersonal theory and interpersonal therapy can be used to blend the best that science and art have to offer, whereas measurement-based care, multicultural responsiveness, and polyvagal theory all combine to enhance the working alliance and group cohesion and to promote positive outcomes. They provide foundations that can be filtered through the lenses of identity, contexts, and cultures, leading toward a client-centered and multiculturally responsive approach that collaboratively promotes client preference and choice. Interpersonal flexibility is a key concept in FBGT, and processes of change are oriented toward that outcome. Chapter 2 explores how these constructs and concepts are organized and structured to optimize mechanisms of change within the time frame.

2 FOCUSED BRIEF GROUP THERAPY STRUCTURE, PARAMETERS, AND MECHANISMS OF CHANGE

This chapter delineates inclusion and exclusion criteria and explores key mechanisms of change. It outlines how those mechanisms operate sequentially but also concurrently, laying the foundations for client success by ensuring evidence-based processes are kept in focus. It also explores how several constructs and techniques became particularly important to focused brief group therapy (FBGT) as a result of clinical learning from therapeutic successes and failures. Key processes that evolved from the challenges of running brief groups is given particular attention: Bookending and inoculation, two major innovations in FBGT, are discussed along with conceptual ideas vital to goal formation and success, such as the quarter turn, homeostasis, and habituation.

CENTRAL PROPOSITION OF FBGT

As already discussed, FBGT listens to what is distressing the client and addresses their self-identified goals. It helps the client to become more interpersonally flexible so that they have more choices in dealing with relationships. It also takes the approach that "if it isn't broken, don't fix it." Preexisting

https://doi.org/10.1037/0000389-003
Focused Brief Group Therapy: An Integrative Approach to Reducing Interpersonal Distress, by M. Whittingham

strategies and interpersonal techniques that work in specific situations and contexts should be continued. FBGT only looks to add new behaviors that can be applied to situations in which the preexisting skills are not working for the client. That idea is the core principle of how FBGT is proposed to clients and forms its central thesis.

The central premise of FBGT therefore consists of

- knowing that your personality is just fine and has many strengths;

- knowing that your cultural beliefs, identity, and contexts are an important part of who you are;

- knowing that you have always done your best to make your way in the world with what you know;

- asking yourself that if you wanted to make some small changes to your interpersonal behavior that might get you closer to getting your needs met in areas that are important to you, if you would want to try them out; and

- asking yourself if you would also be interested in figuring out together afterward how, when, and where to apply those new skills in your contexts and situations so that they can make a real difference.

This premise is the heart of the working alliance, and goal agreement is enshrined in that set of questions (see Chapter 6).

The transdiagnostic nature of the approach is also evident in this premise. FBGT does not assume that everyone will have the same diagnosis; rather, it is understood that diagnostic features emerge from the underlying interpersonal etiology in ways that are idiosyncratic to each client. FBGT also does not assume a one-size-fits-all outcome for each client. The end goal depends on the initial interpersonal goals for each client and is tailored to each one. Therefore, the assumptions of a common mechanism of change and set of outcomes do not apply in FBGT. It is not a common goal for all to be more cohesive or for everyone to be better able to tolerate and manage conflict. Rather, these goals evolve from personalization of outcomes. One member may have a goal of greater assertiveness, whereas another may have a goal of greater connectedness and cohesion with others. Thus, the measure of success is individually based and works on interpersonal flexibility.

The approach therefore is applicable to clients from a range of diagnostic categories, thus allowing for easier referrals and scheduling at a treatment setting. FBGT works on etiology, not symptomatology. So, the inclusion and exclusion criteria are somewhat broader than some therapies, but clear inclusion and exclusion criteria remain.

BALANCING POTENTIAL BENEFITS AGAINST POTENTIAL HARM

A key framework for assessing suitability for FBGT is contrasting the potential for benefit against the potential for harm for both the client and the group. Early research (Rotsinger-Stemen & Whittingham, 2013; Whittingham & Liew, 2020) suggested that clients with interpersonal problems across all scales of the interpersonal circumplex can benefit from FBGT. Moreover, interpersonal problems are universal and cross-cultural. They are part of the human condition. However, the approach is not a panacea, and it requires careful thought regarding client fit, the demands of the treatment setting, and multiple other factors. Some clients come to treatment to work on very specific disorders that may only tangentially be related to interpersonal functioning or may have very different mechanisms of change. For example, anxiety about exams or a specific phobia would fall into both of those categories. Equally, client fit for an eight- to 12-session format that up-regulates and activates client change in session is not suited to everyone. A number of factors affect suitability for FBGT, including treatment duration: the role of fight, flight, or freeze reactions during anxiety-provoking change processes; chronicity and severity of pre-existing conditions; and logistics. Thus, the parameters need to be carefully thought through regarding who is indicated and contraindicated for group.

Equally, although the specific group member's well-being is a primary concern, it is not the only concern. Research has shown that a group's well-being and outcomes are interdependent (Lo Coco et al., 2019). Thus, the whole group can be impacted by a group member's behaviors, so an incorrect referral will affect both that individual client's well-being and the well-being and outcomes of other group members. For example, if a therapist is considering whether to include a member who has sadistic and manipulative tendencies, they should carefully consider the effect of this member on the group as a whole. Whatever benefit that client might obtain from the group must be weighed against the potential for harm to other group members, which, in this case, could be considerable. However, real life is seldom this clear-cut. A less dramatic but no less meaningful example is of a client who is unlikely to attend regularly. Although this may seem more benign than the aforementioned manipulative and malignant client, the impact can also be consequential for the group, as is discussed later in this chapter.

INCLUSION AND EXCLUSION CRITERIA

FBGT does not subscribe to the philosophy of taking on 15 clients and expecting five to drop out. This creates what Yalom and Leszcz (2020) called a *double demoralization*, whereby clients who are already feeling discouraged then feel like a failure at treatment, too. Double demoralization can lead to clients' not only failing to make gains in treatment but actively worsening. Therefore, given the "do no harm" principle of the American Psychological Association (APA) and other medical and psychological ethics codes (e.g., APA, 2017), it is hard to justify an approach that relies on this philosophy as a precondition of a group's beginning.

FBGT is premised on a correct selection of clients, who are then set up to be successful in terms of both process and outcome. The expectation is to keep dropout to a bare minimum, and to carefully analyze every premature dropout to determine how to learn from the situation. The instruments used in FBGT were specifically designed to be used to predict into and prevent early termination and have been rigorously tested for that purpose.

As with the previous section, clinical judgment should not be sacrificed for the sake of strict adherence to criteria. A client should be seen as the totality of their factors and nuance, and clinical judgment should allow for thoughtful decision making if exceptions are to be made.

Inclusion Criteria

Inclusion criteria are also key in understanding how to best use FBGT. The approach is broad based in its application, but it is not a panacea. Clinicians should therefore give careful thought to when and how to recommend it to clients or in terms of how it fits into an overall package of care.

Interpersonal Distress as Etiology

The key referral criterion is that the person being referred has an interpersonal problem that causes them distress and is a main driver of symptomatology. So, a person who is depressed because of loneliness and an inability to form relationships or maintain relationships—or both—would be a good candidate, providing they are not excluded for other reasons.

Interpersonal distress as a central treatment concern can take many forms. It may be the primary cause, when, for example, a client's inability to manage conflict leads to them consequences, such as losing their job or becoming divorced, leading to an episode of major depression. However, interpersonal distress may also be adjunctive or contributory to a primary diagnosis. For example, in their research, Karatzias et al. (2018) showed that complex posttraumatic stress disorder (PTSD) is impacted by attachment style problems, and they suggested that a needed part of treatment is adjunctive treatment to develop social skills.

Consider this example: A returning member of the military has PTSD as their main diagnosis. The client has become increasingly suicidal because a preexisting condition has worsened. As a result, they cannot form healthy social support networks at home and are struggling with their marriage and relationships with their children. In this case, the primary issue is the PTSD. However, problems in managing intimacy or maintaining relationships can lead to mental health problems becoming more chronic and severe. Absence of relationships or poor quality of relationships can mean a person lacks the social buffering that offers protection against mental health issues beginning, continuing, or worsening. Therefore, in interviews, the therapist needs to carefully explore the role of interpersonal distress, including the role it takes as a protective or risk factor in a client's current presenting problems and diagnosis. Careful case conceptualization is essential, and referrers should consider what treatment package or sequential series of treatments are most appropriate.

Ability to Perform the Work of the Group

Clients must be able to perform the work of the group (Yalom & Leszcz, 2020). Can they understand the information provided at intake, move quickly to insight, and function in a group environment in which members are responding to each other in the here and now? Clients do not have to be perfectly functional in every respect; if they were, then there would be no need for a group. However, they do need basic levels of insight, some ability to focus on others as well as themselves, and the willingness to take part in the back and forth of group process. Therefore, some level of cognitive insight, emotional resilience, reasonably advanced interpersonal skills, and moderate resilience at the least are prerequisites.

Ego Strength and Emotional Regulation

Clients must also have a basic level of ego strength (Yalom & Leszcz, 2020). The concept of ego strength is complex and derives from Freud's work (e.g., Freud, 1923/1989)—before being updated by psychodynamic clinicians to explain levels of client functioning. Within FBGT, though, *ego strength* refers to the idea that the person can tolerate the back and forth of the group without decompensating and falling into psychological crisis. They possess enough resilience to manage the demands placed on them by the work. Clients must have a basic level of emotional regulation, adequate self-concept, and the resilience to manage a difficult moment or survive an attack without prematurely terminating. While the ability of leaders to repair ruptures is an important part of therapeutic success (Marmarosh, 2021), if the group member is unwilling or unable to engage after a rupture, then no repair is possible.

Consider this example: A group member with a history of schizophrenia who is on antipsychotic medication is admitted to an FBGT group. After an intense session in which two group members engaged in a conflict, the group member does not return for the next week. The group leader later finds out that the person had found the conflict so upsetting that they had gone home and begun binge drinking, leading to a psychotic episode. The client is hospitalized and drops out of treatment. In this case, the client was highly distressed by the conflict and used maladaptive coping skills that led to serious consequences and group dropout.

Other examples might include someone who is recovering from a trauma, such as a recent sexual assault, that has impacted their ability to achieve secure attachments to others. Trauma has been linked to a variety of problems, including failure to self-regulate emotions, numbness, misinterpretation of innocuous behaviors as threats, and fragmentation of mental processes (Van der Kolk, 2014). In such cases, finding an individual therapist with whom they can begin to slowly build up a trusting, secure relationship would be an important precursor to even considering launching into an FBGT group, where safety will be far more difficult to establish.

Emotionally Down-Regulated

"Up-regulation" and "down-regulation" refer to the two opposing directions taken by the autonomic nervous system when managing emotions and arousal. *Up-regulation* means that the sympathetic nervous system is highly activated such that a person feels intensely aroused and energetic. As discussed in Chapter 1 on polyvagal theory, when this up-regulation becomes overly activated, it can lead to the fight, flight, or freeze response that makes social learning difficult. An example is someone who is in acute stress, having very recently been exposed to intense trauma; is hyperaroused; and is still in fight, flight, or freeze mode; that person will have difficulty attending to others. In this example, the up-regulation is because of a recent event or temporary state, such as a recent trauma or first instance of major depression. However, in other cases, the up-regulation may be more chronic: Someone with severe borderline personality disorder, for example, who is consistently up-regulated will be unable to manage their emotions and relationships. Up-regulation is discussed in more detail later in the section on exclusion criteria.

Down-regulation occurs when the parasympathetic nervous system has activated and puts the body in rest-and-digest mode. In this state, social learning can take place (Flores & Porges, 2017). Down-regulation allows a person to be neurobiologically calm enough to tolerate accommodating an increase in stress that comes with change. For example, a client who has been able to emotionally self-regulate after a major life crisis may now be prepared to undertake the difficult and anxiety-provoking work of interpersonal change.

Suicidality is a concern. It is not uncommon for clients in FBGT groups to have low levels of suicidality, including perhaps some ideation but no plan or intent. However, even these lower levels require monitoring and frequent assessment to detect changes and to determine if concurrent individual therapy becomes appropriate. The presence of such risk factors also suggests the need for more routine outcome measurement to track any increases in suicidal ideation.

Motivated

Motivation to join group therapy is an evidence-based construct linked to successful completion of such therapy (Cox, 2008). However, motivation in FBGT is seen as a malleable construct. Some clients are highly motivated to join before the therapy, pregroup preparation, and screening (TPS) session has even begun. For example, clients with high scores on Scale 8: Uninhibited (see Figure 1.2 in Chapter 1), are extremely desirous of close social relationships so are eager to join. However, other clients, such as those high on Scale 4: Socially Inhibited (see Figure 1.2), perceive the group to be an aversive event to be avoided at all costs.

Each interpersonal style has a complex relationship to motivation with aspects of the group that attract clients to it and aspects that they find anxiety provoking and sometimes frightening. Whether because of their initial interpersonal style, media representations of group therapy (which are typically not positive), or past experiences of rejection, clients will often have mixed feelings about joining group therapy. In most cases, these feelings can be worked through in FBGT. This process of establishing a strong working alliance is a key mechanism of change in FBGT. On rare occasions, though, clients are unmotivated to join or are unable to commit to the parameters. Such factors comprise the exclusion criteria.

Exclusion Criteria

Exclusion criteria are just as important as inclusion criteria. However, because they are inherently more complex, they are discussed at greater length.

No Interpersonal Distress and Etiology

In cases in which clients have little to no interpersonal distress and their symptoms or etiology are unrelated to interpersonal problems, then FBGT is not indicated as a treatment. Conditions and diagnoses need to be considered with respect to their mechanisms of change. For example, research has shown that FBGT can impact a wide range of interpersonal difficulties, such as depression, social anxiety, and interpersonal distress (Rotsinger-Stemen & Whittingham, 2013; Whittingham & Liew, 2020); but, despite those studies showing changes in depression, social anxiety, interpersonal distress, and general stress, the changes to generalized anxiety disorder were of smaller magnitude and only appeared after a longer duration of treatment. Research has shown that generalized anxiety is treated successfully when mechanisms of change, such as muscle relaxation or cognitive change of worry beliefs, take place (Donegan & Dugas, 2012). However, FBGT does not work on those specific areas; thus, the lack of impact on this condition is unsurprising. Therefore, conditions without an interpersonal etiology need a more thoughtful rationale to determine whether FBGT is an efficient and effective means of treating them. Some more clear-cut examples—such as a specific phobia (e.g., fear of spiders) that has no causal relationship to inter-personal flexibility—would also be a poor fit for the model.

On occasion, though, clients have presented with scores on the 32-item Inventory of Interpersonal Problems (IIP-32; Horowitz et al., 2000) measure that show no distress in interpersonal functioning, yet on closer examination and through an in-person meeting, those clients reveal a far greater distress than the instrument indicated. Possible reasons may include, for instance, a client whose narcissism led them to dismiss the whole second half of the assessment and enter zero values in all of the columns. When questioned about this, they stated that the assessment was "stupid and beneath me." In this case, the client's self-presentation and interpersonal responses were more pathognomonic than the assessment itself. Therefore, clinical judgment should always take primacy in assessing suitability for FBGT.

Inability to Perform the Work of the Group

Clients must be able to perform the work of the group and function to some level as a group member across several categories: insight, ego strength, motivation levels, and ability to tolerate up-regulation. Lack of insight and rigid externalization are significant barriers to participating in FBGT because achieving some degree of insight during the initial TPS session is a prerequisite for all future progress in the treatment. As Yalom and Leszcz (2020) described, *rigid externalization* relates to the client's inability to develop insight because of a consistent and unbending externalization of symptoms or causes. For example, the client attributes all their distress to the actions of something or someone outside of themselves and are unable to consider how they might be contributing to their own unhappiness. In some cases, this can manifest itself in somatic complaints in response to feelings questions. For instance, when asked to describe their feelings about a range of situations, the client can only report the physical experiences they are having, such as "a tight stomach" or "warm face."

A required instrument in FBGT, the Group Therapy Questionnaire–Short Form (GTQ-S; MacNair-Semands et al., 2010; see Chapter 5, this volume), has items that screen for rigid externalization that can lead to discussions in the TPS session. This somatization is often linked to poor emotional self-regulation and low insight (Erkic et al., 2018) and will make the work of the group extremely difficult for the client because those qualities are prerequisites for treatment success.

Low Ego Strength

Clients who are considered too emotionally reactive, fragile, or chaotic at a level that could not be contained by the group and group leader within the eight-session format should not be set up to fail (Rutan et al., 2014). Examples of people who may struggle in this way include clients within the severe range of borderline personality or narcissistic personality disorder. They may lack the ego strength to manage themselves in relation to others and may end up decompensating and also potentially causing harm to other group members. FBGT relies on clients' being able to work on their own change processes while maintaining consistent group participation and managing themselves at a basic level in relation to others. Although all clients in the group are expected to have interpersonal difficulties, some emotional reactions to other members, and moments of self-doubt, vulnerability, and anxiety, clients likely to fall into major psychological crisis (e.g., acting out aggressively, using substances, making suicide attempts) because of the stimulus value of the group and the work it entails should be excluded and referred to more suitable services.

Emotionally Up-Regulated

Emotionally up-regulated clients include those with high levels of suicidality, recent acute trauma, current serious addictions, and conditions with psychotic or severely disorganized features that are unmedicated. This is an approach that requires stabilization first and some level of down-regulation such that the person has enough ego strength and capacity to manage their own needs and the needs of others while emotionally and cognitively regulating.

If the client is in major crisis—experiencing high levels of suicidality or suffering a major recent trauma—then FBGT is only indicated as a treatment once the client is sufficiently stabilized (e.g., with medication, if indicated, and with individual therapy). FBGT can be highly anxiety provoking. It is not attempting to down-regulate and relax clients; rather, it challenges them to work on interpersonal change. Therefore, a baseline level of stability is needed such that when stressful change experiences are added, the client is not pushed into levels of distress that are antithetical to change.

The process of change is difficult and is often accompanied by increases in distress. Therapists should always err on the side of ethical care and client safety as well as ensure that any client taken on in group therapy is also receiving regular assessment of their current suicidality. Concurrent individual treatment is recommended in the event of any concerns about safety.

Persistent Low Motivation or Logistical Concerns, or Both

Low motivation can emerge in many forms. For some clients, logistical reasons are a significant impediment to participation. Workplace issues, school schedules, and child care can all significantly impede motivation; however, in some cases, these impediments function as a smokescreen for worries and fears about joining the group or a deeper ambivalence toward treatment itself. Some clients are also highly unmotivated toward therapy. For example, people referred by their human resources departments, the courts, or other punitive bodies are often frustrated and angry that they have to attend treatment. Some also come to therapy at the behest of family members but are only attending an intake to appease that concerned relative rather than out of a sincere belief that they are in need of therapy. Each situation presents the possibility of malleability of motivation as the issues are addressed through techniques, such as motivational interviewing (W. R. Miller & Rollnick, 2002). Some situations, though, remain intractable.

A particular challenge might involve a client who says they can come to group but will either come every other week or will arrive late or leave early. The reasons may be logistical, such as having a job that delays their ability to leave on time, or an ambivalence about the group. The therapist should carefully explore the reasons; in some cases, this exploration can strengthen the working alliance if worked through successfully. However, the group leader should not accommodate requests to arrive late, leave early, or miss multiple sessions.

The boundary of the group must be maintained because the constant "two starts" or "two endings" that happen when someone arrives or leaves separately from the rest of the group, or attends the group intermittently, means the group dynamic is constantly resetting. For example, if an important incident happens in the first 5 minutes that the group wishes to process, and a member arrives 10 minutes late, the group will either recap and move out of the moment, or the late group member will feel left out. While occasional lateness is forgiven, a member cannot be allowed to join the group if they cannot reliably attend every session and arrive and leave on time. The effects on the whole group can be frustration, annoyance, and disjointedness.

Although the group leader may feel a variety of internal pressures (e.g., wishing to be liked, desiring to do good, being unwilling to say no) and external pressures (e.g., the group needs one more member to begin) to accommodate a client's wishes, they should protect the time and space boundaries of the group to ensure a smooth group process and successful outcomes. They need to seek a firm commitment from clients. At times, it is worth emphasizing that the group is only 8 or more sessions long, so committing to a few sessions likely means committing the whole way. However, if at the end of the TPS session, the client remains steadfast that they are not likely to come or will only come with specific conditions, such as late arrival, early departure, or the ability to skip sessions, then they should be referred elsewhere.

Clients With Personality Disorders

The therapist needs to assess on a case-by-case basis whether to include clients diagnosed with personality disorders. The assessment should include consideration of likelihood of a successful group experience, likelihood of harm accruing to the group, perception of the client as being unable to keep pace with other group members, skill of the group leader, and other variables. For example, a client diagnosed with schizoid personality disorder may, in some cases, benefit from multiple iterations of the group but will only change in very small increments. These small changes may be very meaningful to them and should not be dismissed. The group leader must also assess this person's impact on the group to determine whether groups are also benefiting from the client's contributions.

Consider, for instance, the case of a client who had been diagnosed with severe social phobia with features of schizoid personality disorder and would be going through multiple iterations of the FBGT group with different group members each time. In each group iteration, other members consistently showed compassion and understanding and were sensitive to the distress they saw as this client struggled to manage their social anxiety. This holding environment proved therapeutic for the client and was helpful to other members, who learned how to act compassionately and patiently with someone they all experienced as in considerable distress who, yet, showed courage by returning every week.

As this case illustrates, other factors the therapist needs to consider are the client's motivation and their willingness to tolerate the distress. Careful debriefing and interviewing the client again with every new group is necessary to ensure that they are finding the group useful and can tolerate the distress while also benefiting from the group. The client's wishes and preferences need to significantly inform the final decision.

At the end of the six groups, the client described in the earlier example informed the group leaders that they now felt that they may want relationships in their life. This statement reflected the amount of courage, hard work, and commitment that they had shown in working through such a challenging experience.

Other important factors to consider in some cases is the client's prior treatment and readiness for change. For example, a client with severe features of borderline personality disorder who has never undergone treatment would likely be a poor candidate for FBGT, whereas a client with less severe presentation and a prior history of successful treatment with dialectical behavior therapy (Linehan & Wilks, 2015) or mentalization therapy (Fonagy & Bateman, 2006) might be successful with limited and realistic goals. Therefore, careful use of clinical judgment is paramount.

The issue of when and how FBGT takes place relative to other treatment components is a factor in considering the possible benefits and risks to clients. For example, important considerations are whether to use FBGT concurrently with individual therapy, consecutively as a part of a treatment package, or as a stand-alone therapy.

CONCURRENT THERAPY

As a general rule, FBGT works well as a standalone therapy with no other treatment concurrently when used in an outpatient setting. In some cases, *concurrent therapy*—individual therapy taking place alongside FBGT—is permitted, but only if it does not dilute the work of the group therapy and is clinically indicated. For example, a client with specific phobia may wish to work on their fear of flying separately from the work of the group that relates to their problems in relationships. In this case, the specific work has very different mechanisms of change and the two, concurrent treatments would not be contraindicated. However, therapists should communicate carefully to ensure treatments remain discreet and that the client does not begin to dilute their group work by discussing what happens in the group during individual therapy sessions. There are clinical examples of FBGT working well as a consecutive treatment. For example, Whittingham and Liew (2020) described a package of treatment for patients in Singapore involving FBGT followed by individual therapy.

The key elements to consider are whether this is the optimal treatment for the client based on factors such as mechanisms of change, the client's readiness, and the group dynamic. Every case needs to be evaluated carefully to determine whether a client would benefit from this treatment model or whether they would be better suited to a more developmentally appropriate level for them. The therapist must ultimately weigh the risks and benefits of treatment, knowing the parameters of FBGT: that it is brief, designed to impact interpersonal functioning, requires insight, and requires the ability to function within a therapy group. The structure of FBGT is also an important consideration in making these decisions is the structure of FBGT, which is outlined in the next section.

STRUCTURE OF THE MODEL

FBGT is a semistructured model. It has specific tasks at each stage to give group leaders guidance and a clear sense of what constructs need attending to and what tasks need completing. However, the art of the therapy is that this then requires group leaders marry those skillfully to the needs of the individual clients and the group.

Five Steps

As can be seen in Figure 2.1, the structure involves a series of five carefully calibrated sequential steps, and measurement-based care (MBC) dovetails with common factors to promote evidence-based mechanisms of change. Step 1 involves a referral from a gatekeeper, such as an intake therapist; Chapter 5 outlines the process for training referral sources about what makes an appropriate referral to the group.

Once the referral has been made, the client is administered three assessment tools as part of the intake process: (a) the IIP-32 (Horowitz et al., 2000), (b) the GTQ-S (MacNair-Semands et al., 2010), and (c) a quality of life measure that is empirically sound and normed against that population (e.g., the 30-item Outcome Questionnaire [OQ-30]; Ellsworth et al., 2006), which is used in this chapter as an exemplar). The FBGT leader then reviews the assessment tools (see Chapter 5 for an overview of how to do this) and constructs a hypothesis about the client's interpersonal distress; they also consider what goals may be appropriate.

In Step 2, the client and FBGT leader then meet for an individualized session called the TPS session (see Chapter 6). The therapist notices the client's

FIGURE 2.1. Structure of Focused Brief Group Therapy

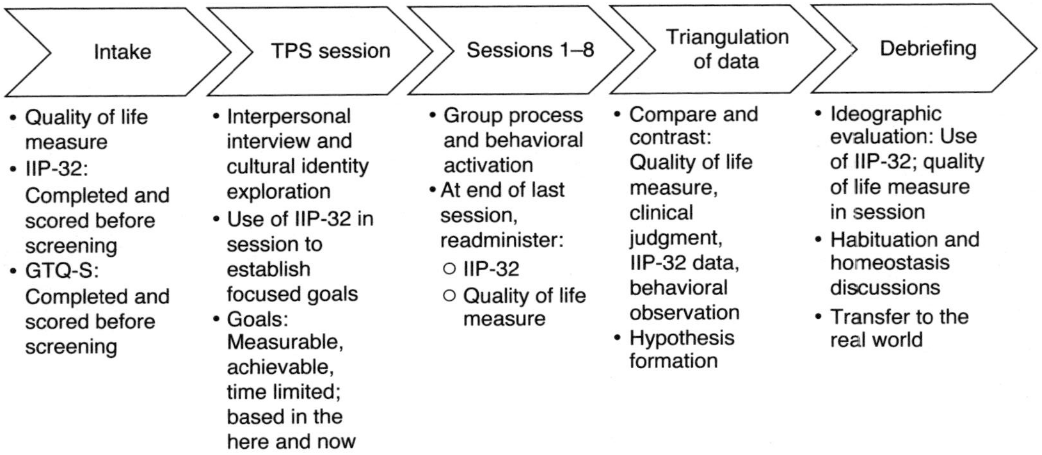

Intake	TPS session	Sessions 1–8	Triangulation of data	Debriefing
• Quality of life measure	• Interpersonal interview and cultural identity exploration	• Group process and behavioral activation	• Compare and contrast: Quality of life measure, clinical judgment, IIP-32 data, behavioral observation	• Ideographic evaluation: Use of IIP-32; quality of life measure in session
• IIP-32: Completed and scored before screening	• Use of IIP-32 in session to establish focused goals	• At end of last session, readminister: ○ IIP-32 ○ Quality of life measure	• Hypothesis formation	• Habituation and homeostasis discussions
• GTQ-S: Completed and scored before screening	• Goals: Measurable, achievable, time limited; based in the here and now			• Transfer to the real world

Note. IIP-32 = the 32-item Inventory of Interpersonal Problems (Horowitz et al., 2000); GTQ-S = Group Therapy Questionnaire–Short Form (MacNair-Semands et al., 2010); TPS = therapy, pregroup preparation, and screening.

interpersonal invitations during the TPS session and notices their own reactions to those invitations. This information adds evidence for or against the hypothesis about the client's interpersonal style. The therapist then shows the client the assessment forms and collaboratively determines a focus for treatment. Both then discuss interpersonal history and current contexts and integrate information about diversity and identity. The therapist establishes a focus for treatment, typically based on the highest score on the IIP-32. The therapist and client collaboratively set goals that follow the MATH (measurable, achievable, time limited, and based in the here and now) formula (see Chapters 1 and 6) and write those goals on note cards.

In Step 3, the client then attends the group and works on their behavioral goals (see Chapters 7 and 8). The therapist tracks the goals and ensures that members are working toward them, offering occasional prompts to do so. As clients complete their goals, the therapist also ensures that immediate feedback is given to ensure each client is able to manage the anxiety that comes with schemas being activated. At the end of the last group session, two measures are readministered: (a) the IIP-32 and (b) the OQ-30; or other quality of life measure; see Chapters 8 and 9).

In Step 4, the data are *triangulated*, which means that the therapist compares and contrasts the prepost data from the repeated measures (i.e., the IIP-32 and OQ-30) to determine if change took place (see Chapters 9 and 10). These data are also compared and contrasted with the therapist's clinical observations about goal completion and witnessing of any behavior changes that accompanied that completion. The therapist uses their clinical judgment to construct a tentative hypothesis about whether change took place.

In Step 5, the client and FBGT leader meet for an individualized debriefing session. They collaboratively and nonjudgmentally explore the data (see Chapter 10) to confirm or disconfirm hypotheses and to collaboratively understand what happened. Transfer of learning to the real world is discussed, and the FBGT leader makes recommendations for discontinuation of therapy or continuation of care.

The FBGT leader needs to remain open minded and keep hypotheses tentative. Assessment data can be highly relevant and, in many cases, generate a clean hypothesis that is also agreed on by the client. However, assessment should never replace clinical judgment but, rather, should augment it (Whittingham et al., 2023).

Adjustments often need to be made to the approach based on clinical judgment, and such adjustments can occur anywhere during the FBGT process. For example, a case may progress without complication until debriefing and then prove surprising in how the client attributed change (e.g., "It wasn't me; it was skillful group leadership"). Or, in other cases, the change may be at the beginning, when the therapist realizes a context is sending the client false information about their typical interpersonal style (e.g., the client is a warm, kind person who is working in a toxic environment with people who are constantly engaging in racial stereotyping and microaggressions and then blaming the client for being "angry all the time" when the client is assertive). In such an instance, a client may sometimes internalize this distress and it may show up on the IIP-32 (Horowitz et al., 2000). Therefore, assessment should be considered part of an MBC that involves collaborative exploration and coconstruction of treatment using the therapist's clinical judgment, informed by the assessment, and mediated and moderated by careful consideration of contexts and systems of power and privilege. Any hypothesis should always be tentative until evidence accumulates from multiple sources, not the least of which is the client. However, finding a balance between structure and clinical responsiveness is greatly informed and assisted by the bookending process.

Bookending

In terms of structure, in FBGT, the TPS session and debriefing session are highly important and should never be omitted. Early in the approach, I began referring to them as *bookending* (Whittingham, 2015) because they serve a similar role: to metaphorically prevent what they were supporting from toppling over. The TPS session serves to set the conditions for success of the group itself by generating rapid movement to insight and creating a strong working alliance, whereas the debriefing session serves to help the client make sense of change and to prepare for transitioning their skills to the outside world. However, both also provide a space where clients can discuss the nuances of their particular situations, identities, cultures, and contexts, thus allowing both therapist and client to collaboratively tailor goals and to ensure that outcomes fit the contexts to which the client would be returning.

The TPS session and the debriefing session proved essential in the development of FBGT and are core to its success. Chapters 6 and 10 explore each end of the "bookends" in more detail.

Inoculation

Inoculation (Whittingham, 2015) is a key intervention that helps manage unintentional early self-sabotage and group sabotage as a result of maladaptive interpersonal strategies being implemented early in the life of the group. Chapter 6 describes inoculation in detail and offers clinical examples. The importance of this technique relates to the convergence of the need to build group cohesion at while simultaneously managing individual group members' phenotypic responses to the stress of being in a new group.

Because people go to their highest individual score under stress, and the first session of therapy is very stressful—lots of people might reject the client, plus one is uncertain about their status in the group—that first session often becomes a place in which extreme behaviors are acted out that are deleterious to all, including to the client who acted them out. Inoculation gives clients the ability to avoid self-sabotage while also allowing the group to cohere so that group members can help the client with their inflexibility within a more trusting climate.

Bookending and inoculation are therefore key processes in FBGT that ensure that clients feel heard, avoid self-sabotage, can set goals, and can move into their contexts in ways that honor their reported distress and the outcomes they are seeking. The other mechanisms of change operate in a stepwise fashion that allow clients and the therapist to move sequentially through the model in ways that maintain the alliance.

FBGT: MAIN FOCUS OF CHANGE

Researchers in interpersonal theory (Horowitz, 2004; O'Connor and Dyce, 1997) have long stated that interpersonal flexibility is central to healthy human functioning. Individuals can experience negative feedback in the form of criticism from a romantic partner, negative feedback at work, or constant rejection from friends. These problems often manifest as interpersonal distress. The person may be confused by this feedback or seek treatment for the symptoms arising from their responses to their distress (e.g., depression, problematic drinking). Sometimes the link between the problem and the symptoms are clear to the client: They feel depressed and understand the reason for it. However, this is not always the case, and it is not uncommon for clients to be completely unaware of their own role in their interpersonal problems.

People tend to misperceive themselves with respect to their impact on others. A recent study showed that only 13% of people accurately match their self-perception with the perception of others (Elsaadawy & Carlson, 2022). Moreover, people tend to misperceive how extreme their interpersonal behaviors can be. To quote a research article, "the fish cannot see the water in which it swims" (Leising et al., 2006, p. 964). People with certain interpersonal styles (e.g., people high in dominance) are unaware of how intensely others experience their behavior and therefore remain unaware of its role in the etiology of their problems (Leising et al., 2006).

People do not always see ourselves clearly, and this lack of clarity makes solutions to the problems we inadvertently cause difficult to enact. This can be compounded by how others deliver feedback. For example, if someone—for either interpersonal or cultural reasons—does not want to offend the person asking for feedback, they may downplay the impact of the other's behavior. Conversely, someone may have a self-serving agenda for complaining that the other person's interpersonal behaviors are worse than they actually are. Gaining accurate feedback on one's interpersonal behaviors requires not only finding someone willing to provide it but also that the person is able to do so accurately. If people are unaware of their role in the problem, how can change even begin?

To work toward change, insight into one's own contributions to situations (both in terms of strengths one brings and how they also sometimes contribute to their own distress) is an important prerequisite. The interpersonal circumplex becomes the central method of tailoring treatment in FBGT because it provides the focus for the approach. The perspective to take within FBGT is to listen for what is causing the client interpersonal distress and to use a measure of the construct to personalize the treatment. Understanding and collaboratively agreeing on the nature of the distress is a first step toward developing *interpersonal flexibility,* the ability to meet the demands of different situations such that one's needs (for either agency or affiliation or some combination of both) are met.

This flexibility is not a wild oscillation between styles but, rather, is the ability to maintain confidence and strengths around a core style or styles while being flexible as the context demands. The idea of mindful selection of interpersonal strategies is embedded in the FBGT approach. Therefore, change is predicated on clients' first identifying the strengths that go with their preferred interpersonal style. Once that is established, the main construct around which change is oriented is to work with the client on their self-selected highest area of interpersonal distress. In many cases, this will be their highest score on the interpersonal circumplex. Remember that this measure captures the client's self-identified distress. Personal preference and client autonomy are key to psychological treatment and are particularly important within FBGT. This score reports how the client experiences themselves and what they feel most strongly about. Looking at this score and collaboratively working on understanding it therefore becomes an important part of the working alliance. Clients typically feel heard and understood when their highest scale is explained to them. Having a chance to explore if and how this applies to their life is then part of the MBC process, which is important in FBGT. Evidence-based processes are linked to mechanisms of change that lead to outcomes, and FBGT has a specific sequence of change processes that generate that change.

Primary Mechanisms of Change in Stepwise Progression

The primary mechanisms of change in FBGT are shown in Figure 2.2. This section provides a description of each.

Rapid Movement to Insight/Working Alliance Formation

Rapid movement to insight is the first mechanism. It involves using the quality of life—typically the OQ-30 (Ellsworth et al., 2006) or a similar, empirically validated, measure of global functioning measure—and the IIP-32 (Horowitz et al., 2000) in tandem to help the client understand the connection between their overall distress and how their interpersonal distress may be causally connected. Collaboratively exploring the IIP-32 allows the client to gain insight into both the specific strengths and problems associated with their highest levels of interpersonal distress and the interpersonal style or styles that may be associated with their distress. Say, for example, a client has a high score on the OQ-30, showing high levels of distress in their life. The IIP-32 shows a very high score on Scale 4: Socially Inhibited and a moderately high score on Scale 3: Distant. The therapist and client explore the history and current role of social inhibition in the client's life. They also explore cultural identity factors and their potential impact. The client realizes that their social inhibition is causing them to feel lonely and depressed and identifies that this might be a helpful area to work on in treatment. This is rapid movement to insight—that the client understands their contribution to their interpersonal distress and begins to construct behavioral options that take the form of goals to remedy that distress. This process strengthens the working alliance because it creates a clear sense of goal agreement.

Behavioral Focus and Goals

The client and therapist then work on establishing behavioral goals using the MATH technique (see Chapters 1 and 6) and refining those goals so that they are calibrated to provide and optimal level of challenge and anxiety to the client. These goals are written on note cards that the client uses every session.

Here-and-Now Experience and Behavioral Activation

Here-and-now activation involves placing the client into the here and now with the group (see Chapters 7 and 8; Yalom & Leszcz, 2020). Doing so provides

FIGURE 2.2. Mechanisms of Change

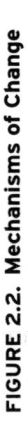

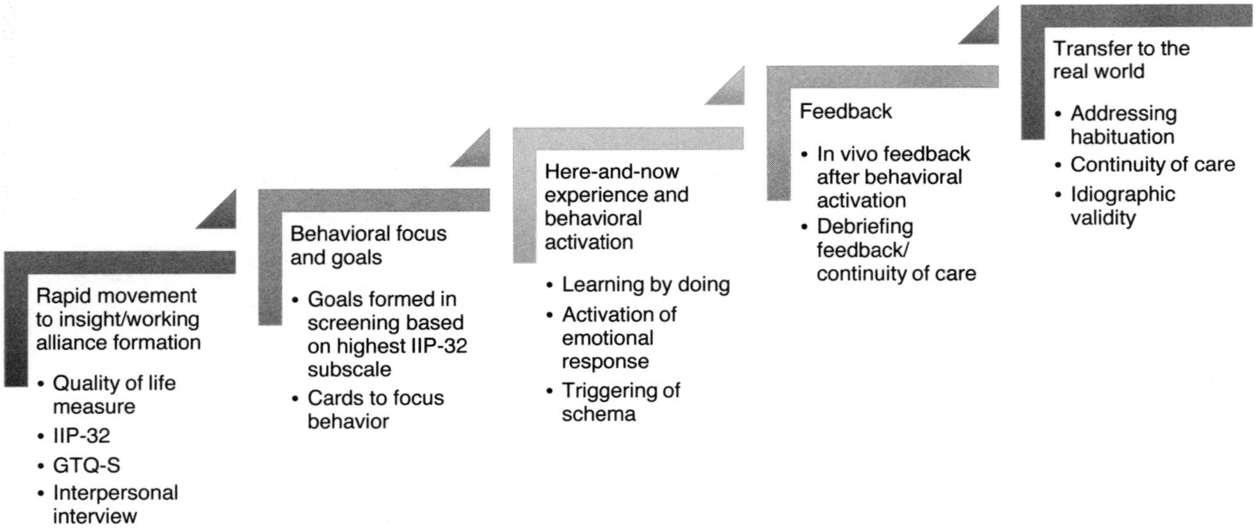

Rapid movement to insight/working alliance formation
- Quality of life measure
- IIP-32
- GTQ-S
- Interpersonal interview

Behavioral focus and goals
- Goals formed in screening based on highest IIP-32 subscale
- Cards to focus behavior

Here-and-now experience and behavioral activation
- Learning by doing
- Activation of emotional response
- Triggering of schema

Feedback
- In vivo feedback after behavioral activation
- Debriefing feedback/ continuity of care

Transfer to the real world
- Addressing habituation
- Continuity of care
- Idiographic validity

Note. IIP-32 = the 32-item Inventory of Interpersonal Problems (Horowitz et al., 2000); GTQ-S = Group Therapy Questionnaire–Short Form (MacNair-Semands et al., 2010).

the therapeutic space for the client to experiment with new behaviors in real time and in the context of the group, whose members share both there-and-then real-life events that impact them and also here-and-now reactions to each other. The here and now provides a space for clients to experience their own schemas, thus activating them emotionally, cognitively, physiologically, and motivationally. As Crocker et al. (2013) pointed out, people's emotions, cognitions, and motivations are inextricably interlinked, and therapeutic interventions need to consider this. Working through their schema's activation of their own polyvagal system becomes a powerful process for clients that mirrors what they will experience outside of therapy. Having an experience in which they are fully activated and can then work through that and realize that the assumed dangerous outcome did not occur becomes a powerful part of the therapy.

Feedback and Fear of Rejection

Research on balanced feedback delivery was first conducted by Stockton and colleagues (Morran et al., 1998) and showed that corrective feedback needs to be delivered later in the group and not in the early stages, and it needs to be preceded and/or sandwiched by positive feedback. This balanced and thoughtful approach to how group members benefit from feedback has been validated in recent research (Kivlighan, Aloe, et al., 2020).

Activating new behaviors is stressful to the system of the whole person. It involves not only thoughts and actions, but neurological and physiological responses that result in the sympathetic nervous system's being activated. During the early phases of FBGT, before the need for immediate feedback became enshrined as key to the approach, clients reported having sleepless nights wondering if a new behavior they had tried in the group would lead the group to reject them when they next met. Others reported considering leaving the group as a means to protect themselves against the anticipated rejection. Fears of rejection when behavior change occurred were very real and impacted not only the client's ability to self-regulate, but also threatened their treatment success.

Feedback delivery immediately after behavior change therefore became a crucial intervention to help clients self-regulate and to prevent treatment dropout. The expansion of restricted interpersonal schemas into more flexible ones requires validation from the group that the anticipated rejection is not occurring in real time. This process also requires leader instruction on, and prompting of, feedback. Interpersonal maladaptive schemas are resistant to change in part because of the fear people have that enacting change will result in rejection, ostracism, and disaster. The stakes are high for social rejection. Research has found that fear of rejection and being alone impede intelligent thought and impact the ability to self-regulate (Baumeister et al., 2002, 2005). This fear is so disabling that people's ability to think clearly and manage their emotions is significantly impaired (Meehan et al., 2019).

This concept is not limited to the United States (Gold & Kivlighan, 2011). Garris et al. (2011) found that when comparing participants from the United States and Japan on concerns over rejection, the participants from Japan (which is considered a more collectivist culture than the United States) were even more concerned about exclusion. The fear of being ostracized and alone can leave people across the world distraught and unable to think clearly. For example, a study by Z. Chen et al. (2020) found that ostracism increased suicidal ideation, surmising that life without acceptance is meaningless and painful. It is no wonder that people retreat into predictable patterns of behavior even when they lead to the same outcomes. The perceived risk of trying something different—potential rejection and increased loneliness—feels greater than the potential for improved relationships. People often prefer the comfort of familiar misery in relationships to the imagined catastrophe of attempting new things. Therefore, the careful training of group members in how to deliver feedback is essential.

Transfer to the Real World

It is not uncommon for group therapies to end with a group celebration and short debriefing for each client. However, FBGT places considerable emphasis on a thorough, individualized debriefing after the group has ended (see Chapter 10). Clinical observations have repeatedly showed that if the group as a whole celebrated and grieved the end of the group, members who felt the group had not met their needs were unlikely to break with the atmosphere of the moment: They shared that they had felt differently. This was far more likely to emerge in the group debriefing.

Equally, how clients made sense of any changes was also illuminating. For some clients, how they made sense of change could be highly idiosyncratic. For example, in the face of therapist observations, outcome data, and behavioral success, some clients still had a difficult time processing that they had been successful. Cognitive attributions for success ranged from being able to internalize their role in the process and achieve a stronger sense of agency to misattributing success to luck or the therapist's skill. Therefore, the role of exploring outcomes collaboratively is essential. However, outcomes are more challenging and sometimes more counterintuitive than they sometimes appear.

A major innovation emerged, though, from Kiesler's (1996) work: the quarter turn on the interpersonal circumplex. The quarter turn is a key mechanism of change incorporated into every goal in FBGT.

Conceptual Ideas Vital to Goal Formation and Success

Several different concepts emerged when developing FBGT that contributed significantly to outcomes. The concept of the quarter turn emerged from learning from both therapeutic successes and trying to understand therapeutic failures. Once instituted, it had a radical effect on the outcomes of clients with certain scale distress scores. The concepts of homeostasis and habituation also came from seeing how clients processed material in debriefing. It became clear that some clients interpreted their discomfort with new interpersonal behaviors as a sign that something was wrong. It also became clear that clients needed help and guidance in being prepared for the systems they returned to, not all of which were going to be positive about the new changes. The quarter turn is considered first because it has a crucial role in understanding goal formation.

The Quarter Turn

The early days of FBGT involved many successes but also some puzzling quandaries. For instance, as many clients succeeded, some consistently failed to achieve their goals. Clinical observation and an analysis of data showed a pattern related to incorrect goal selection: Clients with an elevated score on Scale 6: Focused on the Needs of Others were unable to complete goals related to practicing assertiveness and conflict management skills in group. Because part of the difficulty people with this style have is in experiencing anger and asserting themselves, it seemed that an obvious solution would be to practice assertion and to experience and work through a conflict in therapy. That goal never worked.

Further research on why led back to Kiesler's (1996) work. In that book, Kiesler mentioned the importance of the *quarter turn*, which involves the idea that interpersonal change can only occur when moving clients at 90 degrees— and not 180 degrees—from their starting point on the interpersonal circumplex (see Figure 2.3). For example, if a client begins with high distress on Scale 1: Highly Assertive, they will find goals at 90 degrees on the interpersonal circumplex (e.g., becoming more warm; Scale 7: Warm/Self-Sacrificing), stressful but achievable. However, they will find it significantly more difficult and stressful to achieve those goals at 180 degrees on Scale 5: Unassertive (see Figure 2.3). The same applies to any other scale. Moving 90 degrees from any scale in any direction is easier than moving 180 degrees.

A review of cases showed that whenever a goal was at 180 degrees, it either failed completely, and the client did not achieve success, or the client was successful in their goal but became emotionally flooded and decompensated. While it is sometimes possible to reframe that decompensation as an important

FIGURE 2.3. The Quarter Turn

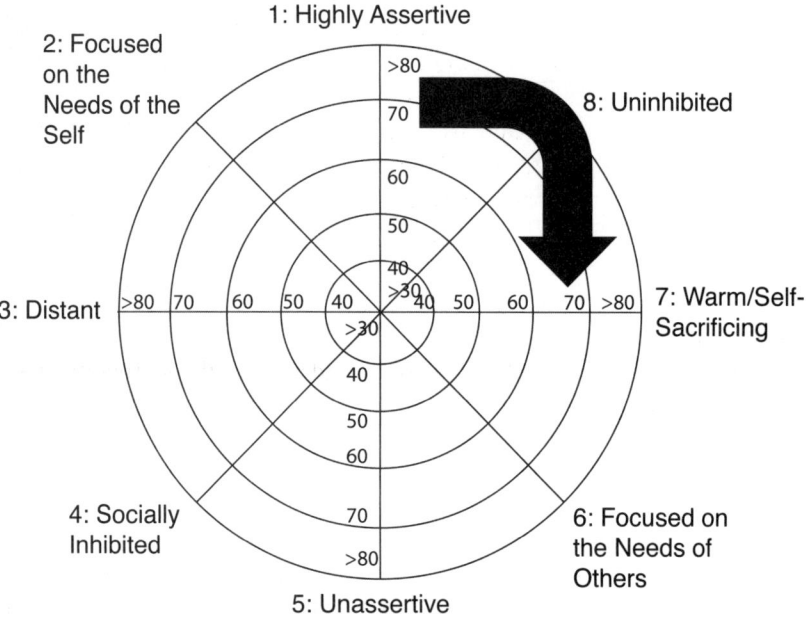

Note. The numbers on the axes refer to distress scores. For example, a score of 55 represents a client's endorsing items that add up to 55. Adapted from the manual for the Inventory of Interpersonal Problems by special permission of the Publisher, Mind Garden, Inc. Further reproduction requires the Publisher's written consent. Copyright © 2000 by Leonard M. Horowitz, Lynn E. Alden, Jerry S. Wiggins, & Aaron L. Pincus. All rights reserved in all media. Published by Mind Garden, Inc., www.mindgarden.com

catharsis, clinical observation revealed that, on balance, the quarter turn goals provided a more successful experience for clients because the social learning taking place was within their polyvagal rest-and-digest state that was more conducive to social learning. Although emotional catharsis is considered central to some therapy approaches, in FBGT, it is sometimes helpful, but it is not essential.

The quarter turn goals represented a smaller step in progress and were therefore found to be more achievable by clients without pushing them into fight, flight, or freeze and shutting down social learning. Thus, for the clients with a problem with elevations on Scale 6: Focused on the Needs of Others, the goal of having a conflict or being assertive was a bridge too far. That was a 180-degree goal. The 90-degree goal was instead a stepping-stone goal: to achieve and articulate a sense that their needs, vulnerabilities, and rights were as important as anyone else's in the group. However, the goals that were 90 degrees involved asking for time, going first in the group, and talking about their own worries and asking for help—that is, making themselves important to both themselves and the group without choosing to engage in an overt conflict around this. The 90-degree goals were far more successful and resulted in clinical improvement at the individual level as well as in a statistically significant change in that group (Allison & Whittingham, 2017; Rotsinger-Stemen & Whittingham, 2013). Another key process that emerged from clinical observation was noticing that homeostasis impacted the therapy at multiple levels, and particularly at the end of therapy when generalizing to the outside world.

Homeostasis

Homeostasis is a term from family therapy and systems theory that discusses how systems and the people within them prefer stability (Jackson, 1981; Seshadri, 2019). It has direct relevance to interpersonal theory as well. Therapists and clients need to understand the impact of homeostasis on the client, the client–therapist relationship, the client–group relationship, and the client's relationship with the systems and people they are returning to (e.g., school, work, family, friends) once they leave therapy. From an intrapsychic point of view, homeostasis works via schemas and interpersonal relationships with the family to generate a sense of internal stability (e.g., a learned role from childhood might be: "I am a peacemaker").

Homeostasis also applies to other constructs at other levels. For example, family systems prefer relationships to be stable and consistent, hence why adults who return to their childhood home for holidays often feel that even though they are now middle-aged, they still feel treated like children when with the older generation. The same can be said of any system the client is in. Friendships, families, workplaces, and other groups prefer relationships to follow expected, stable patterns. Therefore, while, in some cases, changes made by a client might be well received (e.g., someone who was previously nonparticipatory in a group participates slightly more and in ways the group enjoys), in other cases, it may not.

An example is someone who has a rigid focus on the style of focusing on the needs of others. When that person begins to ask friends or family to listen to them or sets boundaries around how much they are willing to listen to others, they may well receive very negative feedback. Systems will try and restore the status quo, so clients must be prepared that not all changes will be met with positivity. FBGT incorporates this idea into treatment throughout. It looks not just at how the client's maladaptive cyclical patterns (a form of internal homeostasis) impact the therapist–client working alliance and the group but also at how pushback from the client's systems (external homeostasis) will impact change as friends, family, and workplaces react to any attempts at interpersonal change.

Habituation

The concept of *habituation* is also an important one in FBGT because it relates to the inevitable discomfort that accompanies change and that is essential to the continuance of social learning (McDiarmid et al., 2019). Habituation to new interpersonal states has been shown to be a key factor in changes in attachment and has been linked to the neurobiological states (e.g., oxytocin) that accompany it (Kiss et al., 2011). In a sense, the client's experience of attempting new interpersonal behaviors is analogous to the therapist's own experience while in training. During training, every prospective neophyte psychotherapist goes through the inevitable discomfort of listening to themselves try to act and sound like a therapist. Skills like reflection of content and interpretation initially feel clumsy, awkward, and foreign. Over time, these skills become more integrated into the therapist's skill set and take on a more natural, socially smooth quality. This is no different for a client who is activating a new skill set. It takes time for a new social skill to become integrated and become smooth, and during that time, the client will feel awkward, anxious, and full of self-doubt and will endure a phase of feeling that their new behaviors and sense of self are not aligned.

It takes time for the anxiety around the expansion of a constricted schema to subside. When reviewing scores from hundreds of IIP-32 (Horowitz et al., 2000) posttests, a pattern became clear. For every improvement on the scale the client was working on, there was a smaller but significant increase in anxiety on the opposite scale. For example, a client who had become less uninhibited became worried on the opposite end of the scale: They now believed they may have become too inhibited. The same was true for all scales: People working on boundaries worried they had become too boundaried and unfriendly, and people who were too aggressive were worried they were now defenseless. Every growth carried with it a subsequent anxiety about the consequences of that growth. However, every feeling of uneasiness also involved the opportunity to make "the growth choice and not the fear choice" (Maslow, 1971, p. 49). Helping the client understand and lean into the uneasiness is a core part of the process of helping clients manage change now and in the future.

Secondary Mechanisms of Change

The mechanisms of change in FBGT are sometimes broader than just cultivating interpersonal flexibility. The interventions are designed to lead the client in a stepwise progression to promote more secure attachment in combination with the promotion of an internal sense of interpersonal empowerment (brought on by realization that more behavioral choices are within their control)—a key factor in healthy coping throughout life. The client's choosing of goals and accomplishment of those goals that are oriented toward improving the client's ability to navigate throughout interpersonal situations are helpful side effects of treatment. Therapy in FBGT is not an opaque process with the therapist providing semimagical insights that the client imbues. Rather, the client is the hero and active agent in this story. It is their courage in attempting new ways of behaving, their work in helping others, and their outcomes that are a direct result of their efforts that drive the approach.

Groups also provide the opportunity for many of Yalom and Leszcz's (2020) therapeutic factors to take place. These include, but are not limited to, universality (the belief that one is not alone in one's misery), altruism, social learning, modeling, and cohesion. The approach is strengths based: Aspects of interpersonal style, culture, and identity are seen as strengths and are reinforced throughout the groups.

SUMMARY

FBGT is an integrative model with clear mechanisms of change that operate in a stepwise fashion. Mechanisms of change begin with rapid movement to insight and then progress to the activation of a strong working alliance, followed by clear behavioral goals. Once behavioral activation takes place, feedback should follow. Transfer of learning to the real world is the final mechanism of change that follows triangulation of data.

MBC is woven into every stage of the approach. The inclusion and exclusion criteria for FBGT involve carefully considering each individual's likelihood of benefiting from the treatment compared to a potential for harm to that individual or to the group. An interpersonal etiology is the key consideration for inclusion, while other more specific factors also impact exclusion. Processes and techniques embedded within the approach, such as inoculation, bookending, the quarter turn, and the use of homeostasis and habituation to understand and explain change to clients are a vital part of this process.

3 INTERPERSONAL SCALE DESCRIPTIONS

Understanding and interpreting scale scores are an essential part of focused brief group therapy (FBGT). Because these scores form the focus for treatment, being able to collaboratively explore their meaning with a client represents a key step in successful outcomes. However, failing to accurately capture the client's meanings and life experiences using these scales and then setting inappropriate goals can lead to treatment failure and dropout.

It is vitally important for the therapist to focus on the strengths of each style before addressing the challenges a style also brings. As a strengths-based approach, the FBGT process should always involve keeping clients rooted in the positives offered by each style. Thus, the approach works on reinforcing self-compassion and keeping the client focused on their personality and cultural identities as strengths to be built on. FBGT reinforces the importance of trait-level personality and cultural identities as being a source of pride, self-worth, and celebration. No matter what the person is inviting from the therapist or how maladaptive the extremity of the person's style may be, underneath that series of invitations is a series of strengths. For example,

https://doi.org/10.1037/0000389-004
Focused Brief Group Therapy: An Integrative Approach to Reducing Interpersonal Distress, by M. Whittingham

someone who is aggressive and domineering is someone who is also well equipped to defend themselves and others. Defense attorneys, surgeons, and chief executive officers all need the skill set of being able to take decisive action under pressure to be able to defend their positions and maintain control over groups of people.

Therefore, once a client identifies that their distress score accurately represents their overall style, the therapist shifts the conversation to the strengths of that style first. The therapist must also maintain a focus throughout the therapy process—and particularly at debriefing—that emphasizes the strengths of the scale style and to continue to use behavioral strategies in the arenas in which they are working. Clients are often so energized by the changes asked of them that they overgeneralize and insert new strategies where they are sometimes unhelpful and the old strategies did not need fixing. For example, a mechanic who is used to aggressive banter with their colleagues overgeneralizes the work on empathic encouragement they have been doing to improve their marriage, and they are met with ridicule by their workmates. The therapist must help clients maintain focus on their strengths throughout while emphasizing that behavioral changes that take place during therapy are only intended to widen possible choices in any situation and do not serve as a replacement for existing strategies that work.

The focus of FBGT is defined by the use of scales. The process of using those scales to help therapist and client understand and define the presenting problem is what defines the approach.

SUBTYPES IN FBGT

This section explores each scale. The scales do not represent a definitive description of anyone with scale distress; rather, they form *phenotypes*, exemplars of the way the scales may be considered if they represent a clear example of that style. Thus, in the following descriptions, scales are presented as the starting point for considering how to contextualize and add in cultural and other identity variables. The therapist must only use these phenotypes as a list of possibilities that need affirming by the client.

Equally, distress is not defined by the presence of all of these criteria or none of them. The therapist must listen carefully to the client to determine the degree of fit. The examples that follow illustrate the kind of qualities and person–environment fit that are possible for a scale. The therapist's skill and judgment are crucial in interpreting the results in collaboration with the client. Group leaders may also find it useful to compare and contrast styles by exploring how they differ from adjacent styles. For example, someone with an archetypal Scale 3 score might behave in ways that discourage connection and are low in warmth. However, someone with an archetypal Scale 4 distress might be less overtly aloof and more obviously socially anxious, deferential, and self-critical. Someone with an archetypal Scale 5 might be slightly less anxious, giving eye contact and appearing more able to connect but having a chronic lack of assertiveness and showing deep concern at displeasing the therapist.

By understanding the basics of a subtype, therapists are then able to use this information to develop increasingly sophisticated conceptualizations. Sometimes the archetypes capture the essence of a client's problems in clear and unambiguous ways. A simple interpretation using a high score can sometimes also allow a client to grasp the essence of a problem in a way that feels authentic to their experience and also captures the problems that have brought them into therapy. However, not all interpretations are simple, and the therapist must use considerable skill in forming hypotheses and listening to how the client interprets the findings. Any hypothesis about a client's interpersonal style should be held as a tentative one. Collaboration with a client on understanding the score is a key part of any formulation. The therapist must remain simultaneously rooted in the theory of subtypes while also listening to the client's interpretations and descriptions of when and where the distress takes place.

Scale Differences in Awareness of Others' Emotions

Some generalizations about styles in the broader sense are worth considering. As Moeller et al. (2011) pointed out, people higher in dominance tend to be less attentive to and have more difficulty noticing and interpreting others' emotions. The authors noted that people on the opposite end of the scale tend toward being much more sensitive to others' states and emotions and much more able to interpret them. Therefore, people with scale scores that are high at the top end of the interpersonal circumplex (Scale 2: Focused on the Needs of the Self, Scale 1: Highly Assertive, and Scale 8: Uninhibited) will have more difficulty with noticing others' reactions, and those on the lower scales (Scale 4: Socially Inhibited, Scale 5: Unassertive, and Scale 6: Focused on the Needs of Others) will be more attentive to others' states. This will have an impact on the group dynamic as well. Groups that are heterogenous on one end of the scale or another will either be highly attuned to each other or oblivious to each other's feelings.

Scale Difference in Internalization and Externalization

Equally, as Girard et al. (2017) pointed out, internalization tends to fall on scales more associated with being lower in dominance—those on the lower half of the interpersonal circumplex (Scales 3 through 6). They identified that depression tended to fall more frequently within Scale 4 and Scale 5 (Socially Inhibited and Unassertive, respectively), whereas dependent personality disorder fell more on Scale 6: Focused on the Needs of Others. Scores more characterized by higher agency included borderline personality (which straddled Scales 2 through 8); antisocial personality disorder (Scale 2); and alcohol and drug dependence, which clustered around Scales 2 through 8. These are, of course, phenotypic. For example, depression may most typically occur with Scale 4 and Scale 5, but that does not mean it is not present in other scales as well. Equally, a high score on, for example, Scale 6: Focused on the Needs of Others does not diagnose dependent personality disorder by itself. That would need a full set of diagnostic considerations based on a more thorough evaluation. However, the occurrence of these diagnostic categories on the scales does tell us something important about the interaction between interpersonal style and predicted symptomatology.

Understanding how people with different interpersonal styles cope with problems can establish links between distress and diagnosis in ways that can help clients feel understood. For example, being able to link distress with negative feedback from important others to the use of alcohol to cope can help identify problems and maladaptive solutions in a way that the client feels connected to. This presupposes that this working alliance is formed nonjudgmentally and without shaming, as described in Chapter 6 on therapy, pregroup preparation, and screening (TPS).

SCALE DESCRIPTIONS

The following subtype descriptions are based on the work of Horowitz et al. (2000), with the addition of information on how each scale plays out in therapy. These scale descriptions break down the style into a brief descriptor. It is beyond the scope of this chapter to explore every possible combination of person–environment fit or to consider every cultural and identity variable that might occur to inform the scale. Equally, some scales are combinations of the two main axes; for example, Scale 8: Uninhibited is a combination of Scale 7: Warm/Self-Sacrificing and Scale 1: Highly Assertive. Therefore, as mentioned in the chapters throughout this book, these scales need to be considered as phenotypical, yet in need of thoughtful clinical judgment. For example, the term *shared conceptual space* is used at times during the descriptors to describe instances in which a scale score is also a place where someone with a personality disorder or other mental health issue might be present on the interpersonal circumplex. It is important to remember that sharing this same interpersonal space does not necessarily mean that these diagnoses are present. Clinical judgment and correct diagnostic procedure are required to accurately assess each construct, and the interpersonal circumplex profile should not be used as a sole diagnostic criterion. Rather, it should be thought of as a set of overlapping Venn diagrams (or, in some cases, of separate circles altogether) with each person capable of significant overlap or little to no overlap on each category.

The scales are now each addressed in turn. The discussion of each scale provides an overall description, a consideration of the client's place in the group dynamic, comments on how to manage the working alliance, an explanation of goals, and notes on debriefing issues.

FBGT Scale 1: Highly Assertive

Being highly assertive can be helpful in life but depends on how adaptive it is to each situation and context. Remember that different cultures, subcultures, and contexts ascribe different meanings to this set of behaviors, depending on what is considered "normal" in each place. Therefore, for this scale, as with the others, it is important to note how this phenotype may be seen positively or negatively, depending on factors such as time, place, context, and identity variables (e.g., gender, race, ethnicity) of the person who is involved. The following phenotype therefore serves only as a starting point from which the therapist and client can consider what is true, not true, and somewhat true for each specific client.

Overall Description

People with this style might describe themselves as highly assertive and as leaders. Confident and talkative, they are most comfortable in a leadership role: giving advice, telling others what to do, and making decisions for everyone. In times of certainty, groups can find this take-charge attitude comforting, but it can lapse into others' feeling controlled and becoming resentful. Those with a Scale 1 high score can be very focused on realizing their own goals and getting their own needs met, and they can be single-minded in doing so. They are often able to tolerate high levels of conflict and may enjoy the stimulation that comes with argument. In extreme cases, particularly when paired with a peak on Scale 2, people with this profile may be overly aggressive and vindictive, and they may take pleasure in the pain of others. They may also be highly suspicious of others and dismissive of attempts to generate affection or love.

People with this style occupy a shared interpersonal space with people with substance and alcohol abuse disorders as well as with people diagnosed with antisocial personality disorder. People with borderline personality have a common profile that shares aspects of both Scale 1 and Scale 2, both of which are disinhibited. However, people with borderline personality disorder tend to be more internalizing (Girard et al., 2017).

Place in the Group Dynamic

Within the group, people with this style are likely to engage in controlling behavior and may be more talkative and domineering than other members or may seek to steer the conversation and topics to areas they believe are important. They often give advice and suggestions to other group members on how to improve. However, this advice may not fit with the other group members' needs, wishes, identity, or personality; therefore, they may perceive this advice as overbearing.

People with a domineering style may also become resented by the group. This style invites a complementary style of unassertiveness and submission. However, those with some degree of dominance are likely to fall into non-complementary interactions, creating tension in the room as they compete for time, attention, and status. Those people with styles that are in the lower half of the interpersonal circumplex often fall into quiet resentment because they realize they are unable and unwilling to challenge the domineering person's overbearing style. For them, the complementary style is familiar but unhappy and full of suppressed resentment.

The domineering member supplies a significant amount of dynamism and energy to the group. They are unafraid of bold statements, will initiate conversations, and will provide depth and challenge to the group. They also have no fear in calling out issues, such as lack of engagement or avoidant behavior in the group. They are likely to see more avoidance than is actually present, generating the self-fulfilling prophecies that drive their interpersonal problems (Kivlighan & Angelone, 1992).

Working Alliance Formation

The *hooked position* (i.e., the expected, complementary response to the invitation; Kiesler, 1996) is to feel the pressure to accept or reject the urge to submit and take an unassertive role. Behaviorally, a client with this style may enter the TPS session and take control of the situation, appearing confident and sure of themselves. They are ambivalent about expressing distress, preferring instead to display competence and strength. Therapists should be careful in using language focused on emotions or being too kind or compassionate in their language. Rather, they should focus on client strengths and explore vulnerabilities carefully, knowing the client will reject any insinuation of "weakness."

The working alliance should typically take place from the *unhooked position* (i.e., adopting a stance that is acomplementary) because attempts to be more direct with this client may cause an alliance rupture. Unhooking involves matching carefully along acomplementary lines, which involves what FBGT has come to describe as the *dance with dominance*: The therapist alternates between careful listening, support, and agreement while interspersing comments that carefully open the door to possible distress.

Equally, interventions tend to work best when the client feels in charge. Therefore, offering choices and exploring ambivalence can be helpful. Use of disqualifiers (e.g., "I wonder if it is possible that . . .," "I could be wrong but . . .," "What do you think about the idea of doing . . .") leaves the client in a dominant position but allows the therapist to guide treatment. However, in some cultures and regions, these techniques may be ineffective, and therapists should carefully consider whether they are able to successfully maintain the alliance with other, more direct strategies.

For example, the therapist takes a more dominant role, saying,

> I hear what you are saying, and I get that you feel like these issues are not a problem for you. Yet I also hear that several family members and people at work are really giving you strong feedback that this is not working for them.
>
> I am guessing that you are okay with how you feel about it to some extent and that it is something you don't want to give up completely as it probably works pretty well at times. However, I also wonder if all this negative feedback is making you pause. I wonder if you have considered whether you need to develop some other ways of helping other people feel okay about their time with you? Maybe some interpersonal behaviors that will help them feel better and so lead to less negative feedback for you. What do you think?

Goals

The quarter turn involves goals at 90 degrees on the interpersonal circumplex that build on the strengths of those scales. So, for a client working on being more flexible with their highly assertive behaviors, a Scale 1 goal, being more warm is achievable and valuable as is going the other direction on the quarter turn toward Scale 3: Distant, meaning exerting less control over discussions and the actions of others. The client's 90-degree goals typically move to warmth (Scale 7: Warm/Self-Sacrificing) or distance (Scale 3). Scale 7 goals might be to ask follow-up questions, be encouraging, and to work toward complements and positive feedback. Goals on Scale 3 relate to inhibiting the desire to control or overwhelm others with advice, and these goals require inhibition. As with Scale 2, clients with this style struggle with being unassertive, passive, and quiet. Inhibition is difficult but not impossible. They tend to perform well and feel less constrained when moving toward warmth, such as by asking follow-up questions and offering encouragement. As they enact their goals, they worry that being warm will open them up to being exploited or seen as soft and vulnerable.

Clients also need feedback on two levels. First, despite their seemingly uncaring attitude toward others' opinions, when they attempt new behaviors, they feel just as vulnerable as other members do. They need to hear that the goal achievement did not result in rejection. Second, during the debriefing, they also need reassurance that their highly assertive behaviors can still be useful, depending on the situation. For example, a CEO may need to act like a formidable presence to defend their company. They should be reminded that adding skills does not mean removing existing behaviors when they are useful or were working perfectly well.

Inoculation (defined in Chapter 2) is important with clients with this style. Some clients with a very strong domineering style may be tempted to dominate the time in the group completely. For example, if the therapist feels overwhelmed and finds it difficult to intervene and talk during a TPS session, that is an indication that under conditions of anxiety, the client is likely to repeat this strategy immediately in the first session. The client may also be tempted to verbally attack other group members to gain control.

Collaboratively exploring what the client's typical strategy is and developing goals to prevent it and redirect the anxiety is important. A set of goals for the client could include these:

- Encourage other group members at least twice during the life of the group.
- Ask for feedback from other group members about how well you are letting others talk and contribute.
- Ask follow-up questions of other group members.
- Avoid attacking other group members early in the group.

This set of goals presupposes that the client has identified these as likely events. However, the fourth goal is an example of one that would only be included if the therapist has clear evidence that this would be a likely occurrence— for example, the therapist notes that some people with this style attack others when they feel anxious. The therapist then asks themselves if this is something this client is likely to do. The therapist also could gain evidence from asking the client to describe typical peer or friend interactions and by noticing if the client is engaging in criticism or covert or overt attacks on the therapist during the TPS session.

Debriefing Issues

Clients on this scale may express concern about when to use new behaviors versus old ones. They will need reinforcing that they should not give up their typical style but, rather, should continue what has previously worked and implement new behaviors only when it makes sense to do so. For example, a client in a role as a business owner may be tempted to overgeneralize the behavioral changes they have been seeking with a romantic partner, such as listening and asking follow-up questions, into their workplace. If the workplace is organized hierarchically and requires swift, decisive action by the leader, and their previous style worked well in this context, then inserting new behaviors may be unhelpful.

The client should be reminded to not replace behaviors that were previously effective with new ones. And because clients will often ask, they should also be reminded that they are still able to defend themselves in any way they see fit in the situation and that they should integrate new behaviors selectively and carefully. The person with this style often worries that becoming more warm will leave them vulnerable and open to exploitation. Care must be taken to ensure that they are aware of the risks of being more open but also clarify that defense mechanisms are still available. The client with this style also needs reminding that the group is a starting point for awareness and that, over time, they may need to explore other, new strategies to be effective in situations they see as challenging. Remember that FBGT does not offer a wide array of options that can meet every situation, but that the behavioral change the client achieves is a step in the right direction that eventually, with a willingness to continue exploring new behaviors, could result in significantly more success in achieving their life goals.

FBGT Scale 2: Focused on the Needs of the Self

This scale is different than Scale 1: Highly Assertive because it is closer to distance and farther away from warmth. Therefore, the behaviors that go with this tend to be highly assertive but with a more aggressive, attacking, and distant feel to them. While certain contexts and cultures value this skill set, and they can be very valuable, they become problematic when rigidly applied or extreme. The person coming to treatment may well be experiencing distress because family members are stating that the person is unsupportive or unloving or because a workplace complaint has led to human resources requiring treatment.

Overall Description

People with this style are described as decisive, assertive, commanding, and able to exercise control over situations and people. They are not averse to speaking the truth, albeit in sometimes excessively harsh ways. They may also do well in leadership roles that require toughness, assertiveness, and aggression. They can energize groups with drive, forcefulness, and task focus, and they may well be considered someone who "rules with an iron fist." People with this profile can be very single minded in accomplishing goals and are very focused on their own needs. They set strong personal boundaries and can act with hostility and vengefulness if attacked or if they feel that their boundaries are being violated or wishes being ignored. They have little empathy for others' feelings, but this may be a strength in situations in which a task focus is necessary. The detached nature of this style enables a degree of ruthlessness and decisive action that can be useful when dispassionate judgment is required in some business or combat situations (e.g., when survival of an organization or life and death decisions must be made).

The brutal honesty and behavior that maintains status can provide energy and directness to a group while also act as a source of confrontation, conflict, and telling of difficult truths that may drive the group forward. However, the harshness of the feedback can sometimes impede the message. Equally, if left unfocused, the degree of competitiveness among people with this style can prove challenging for groups. In particular, early in the life of the group, aggressive or insulting body language, comments, and insults can be a threat to group cohesion.

Place in the Group Dynamic

The directness and critical feedback provided by people with this style can adversely affect some group members, particularly those who are already prone to internalizing and are sensitive to rejection. If left unchecked, the aggressive outbursts can damage group cohesion and eventually cause some members to leave. If these clients are paired with other dominant members or leaders, competition for status may become a barrier to progress in group. Constant conflict may be energizing for this group member but eventually has a deleterious effect on other group members who may fall into fight, flight, or freeze, a position from which little social learning will occur in a short-term group.

People with this style share a space on the interpersonal circumplex (when in extreme form) with people with narcissistic personality disorder, paranoid personality disorder, and antisocial personality disorder (although this seems to operate in tandem with Scale 1). People with borderline personality disorder typically have scores that are extreme and share a space with Scale 1. They also tend to be internalizing. People in this same conceptual space are also described as disinhibited, sharing that same conceptual space as those with substance and alcohol dependence (Girard et al., 2017).

People with this profile may seek to control the group using direct insults, making fun of others, and sometimes being verbally aggressive. This is entirely self-protective. They take comfort in being in control and feeling that they can both control their own boundaries and eliminate potential threats. They experience vulnerability as dangerous, often as a result of parenting that may have involved their being ignored, dismissed, or having had vulnerability treated as weakness. Once inoculated, they may still revert to aggressive and sometimes overtly hostile attacks on other group members. Under stress— for example, when someone seeks to dominate them or attacks them—they may revert to aggression as a tactic. Acts of overt aggression from others may sometimes be met with escalation of aggression in reply in a process of reciprocal escalation.

Working Alliance Formation

If the therapist feels demeaned, intimidated, frightened, or inadequate or has the desire to be quiet and give in to the hostility, they have been hooked into complementary hostile submission. A therapist high in dominance may feel the desire to compete against, crush, demean, control, or punish the member.

The unhooked position is to notice the client's attempts to seek safety, and then assert dominance and take a calm, nurturing position from which to be helpful. The therapist's first task is to remember that this style evolved in response to failed attempts to get love and attention from parents. The challenge is to provide unconditional positive regard for the client by looking toward their intentions. Specifically, it is important to remember that the client is always doing their best with what they know. Their maladaptive techniques to connect via dominance make sense in terms of their life history and upbringing. Use of disqualifiers is essential for the working alliance. It is possible to direct and lead the conversation with someone with a style that is focused on the needs of self, but that effort requires some verbal gymnastics to do so. Like people with the style of Scale 1 is the use of "I wonder if it could be that . . ."; "I could be wrong, but what if . . ."; "What do you think about the idea of . . .?"; and "Is it the same as what I just said or different?"

Goals

Goals on the quarter turn are on Scale 8 or Scale 4. On Scale 8, they involve listening, asking follow-up questions, encouraging others, and sharing about oneself at a slightly deeper level (e.g., what it was like growing up and what you learned about relationships). Goals toward Scale 4: Socially Inhibited, tend to be challenging for clients with this style because they are often more comfortable staying active in the group but being warmer. However, inhibiting the desire to attack others is an important goal as well as an inoculation against self-sabotage and simultaneous damage to the group cohesion and to its individual members.

Debriefing Issues

Debriefing issues typically revolve around reaffirming that the client may return to previous modes of functioning whenever those modes fit the situation. Movement toward warmth and encouragement is typically accompanied by worries that this may mean losing power or being taken advantage of. While some of this may be founded in past experiences and may be a maladaptive belief, it also may be reality based in some circumstances the client finds themselves in. For example, if they function in a work or home culture defined by power plays or in which they must maintain an "alpha" status (e.g., a military officer, an executive in a highly competitive company), then acting in ways that are warm, may, in some instances, be perceived as weakness by others and lead to negative outcomes.

Clients with this style need to be reminded to be thoughtful in considering when to use which strategy. If their prior choices were already working—for example, being sarcastic and making fun of others was perceived as funny and consistent within their work culture—then they should continue that strategy. However, if the same strategy, when applied rigidly to their romantic relationships, has repeatedly been proven unsuccessful, then they may wish to either explain the meaning behind sarcasm; find a partner who enjoys sarcasm; or attempt new behaviors, such as offering encouragement and listening. Ultimately, the client has a choice as to how to behave to better meet their goals in life, but they should not completely give up old ways of behavior. Rather, they should build on strengths.

FBGT Scale 3: Distant

The Distant scale is less aggressive and assertive than Scale 2: Focused on the Needs of the Self but less shy than Scale 4: Socially Inhibited. People with distress on this scale are motivated to maintain distance between themselves and others to keep themselves safe. As with other scales, cultural differences can cause misunderstandings about the meaning and purpose of behaviors associated with this scale. For example, different expectations around how close to stand to someone, how to greet them, or how to express emotions in a discussion can lead to difficulties in social interactions, leading to distress.

Overall Description

Clients on this scale are typically able to set and maintain strong boundaries. They can keep emotional distance, which allows them to observe others with intensity. They may value the internal working of the mind and appreciate alternate means to achieve stimulation. They are adept at self-protection and can keep others' attempts to connect at bay. They are thoughtful and analytic and may offer searing and honest insights to the group at times, if given the opportunity.

They may find forming and maintaining meaningful connections with others difficult. Their difficulties with expressions of intimacy can result in challenges in their romantic life or with people with whom they wish to have a loving relationship. People with this scale score experience any cohesion between other group members as aversive. In particular, if they are the only person with a distant style in an otherwise cohesive group, they experience the group climate as toxic and dangerous. This makes them a strong candidate for premature termination and poor outcomes (Kivlighan et al., 2017).

Place in the Group Dynamic

People with this style are frequently perceived by other group members as aloof and unfriendly. Because their inhibition is one that often involves masking emotions and responses to remain hidden, others sometimes perceive this as lack of engagement or of negative judgment of the group. They may also frustrate the group with their inability to connect, particularly if the group is highly cohesive. Highly cohesive groups will sometimes scapegoat this person because group members are feeling frustrated that this person is excluding themselves from the warmth of the group. Individual group members, therefore, may experience that exclusion as a collective rejection, which can bring up painful feelings for the group. Group members may then struggle to articulate those feelings but, instead, become frustrated as their warm advances are rejected. It is important that the group leader intervene to help the group manage that moment.

The person high in distance is also an effective model for how to set clear boundaries and to protect themselves. The warm members of the group will learn much from this model if they can "work the axes" (see Chapter 8) and come to understand and appreciate the client, thereby making amends with a part of themselves that they have cut off from their self-schemas. Equally, the client's efforts to both actively listen and give advice while simultaneously keeping a boundary by holding back from deep emotional sharing and warm encouragement also need validating. These are difficult goals for this member and need to be acknowledged as such.

Homogenous groups of distant members are a particularly interesting challenge in that the group members have immense difficulty in showing empathy for each other despite, at times, feeling they would like to show empathy. Their lack of skills in offering compassion or support makes for some awkward moments that exhibit when any group member expresses vulnerability, such as sadness. Instead of showing empathy by expressing condolences or support, the group may instead shift away from the emotionally charged moment by deflecting, becoming silent, or rapidly changing the subject. However, that moment provides a rich opportunity to process comments, thus allowing members to return to difficult moments and attempt a brief 180-degree goal of offering a supportive statement. Providing that the therapist reframes and contains the experience, even this more distant goal can be achievable as a one-off for the group.

Working Alliance Formation

The warm group leader may feel disconnected and unable to establish a warm bond. Because the client is in a distant position, this invites therapist distance. Attempts to form a warm connection are rebuffed and may prove frustrating to the warm, dominant therapist if not recognized as typical of the hooked position. A warm therapist may experience this distance as rejection and failure of the alliance. However, the unhooked position involves working from a distant position to introduce small amounts of warmth into the interaction. Overall, though, the stance must remain one of interested distance. The working alliance is formed by working on goals related to the quarter turn (i.e., advice giving and active listening) while maintaining a core posture of distance and slight warmth.

Goals

Goals for this client are not ones group workers typically set for clients. Some group therapy models see the end goal of group as all members achieving the same levels of intimacy and disclosure. FBGT does not take this position. It looks at what is challenging for every client and assumes that challenges are different for every person based on the 90-degree turn. So, the goals for people who are distant are advice giving and silent but active listening.

On occasion, a distant member may undertake more intimacy and closeness with greater self-disclosure. For example, having the distant client explain to the group that it is hard to connect and that this is the best they can do may be helpful for the group because it allows them to develop theory of mind and empathy. However, the group leader should be mindful that this is a 180-degree goal—disclosing about the self—that may be too difficult for the client or may result in the client's desire to not return the next week. Therefore, the therapist should be ready to help the client protect their boundaries. This can be a therapeutic opportunity for others to work on how they are experiencing how someone else manage their own boundaries and what it means to them to not have to help or to be closer.

Debriefing Issues

Debriefing issues include considering how to maintain boundaries in places where they are appropriate. Discussion also needs to take place around how intimate relationships might eventually need, at times more closeness and self-disclosure. In addition, discussion is needed about the eventual translation of new skills and an awareness of how those skills are being received; for example, the therapist may note that active listening and advice giving will help reduce distance for some, but others may need more self-disclosure or may push back against advice.

FBGT Scale 4: Socially Inhibited

The Socially Inhibited scale is closer to the Unassertive Scale and farther away from the Focused on the Needs of the Self scale. When this type of distress is a style, the people who exhibit it tend to be withdrawn and socially anxious, struggle to assert themselves, and are more preoccupied with being judged by others.

Overall Description

The strengths of introverts and people described as "shy" are myriad. Such people can be highly analytical, thoughtful, and insightful because they spend considerable time considering options. They tend to inhibit well and are cautious and thoughtful in how they move through life. They are attentive to group processes and considerate of others' needs and wishes. They follow direction and attempt to minimize conflict in the group. They track the emotions of people in the group well and are highly sensitive to conflicts, upset, and others' emotional states.

Yet, the question is one of degree. For example, although they are analytic and thoughtful—both of which are positive—when, taking those to extremes, the client can become overly focused on worries about the self in relation to others and overly preoccupied with fear of social embarrassment and judgment. Anxiety about social situations can be very high and, in some cases, can lead to a diagnosis of social anxiety disorder or, in extreme situations, schizotypal personality disorder.

Place in the Group Dynamic

People with social inhibition are sometimes mistakenly perceived as aloof or distant. Their quietness is easy for others to project onto and can be mistaken for disdain or disinterest. It can sometimes be helpful for members to understand the inner state of someone with social inhibition so they can understand their motivations. For example, understanding that quietness means they are worried about being judged for saying the wrong thing rather than ignoring or judging others can be helpful for the group. However, this represents a risky 180-degree goal for the client, so the client should not be held in this space for long, and the group leader should be mindful that the client may need to recover boundaries afterward. Venturing into a 180-degree goal runs the risk that the client seeks considerable distance to recover, including the possibility that they may skip a session. The client should be encouraged to set their boundaries within the group rather than by leaving it.

Boundary setting inside the group—a Scale 2 goal—can also provide goal completion while simultaneously preventing premature group dropout. Clients on this scale typically take a reserved, quiet role during the group: They wait for other to speak, may hold off on goals until late in the life of the group, and may otherwise inhibit their own responses. They avoid conflict and may respond to conflict among other group members with silence and avoidant behavior.

Working Alliance Formation

The working alliance is complex. Clients with this style tend to respond with a strongly stated wish to *not* take part in group. People with this style are typically afraid of other peoples' judgment; therefore, the idea that they should join a group is equivalent to asking a person afraid of heights to sit on a mountaintop all day! The exposure to these feared stimuli is by itself curative, however, because it represents exposure to the feared stimuli. Outcomes for clients with this scale score are particularly strong (Yutrzenka, 2012).

However, persuading someone to take on the challenge of joining the group requires a degree of persuasion and skill. Customarily, the group leader's response to the client's initial hesitation or outright refusal is to state that the group may be the thing that the client is most fearful of, but that is exactly why the group is helpful. While empathizing with the client's fear of the group, the leader can explain that, over time and as goals are acted out, the anxiety will diminish. The leader can also point out that this is what the client came in to do and that joining the group represents facing their fear. Mere attendance requires bravery on the part of the client.

Clients with this profile (i.e., distant, submissive) often elicit the therapist's feeling a need to talk more and be directive (i.e., distant, dominant). Although some therapists are warm and dominant, they may find themselves becoming slightly more distant over time as they adjust to their invitation not being met with warmth in return. The unhooked position takes place partly in the group and partly in the TPS session. Overall, the therapist should adopt a position of warmth with slight dominance that allows for the client to make decisions. Although some persuasion will be needed that involves the therapist's making recommendations from a dominant position, as many decisions as possible should come from the client. Equally, warmth can be communicated through empathic understanding during the information-gathering portions of the session. Therefore, overt warmth can take place—but in smaller doses that do not overwhelm the client.

Goals

Goals that are most effective for clients with social inhibition (Scale 4) are at a quarter turn to this scale, namely, Scale 6 goals and Scale 2 goals. Goals on Scale 6 typically include asking others follow-up questions and offering encouragement and support. Feedback on these goals is particularly important for people with this profile because they often have heightened anxiety about being perceived as nosy or intrusive when they attempt the goal. Failing to have the group give feedback after they have attempted their goal can lead to premature dropout because they worry about the impact of their new behavior and assume it has led to rejection. Goals on Scale 2: Focused in the Needs of the Self may involve explaining to others that they are not aloof but are merely very focused on what they should say next. It may also involve explaining any cultural or family aspects related to inhibition, if this is salient. However, self-disclosure is typically a Scale 7 or Scale 8 skill, so represents a 180-degree turn; therefore, it should only be lightly touched on.

Debriefing Issues

Clients need help understanding habituation. After behavioral change takes place, clients typically experience reductions in their targeted scale score— Socially Inhibited. It is also typical for clients to experience distress related to this change (as is the case with all scales) that comes out as an increase in distress on scores that are opposite to their profile (in this case, Scale 8). This increase in distress can also come out as increases in scores directly next to the opposite score (in this case, Scales 1 or 7). Explaining and normalizing these increases as being part of adjusting to a new normal helps clients understand that discomfort is part of growth and will eventually subside with practice. Clients also should be reminded of the importance of a Scale 2 goal: seeking and being able to assert the need to have alone time and personal space to recover from social situations.

Discussion needs to take place about the places and contexts in which to try out new behavior. In particular, pay attention to finding a balance between connecting and distancing and where, how, and with whom to do this. Remind clients of the need to see this as a beginning and to continue to grow in the real world. In some cases, clients may be tempted to only try new skills in online places. Although doing so has some benefits, the client should strongly be encouraged to continue to try and connect with people in real life.

FBGT Scale 5: Unassertive

People with high distress on this scale are in considerable emotional pain. There is tremendous internalization, guilt, shame, self-doubt, and embarrassment that accompanies and underlies this interpersonal style. It is an act of considerable courage for these members to even attend a group. Doing so risks everything that they are most worried about: being judged by others and feeling inadequate. However, seeing others struggle also allows them to learn that others also have problems and are not always coping well or able to function perfectly. Therefore, creating a safe, cohesive environment is particularly important for people with this style.

Overall Description

People with this style can be effective at following and being an effective team member. They may tend toward a quieter style and have a tendency to defer to others, which can be helpful when groups require consent to move quickly. They may be seen as loyal, dependable, helpful, and willing to serve others. In workplaces, families, and cultures in which this kind of service is important, they may be highly valued.

Clients with this style may describe themselves as struggling with feeling confident to engage in agentic, self-motivated behavior and as being full of self-doubt. They often report having low self-esteem and feeling inferior and inadequate. In addition, they report avoiding situations that require them to exercise power or leadership. Although often avoidant of others, they may feel incapable when alone because they lack the belief that they can exercise self-care, and they feel unable to look after themselves. They also avoid making their needs and wishes known to others.

When paired with high scores in social inhibition, a person should be evaluated for avoidant personality disorder. When paired with the style focused on the needs of others, the presence of dependent personality disorder is possible (Horowitz, 2004). As with the other styles, cultural role expectations and variables may also play a part in the formation and maintenance as well as the continuation of this style, and they should be assessed.

Place in the Group Dynamic

During times of distress and conflict, people with an unassertive style become quite silent and withdrawn. They take advice from others readily, and thus are seen as valuable by some group members; however, this is contrary to what they most need: to achieve distance or warmth. People with this style have a tendency to fade into the background and be ignored by the group. In groups populated by people with scores high in dominance, those with this style may tend to be particularly anonymous because they perceive others' confidence as a verification of their own felt sense of inadequacy.

Working Alliance Formation

Clients with this style are inclined to follow whatever recommendation the therapist gives. They behave in ways that are ingratiating and unassertive during the TPS session, leading to the therapist's hooked feelings of the urge to instruct, tell, and teach. The unhooked position is to maintain warmth and energy while moving between slight dominance and moments that promote giving choices.

The client may be quite reluctant to accept the validity of those choices and may continue to seek to determine what the therapist wants, taking a dependent position in the face of the therapist's perceived and actual authority. Thus, the therapist must carefully position themselves to motivate the client toward goals that will be helpful while allowing the client to maintain choices. For example, goal selection and calibration are important moments to provide information from which the client can select meaningful goals. However, the therapist must stay vigilant to the power dynamic in the room and remind the client of their choices and autonomy—something the client may struggle to accept.

Goals

Goals on the quarter turn reflect working on the strengths associated with styles that are two scales away from the scale that is the focus for treatment. In other words, people with distress on Scale 5: Unassertive will be working on strengths that are related to Scale 3: Distant and Scale 7: Warm/Self-Sacrificing. Goals that are on the quarter turn include expressing needs, wishes, and feelings, providing an opportunity for the client to also later express their needs and wishes as being as important as any other group member's (i.e., Scale 7). While the client is unable to engage in a serious conflict (i.e., a goal that is 180 degrees), they may be able to define their own needs as of being importance to the group. For example, asking for time from the group to talk about an issue of importance to their life is, if achieved, a significant accomplishment. Equally, using distancing behavior, such as saying no to an invitation by another group member, is another challenging but potentially worthwhile goal because to do so requires that the client establish a boundary and risk not being liked. This goal is difficult for the client, and the therapist should take care to not overstep and demand too much of the client. Therefore, the therapist should carefully calibrate this goal with the client.

Debriefing Issues

Becoming more agentic and warmer or distant has consequences in systems. While some may welcome increased distance as seeing someone stand up for their boundaries and may see increased warmth as a positive thing, others may not. Setting boundaries is not always well received, so the therapist should work with the client on timing and context of when to use new strategies. Equally, even increasing warmth may be welcomed by some but may upset other, more delicately balanced or negatively valanced environments. For example, if working in a setting defined by aggressive, domineering people, increasing warmth may be anticomplementary to the client's style and be dismissed and ridiculed by the group. Therefore, it is wrong to assume that any change will be universally well received. In particular, the therapist should encourage "small victories" in low-stakes environments as a beginning and encourage a test-and-learn philosophy.

FBGT Scale 6: Focused on the Needs of Others

Being focused on the needs of others is a double-edged sword. It typically (but not always) engenders considerable positive feedback from others, with friends, family, and colleagues considering this person a "true friend" or suggesting that they become a therapist due to their listening skills and helpful suggestions or action. However, when extreme and rigid, people with this style can eventually burn out and become resentful. This style is particularly risky in groups because the group and therapist welcome them as promoting cohesion and providing valuable modeling. However, these are also clients who are highly likely to drop out because they secretly harbor resentment that, again, no one is looking after them or letting them be seen—a fact that they try to hide from the therapist so as not to disappoint them, either. Goal selection is therefore extremely important.

Overall Description

Clients may describe being seen as the glue that holds friends and family together. They are often prized by groups and individuals for their selfless and seemingly tireless attempts to look after others' needs. In work or volunteer settings, they may receive praise and recognition for their selflessness and commitment to the workplace, religion, or population being served. Friends experience them as an endless source of support and constantly available to help and assist. The praise received for this role is considerable. Those with this profile may be seen as a peacemaker or pseudotherapist by others and may end up in a helping profession.

However, this role is exhausting for the person involved. They may report dysthymia, exhaustion, lack of sleep, anxiety, and a constant feeling of being on edge. They may describe symptoms of burnout and sometimes express a feeling of being emotionally "broken." Feelings of being used, taken for granted, and taken advantage of are common. Because they have considerable difficulty expressing anger and being assertive in defending their boundaries, they may instead become resentful and bitter. Typically, clients with this style report that friendships feel unidirectional—that friends seek their support at all times of day and night but fail to reciprocate. People with distress on this scale seldom ask for help because they have low expectations of their needs getting met and often have buried their needs so deeply that, at times, they cannot even identify them.

Place in the Group Dynamic

This person is often beloved by the group. They serve as peacemaker, support, warm encourager, and effective listener. The group gives them the same praise they receive in the real world for prosocial behavior. The group leader may also be lured into seeing them as a favored group member and may allow them to persist in this role because they help with group cohesion. However, the group member with this style continues to not get their own needs met, thus replicating the same problem they brought to the group from outside. Without goals that are clearly motivating the person away from this typical pattern, they are at risk of either dropout or poor progress in therapy.

At some point, if a person with the opposite style—Scale 2—is present in the group, they may target for attack the person focused on the needs of others. It is a common occurrence in groups for someone with a high score on Scale 2 to attack someone with a high score on Scale 6, calling them "weak" or "pathetic." This can be quite a shocking moment to the individual and the group.

Working Alliance Formation

Therapists frequently misunderstand the working alliance with individuals with these scale scores. When asked if they are motivated to join and would like to be a part of the group, the answer is often yes. Because they are focused on the needs of others, they likely are eager to please the therapist by agreeing to their treatment suggestions. However, in actuality, the client is likely highly ambivalent about joining a group. In the group, they feel they must take care of everyone, and they quickly fall into this role. However, even when they are successful in taking care of everyone, they are left feeling empty and resentful because they did not ask for their needs to be met.

The therapist must be the one to point out to the client that they should also get their needs met and keep a focus on meeting those needs. The therapist must also be careful to notice if they are becoming too pleased with how well the session is going and how the client is agreeing to all requests. Underlying this acquiescence and warmth is a significant risk that once they fail to get their needs met or feel burdened by the group's demands, the client will leave the group. The hooked position is for the therapist to take a warm but dominant stance to the client's warm submission. The unhooked position is to give the client choices and to notice the balance between offering choices and suggesting options. The therapist must carefully balance the need to sometimes remain dominant with the need to give the client choices, thereby placing the client in the dominant role.

Goals

It is key for the leader and the group to stay focused on the group member's goals, which should relate to asking for their needs to be met (Scale 8) and occasionally passively refusing to meet others' needs (Scale 4). Asking for their needs to be met is a crucial goal. The client will have tremendous difficulty with highly assertive behavior (Scale 2) but will benefit from a quarter turn toward more agentic behavior. Consider that to disagree with someone or refuse to acquiesce to a demand requires that the person first believes that their needs and wishes are also important. The person with distress (Scale 6) may not acknowledge or know they have needs.

An important middle step, therefore, is for the person with this profile to name needs and attempt to get them met. The goal might be for them to go first in the group or to ask for help from the group in talking about an issue important to them. The act of asking and having a need met is vitally important because it presupposes that their needs are as important as anyone else's. Obtaining immediate feedback from the group that this was okay is then essential to prevent the maladaptive schema from overwhelming the moment with negative self-talk and physical reactions that suggest a disaster has occurred.

Debriefing Issues

Debriefing should take place around selection of people, places, and times to attempt new behaviors. It is important to remember that people with this style are highly likely to receive adverse consequences to changes in behavior and that they therefore need to be prepared for this and to think it through in advance. Whole systems may well depend on the client's continued overfunctioning and willingness to give until they have nothing left. People label those with this profile as "always dependable," "a true friend," and "utterly selfless." Attempts to set boundaries or get their own needs met do not always go well. Some friends and workplaces may be quite resistant to a new status quo. For example, the friend who calls at 3 a.m. to talk about trivial problems and does not reciprocate may well react badly to being told that the time is not appropriate. Some friendships may end. The therapist should not pretend that all changes, although healthier in the long run, will not also result in the changing or ending of some relationships that cannot tolerate a more equal footing. Thus, debriefing must be honest and must prepare the client for what is to come.

In many instances, follow-up sessions or even a follow-up group may help with generalization and transfer to the real world. Even the presence of a simpler support group or booster sessions in which the client talks about their issues may be helpful. Continuity of care needs careful consideration given the potential turmoil that may ensue. While there may be considerable benefits to the client in the long run, the client should carefully select when and with whom to place boundaries so that their early attempts are met with success and not rejection. The client may well wish to enlist support from others they believe may be supportive by explaining the process they are undertaking.

FBGT Scale 7: Warm/Self-Sacrificing

In countries and contexts that prize warmth, it is not uncommon to see this trait as unproblematic. It can facilitate satisfying relationships marked by enjoyment, fun, and intimacy. However, when rigid and extreme, the lack of boundaries, an inability to tolerate conflict, and a lack of self-care can sometimes result in very negative outcomes and high distress. Loneliness is not just an absence of relationships, but is also the presence of low-quality relationships. Clients who are unable to set boundaries or embrace conflicts when needed may eventually begin to feel "lonely in a crowd," undifferentiated from others, unable to set boundaries, and unable to express anger as they feel it.

Overall Description

People with this style are typically outgoing, lively, enjoy social mixing, and are extraverted and able to connect well with others. They tend to be successful in relationships and are often regarded as socially adept in cultures that prize warmth. Those with this style typically have more secure and attached relationships with others. They are often seen as fun, caring, and people oriented. However, people with high levels of distress on this scale may report having difficulty setting boundaries. For example, they may indicate being unable to refuse social invitations even when important due dates are impending or getting into difficulty with other issues around limit setting for themselves or others. Refusal and assertiveness skills may be particularly challenging when social pressure to conform is high and a potential loss of social connections is at stake. They dislike conflict and struggle with being assertive.

Place in the Group Dynamic

The place the person likely takes is to be the warm, connected model for the rest of the group to emulate as they move toward cohesion. The group values this person's warmth and connectedness, enjoying their use of humor and ability to both initiate and maintain conversations. The positive feedback for their overall presence in terms of establishing and maintaining group cohesion likely makes them a valued group member. People with this style can become frustrated with those in the group who keep strong boundaries or who engage in conflict. They attempt to befriend others, but if those advances are rejected, either passively or assertively, they may become sad and frustrated.

Working Alliance Formation

Working alliance formation involves being warm but maintaining boundaries. The client is likeable and easy to talk with. Being hooked involves the therapist's feeling amused, feeling connected, and having a desire to loosen boundaries; for example, they report to a colleague later that they could imagine being friends with the client. The initial contact might involve feelings of liking, being connected, or feeling entertained. The unhooked position is to maintain a clear boundary while also acknowledging the client's need to be taken seriously and have their own boundaries. The unhooked position also involves becoming more distant: acknowledging that the client is likable but also honoring the part of them that would like to be taken more seriously.

Goals

Goals include moving toward Scale 1: Highly Assertive and Scale 5: Unassertive. Scale 2 goals involve taking a leadership position and directing the group or disagreeing. The client's goals could include asserting themselves, engaging in a conflict and surviving it, or leading the conversation in a different direction. Therefore, client may, at some point, choose to say no to another group member's request or to resist pressure to join with the group on a topic or idea. This may feel forced and challenging for the client. In effect, they are waiting to find a moment to disagree or may take a position that is a contrary one. They may also choose to say no to a request or an invitation to join with someone in a more connected way. This can feel quite artificial to the client attempting it but may still feel genuine to the group. The group can therefore be helpful to the client by giving feedback and helping the client understand that they can disagree and still be liked.

Equally, by removing themselves from some discussions, the client can learn to see themselves as autonomous and able to function as an individual separate from the group. Clients in this octant also sometimes look to engage with members of the group outside of the therapy session, sometimes forming a friendship or even romantic relationships with other members. Group goals might also include the idea of keeping the group boundary sacrosanct as a way of learning to inhibit that urge.

Debriefing Issues

Debriefing is crucial in identifying specific areas in which employment of these new skills might helpful. Overgeneralizing could result in the deterioration of important relationships, so it is essential to remember that warmth is, in most instances, adaptive for the client. However, judicious use of boundaries may be necessary to establish a clearer vision of when there is a need to assertively or unassertively disengage from social connections to improve a needed boundary. Discussion should take place on what the client's goals are in terms of meeting their own needs while also being able to form connections with others. Discussing the need to be liked as both a positive force and also one that can sometimes be problematic in one's life involves a careful analysis of each area of their life to determine where changes are appropriate.

FBGT Scale 8: Uninhibited

The uninhibited scale score for distress is one that was particularly important to understand when FBGT was in its early stages of development. In fact, the technique of inoculating clients largely developed from learning from case studies with this particular style (as well as with Scale 2). Clients with this style could be entertaining, warm, and extraverted and often set the tone in the group. However, when rigid or extreme, they could overdisclose too early and be so intrusive so quickly that the group could quickly derail. Their desire for close relationships was so strong that they would inadvertently self-sabotage by moving too quickly into depth, scaring the other group members. This would also take place in the TPS session, where clients would push boundaries, immediately seeking intimacy beyond the scope of the professional therapist role. The techniques for managing this both in individual sessions and in the group became a key innovation in FBGT.

Overall Description

Clients with this style are sometimes the most dramatic and interesting clients in the group. Outgoing, vivacious, and larger than life, they can offer the group a great deal. However, along with clients with scores high on Scale 2, clients with this profile also offer the most significant risk of poor outcomes and also of negatively impacting the group, leading to premature dropouts of other members. However, in FBGT, the technique of inoculating has proven highly successful in ameliorating harm and generating success with these clients. Inoculation developed from working with clients with peaks on Scale 2 or Scale 8, and this technique became a cornerstone technique within the approach.

Warm leadership, good interpersonal skills, and a genuine interest in other people are all hallmarks of people with strengths in this area. At their best, people with this style can be compelling public speakers and good listeners; can attune well to others' needs and feelings; and can be charismatic, funny, and charming. They value deep personal connection and divulge personal information quickly and expect the same of others. Over time, if in balance, this person is attentive to maintaining relationships and is warm and active.

However, with very high scores on this style, these qualities become out of balance and morph into a more extreme version of the positive qualities. Attentiveness become intrusiveness: Others experience the person's interpersonal strategies to become closer as "too much too soon." That person may have a series of immediate rejections as people distance themselves and place firm boundaries or have other experiences of starting relationships very intensely and positively before they burn out, and the friend or romantic partner steps away.

Place in the Group Dynamic

Members with this style often take a leadership position and are experienced as supportive and curious about others. However, those with high scores on this scale are also very challenging to early group cohesion. Their attempts to quickly connect and to deepen relationships feel premature and forced. They may overdisclose very personal information extremely early in a relationship or quickly on meeting people. This overdisclosing is sometimes called being an "early provocateur" (Yalom, 1966, p. 409; see also Cox, 2008) because it can involve dramatic and startling revelations or questions that heighten the drama of the group but end up leading to premature terminations instead. These overdisclosures or overly intrusive questioning of others can leave group members feeling overwhelmed and shocked. For example, when the leader asks the group members to share something small about themselves in less than 5 minutes, the group member with this style offers a lengthy description of a recent sexual conquest, briefly mentions a prior suicide attempt, and then asks other group members if they have ever felt suicidal. These early, intense disclosures (too much or too deep too quickly) can lead not only to members' feeling overwhelmed, but also feeling pressured to match the level of self-disclosure. As a result, members sometimes leave the group and do not return. The client with this style may perceive this departure as a rejection and then feel shamed and also leave the group.

Working Alliance Formation

Clients with this style may typically enter the room and immediately comment favorably on the office, the therapist's appearance, or the therapist's marital status. They may ask intrusive questions, play with the boundaries of the session ("Maybe we could hang out after the therapy is over"), and immediately disclose at the deepest level. The therapist may well feel a flood of emotions from the invitations: flattered, concerned, overwhelmed, and immediately worried about how to set boundaries without breaking the alliance that has not even begun to form. These feelings can leave the therapist feeling relieved when the client leaves and upset and agitated as they wrestle with all the competing feelings. Remember that this is how everyone who encounters this client will feel: overwhelmed, confused, and with a desire to escape. However, it is also important to remember that this client is doing their best with what they know. They are seeking to form good connections, but are going about it too quickly.

The working alliance is typically formed through unhooking and nonjudgmentally exploring the client's interpersonal distress in terms of recognizing the appropriate desire to connect while tweaking the techniques to get there by slowing down a little. A graduate student of mine used the analogy of two people reading a book, but one person wants to skip to the last chapter immediately. The key is to slow down and match the other person's pace. The unhooked position involves noticing the urge to set strong boundaries and experiencing the alternating feelings of liking and wanting to push the client away and keep them from intruding. The therapist must notice the underlying desire that the client has to connect and acknowledge to themselves that this client is doing their best with what they know. They should acknowledge the client's strengths and desire to connect and encourage exploration of the pacing of connection. The unhooked position involves noticing the urge to set strong boundaries and experiencing the alternating feelings of liking and wanting to push the client away and to keep them from intruding. Setting consistent boundaries is important while also acknowledging the person's likeability and strengths.

Another key concern for this style is that once insight is obtained, the person may then look back at their life and feel shame that they may have contributed to the ending of relationships by moving too fast. It is important for the therapist to notice and ensure that the client recognizes they were always doing their best with what they knew and that any attempts to connect were well intentioned. The therapist then needs to focus attention on how to move forward with success.

Goals

Goal selection for clients on this scale involves inhibiting the desire to over-disclose too quickly or in too much depth and also to avoid asking penetrating questions too early. The goal is to have the client slow down their interpersonal communications so they can better meet their ultimate goal of more meaningful connections that have the potential to be longer lasting. Therefore, goals, such as matching to the middle-most disclosing person in the group in terms of length of comments and duration of comments, serve that effort while also acting as an inoculation.

Debriefing

Debriefing clients with this scale is a complex process. They often struggle with the process of slowing down, and so processing how the group unfolded and whether slowing down helped is a key aspect to this session. Clients also experience considerable anxiety that they do not feel "known" by the group because they did not disclose at their normal depth. Discussing the speed and depth of relationships and returning once again to a book or movie metaphor are important steps. Showing them that their interpersonal distress reduced but that they are now anxious about not being seen can be translated back to the metaphor that the book is still to be read. It is not on the last chapter, so the feelings of intense connection are not there yet, but the other person is still reading with you, so it has not ended prematurely.

The client may also try and reinitiate an unboundaried connection with the therapist, suggesting going out for coffee or lunch. It is important to anticipate this request. This is not a sign of treatment failure but, rather, another opportunity to set a warm boundary. Explaining how much you have appreciated their work and courage while also maintaining the professional boundary gives the client an exemplar of how a relationship can be healthy and positive and yet have boundaries and an ending. This can serve as a template for the client with respect to other relationships in their life as they negotiate through different contexts.

CONSIDERATIONS WHEN SELECTING GOALS

There are many considerations when selecting goals, ranging from the technical (e.g., understanding the quarter turn, keeping goals behavioral) through to an integration of cultural, contextual, or other factors. Remember that distress can come from interpersonal sources (a person's distress is across all situations), contextual (a person's distress is activated by specific contexts or cultural interactions, e.g., dealing with a microaggression), or combinations of both (e.g., someone identifies as being socially inhibited and also has the most difficulty expressing their identity as different than others around them when in different cultural spaces). Therefore, the role of the therapist is to consider the important role of phenotypes while also determining if goals need to integrate cultural data or not. This is done in combination with the client, being careful to elicit cultural data and to collaboratively explore this with each client. It is important to listen to the client while doing so and to determine what they feel is important.

It is also important to integrate technical factors into goals. Table 3.1 shows the focus of treatment, the two possible quarter turn directions, and the possible goals for each turn. Research by Rodrigo et al. (2022) highlighted the idea that cognitive control is an essential part of interpersonal functioning. This has been borne out in FBGT in which control for some styles involves metaphorically stepping on the social accelerator (e.g., by behaving in ways that are warmer), whereas for others, control involves inhibition (e.g., slowing down self-disclosure or holding back from rescuing others). This personalization or tailoring of goals is central to FBGT and also requires a more sophisticated and nuanced leadership style that permits and supports differences in outcomes based on what is increasing interpersonal flexibility for each client.

FBGT does not subscribe to the idea that every therapy group should involve having all members disclose deeply and find ways to be maximally cohesive with each other. Rather, FBGT suggests that each client should work on their

TABLE 3.1. Typical Goals for Each Interpersonal Scale Distress

Highest client scale: The focus of treatment	Scale attribute client is seeking to work toward: The quarter turn goal	Possible goals for the quarter turn
Scale 1: Highly Assertive	Scale 3: Distant	Listen to others without commenting at least ____ times. Hold back from offering advice or telling people what to do at least ____ times.
	Scale 7: Warm/Self-Sacrificing	Ask follow-up questions about what someone else is saying at least ____ times. Offer encouragement and support at least ____ times. Self-disclose about something you feel slightly vulnerable about at least ____ times.
Scale 2: Focused on the Needs of the Self	Scale 8: Uninhibited	Offer encouragement at least ____ times. Ask follow-up questions at least ____ times. Talk about your own problems at least ____ times.
	Scale 4: Socially Inhibited	Listen carefully at least ____ times to what others are saying. Hold back on offering thoughts and advice at least ____ times. In the first three sessions of the group and after that, seek feedback on any criticism you give. Consider what others are thinking and feeling at least ____ times.
Scale 3: Distant	Scale 1: Highly Assertive	Offer advice at least ____ times. Suggest a topic or frame the topic at least ____ times.
	Scale 5: Unassertive	Listen quietly and give nonverbal encouragement (nods, "uh-huh," eye contact) at least ____ times. Attend every group.
Scale 4: Socially Inhibited	Scale 6: Focused on the Needs of Others	Ask follow-up questions at least ____ times. Offer encouragement at least ____ times. Offer help to another group member at least ____ times.
	Scale 2: Focused on the Needs of the Self	Ask for feedback on how you are coming across at least ____ times. Speak without thinking too hard about the consequences to yourself or the group at least ____ times. Assert yourself if you disagree with someone at least ____ times.

Scale	Behaviors
Scale 5: Unassertive	Find something you have in common with someone in the group and comment on it at least _____ times.
Scale 7: Warm/Self-Sacrificing	Offer supportive encouragement at least _____ times. Ask follow-up questions at least _____ times. Ask for time to talk about yourself at least _____ times.
Scale 3: Distant	Hold back from involving yourself in a discussion or agreeing if you don't feel you believe in it at least _____ times.
Scale 4: Socially Inhibited	Hold back from offering to serve the group at least _____ times.
Scale 6: Focused on the Needs of Others	Listen quietly without trying to help, support, or encourage another group member at least _____ times.
Scale 8: Uninhibited	Ask for time from the group at least _____ times. Go first in the group at least _____ times. Ask for help from the group at least _____ times.
Scale 5: Unassertive	Follow along with a group decision at least _____ times. Listen, but don't add anything to the discussion at least _____ times.
Scale 7: Warm/Self-Sacrificing	Explain yourself to the group if you are feeling misunderstood at least _____ times.
Scale 1: Highly Assertive	Take charge of a topic or conversation by setting the agenda at least _____ times. Maintain a sense of distance from the group by holding back on emotional support at least _____ times.
Scale 2: Focused on the Needs of the Self	Hold back on offering warmth at least _____ times. Maintain a boundary by not asking questions of others at the beginning of the group for at least _____ times.
Scale 8: Uninhibited	When I share, I will match the depth and intensity and time spent speaking of the person in the group who is disclosing an average amount. Ask for feedback on how you are coming across from others in the group after three sessions.
Scale 6: Focused on the Needs of Others	Ask others questions (but only at the same level others are asking) at least _____ times. When I notice I am talking too much, I will pause and say, "I will stop there" and wait for someone else to speak at least _____ times.

own 90-degree goals within the context of the here and now and within the context of sufficient group cohesion to act to promote retention.

For some clients, their goals may mean moving toward more cohesion; for others, it means growth in their own interpersonal flexibility that involves the opposite: putting boundaries in place or becoming slightly more distant than they might typically have been. Remember that the goal of therapy is to reduce feelings of distress about relationships. For one person, their distress relates to lack of connection and closeness, but for another, it may relate to problems setting boundaries, asserting themselves, or being quiet and allowing others to speak. Loneliness is not just the absence of relationships, but also the presence of relationships that are unsatisfying. Group members can learn that setting more boundaries or becoming more assertive does not have to end in disaster; they can sometimes tolerate a loss of warm connection in return for greater feelings of agency and autonomy. This may also mean losing some friendships or relationships that are so unsatisfying and so unlikely to change that they are not worth preserving. This does, however, risk exchanging one type of loneliness (an unsatisfying relationship) for another (no relationship); therefore, choices to do so should be addressed with informed consent and considerable support.

Therapists must be aware of another caution: In cases of abusive and violent relationships, care should be taken not to proscribe that a client increase their assertiveness with that abuser. Evidence shows that abusive and violent partners respond to assertiveness or their partner's leaving with increased violence (Campbell, 2004). Therefore, clinicians should ensure people at risk of domestic violence are given individualized treatment by trained professionals with awareness of the risk factors involved.

Goal development is further elaborated in the next chapter, which explores in more detail the cocreation of tailored goals. Goals are sometimes boilerplate; however, in many cases, it is important to understand the 90-degree turn but then develop goals accordingly. For example, some clients with social inhibition find initiating relationships easy, but continuing and deepening them is more difficult; for others, it is the reverse. Exploring with the client what specifically it is that they find difficult is a key step in tailoring treatment. Remember that identity issues can be woven into goals if this is something that the client wishes to work on. For example, a client who wishes to become more assertive (starting off at a high score on Scale 4: Socially Inhibited or a high score on Scale 8: Uninhibited) might choose: "To assert myself at least once around an issue important to my identity."

Equally, it is important to understand that combinations of styles can provide very different understandings of a client. For example, in the scale descriptors discussed earlier, it is possible to see that Scale 5: Unassertive when paired with Scale 6: Focused on the Needs of Others can sometimes lead to a diagnosis (if other criteria are also present) of dependent personality disorder. If Scale 5 is paired with Scale 4, it can sometimes—subject to other diagnostic variables being present—lead to a diagnosis of avoidant personality disorder.

Many profiles involve more than one peak; therefore, the therapist should carefully assess what the combination of scales indicates and suggests. This is also where the art and science of FBGT meet in collaboration with the client's explanation. Profiles are sometimes very distinct, but, at other times, can be confusing until one asks the client and listens to their explanation. Therefore, assessment should inform and not supplant clinical judgment, and the client should always be a key source of that understanding.

SUMMARY

Each interpersonal style carries with it the potential for considerable good while also containing the possibility of causing distress if misapplied to the wrong context or in extreme and rigid ways that are inconsistent with the demands of the situation. Understanding interpersonal styles can also augment the clinician's skill set immeasurably because there is potential to understand and intervene more effectively based on the client's strengths while also predicting potential pitfalls and self-sabotage. Clients seek self-understanding, so helping them become more self-aware about both their strengths and their impact on others can offer them the opportunity to not only feel more congruent, but also to become more flexible in how they manage themselves in relation to others.

4 LEADERSHIP ATTITUDES, FOCI, AND SKILLS

Focused brief group therapy (FBGT) demands a great deal of the group leader and offers those who are willing to undertake a lifelong process of learning the opportunity to challenge themselves to continue to grow. FBGT also requires an understanding of one's own interpersonal style, an ability to adjust and match to each client and the group, an ability to decode and intervene in group dynamics, a willingness to embrace complexity, the courage to confront mistakes and treatment failure without self-recrimination, and the ability to retain a willingness to continue to learn and grow. Overall, FBGT offers a rich opportunity for professional and personal development for the therapist who is willing to embrace the process of continual growth.

FBGT LEADERSHIP

To learn the FBGT approach, consider the several connected skill sets that are assumed within FBGT. First, prior training or acquisition of knowledge, skills, and supervision described in Yalom and Leszcz's (2020) work on interpersonal process is helpful in practicing the approach.

https://doi.org/10.1037/0000389-005
Focused Brief Group Therapy: An Integrative Approach to Reducing Interpersonal Distress, by M. Whittingham

Second, therapists need to be committed to exploring the nuances of the assessment tools in FBGT, particularly with respect to how these tools intersect and combine with multicultural and cross-cultural data. This exploration of results through the lens of both interpersonal theory and multicultural theory, as is discussed throughout this book. The relationship between the two is complex, and client distress unfolds from the notion that between-group differences and within-group differences are present within everyone. Groups can differ in very meaningful ways, but people can also be different within groups, and the two categories are not mutually exclusive. Engaging with the complexity of how culture interacts with personality and how individuals achieve what they want from relationships is a key aspect of conceptualization in FBGT.

Third, that the therapist must be committed to lifelong improvement and learning. FBGT is designed to allow practitioners to get feedback from data at the local level, an empirically supported strategy (Wampold & Imel, 2015). The model is therefore well set up to encourage clinical curiosity about the connection between process and outcomes and to facilitate the opportunity for continuous improvement and lifelong learning. Each of those innovations came from learning from successes and mistakes. I hope that the spirit of continual learning that goes with FBGT remains a part of any future iterations or adaptations of the model. It should evolve in a thoughtful and considered way with plenty of data supporting decisions and adaptations carefully monitored to ensure they are successful.

LEADER ATTITUDES

The leader's basic stance should always emanate from engaging in unconditional positive regard and person empathy (Rogers, 1957), a construct that has not only stood the test of time but has been found to be highly predictive of treatment outcome (Wampold & Imel, 2015). When engaging in *unconditional positive regard*, the therapist seeks to find the core loveable person—who has made every effort to do their best with what they know—by exploring that person's past history empathically. What did it feel like to be this person as they grew up and became the person they are today? Regardless of their presenting behavior and what it elicits, the leader's task is to find a person to care about by understanding their story.

That means therapists should be honest with themselves about what they are feeling. If they feel antipathy toward a client, they should engage in self-exploration and uncover what it is about feelings of dislike that emanate from them and from the client. In some instances, it represents a hooked response to a client's behavior. An important empathic step that can be part of the interpersonal interview is taking the perspective that this person is doing their best with what they know and also exploring how that person first came to this strategy. Equally important is to remember—whether the client is expressing pain or vulnerability or not—that this person is in therapy because they are suffering. The therapist's ability to achieve *person empathy*—to walk in that person's shoes and to consider the deeper, underlying motivations, fears, and worries—is a vital step in basic liking of the client that is so essential to the alliance. Part of the process of disentangling positive and negative countertransferential feelings involves self-exploration, ranging from personal therapy and understanding how early attachment experiences impacted one's own attachment and interpersonal style to considering how both trait-level and culturally embedded understandings of the world influence feelings toward other people.

This process must be undertaken with considerable self-compassion. Therapists should treat themselves with the same levels of compassion and unconditional positive self-regard with which they treat clients. The purpose of therapist self-awareness should be built around acceptance of interpersonal traits, self-compassionate viewing of early childhood, and a willingness to understand how cultures and identities are both similar and different to our own experience. The idea that clients are always doing their best with what they know is one that therapists also need to embrace for themselves. However, that does not mean that change cannot take place. Rather, the process should be one of self-acceptance combined with nonjudgmental self-improvement and growth, not as a shame-based destination for a therapist to become stuck in.

LEADER CULTURAL AWARENESS

Leaders should also take every opportunity to undertake work that allows them to explore issues of power, privilege, and oppression with respect to their own identities and the marginalized identities of others. Being aware of culture and how it intersects with power and privilege is an essential part of effective group leadership and is important across a wide range of outcomes (Falender et al., 2014). Research has shown that the group leader and the group members' ability to manage rather than miss multicultural opportunities is an important factor in outcome (Grimes & Kivlighan, 2022).

Multicultural awareness, humility, and willingness to broach issues related to power, privilege, oppression, and cultural difference are noteworthy factors in effective group leadership. Research shows that diversity awareness and actions based on that knowledge are still insufficiently practiced, however (e.g., Wilcox et al., 2020).

Developing cultural comfort and risking broaching these topics are therefore crucial leadership skills (Owen et al., 2011). The same spirit of humility and self-development that goes into work on becoming more mindful and self-accepting of one's interpersonal baseline must also go into becoming more aware of one's own interpersonal cultural baselines and becoming curious about how other cultures may differ. Learning about other cultures and differences in cultures across either wide, nomothetic groupings (e.g., Kitayama et al., 2022) or smaller regions as well as learning about populations and cultures across diversity variables, such as gender, sexuality, ethnicity, spirituality, and race, can all add to a therapist's cultural comfort.

GROUP LEADER AS PARTICIPANT-OBSERVER

These attitudes on the self, mindful self-awareness, and cultural humility are vital because they relate to the leader role during all phases of group. The leader takes the role of *participant–observer* throughout the experience; this role entails a combination of self-awareness and mindful experience of one's own emotional responses as a form of data. Thus, the therapist must notice and monitor their own feelings, using their reactions to the client as information to add to the data already collected.

To be successful with this approach, undertaking one's own therapy is strongly recommended as is having a keen understanding of one's own basic interpersonal style and tendencies. The group leader must be able to separate their own material from the material of the group and its members. This is a contentious issue in the psychotherapy literature (Safran & Muran, 2006). Some have argued that the therapist can never truly be objective and should not assume they have a completely clear viewpoint on the client. However, FBGT takes a position on this issue with respect to both clients and leaders. First, it posits that the therapist needs to have undergone sufficient personal work to be able to step back and notice their own emotional reactions to members and the group without being consumed by their own therapeutic issues based on past experiences. A leader who cannot notice and retain control of their emotions and retain a therapeutic stance is unlikely to lead purposefully and with intent.

Second, FBGT assumes that the therapist has taken the 32-item Inventory of Interpersonal Problems (IIP-32; Horowitz et al., 2000) themselves and has undergone a period of reflection and learning regarding the implications for themselves as a person, therapist, and group leader. The therapist should understand not only how they will likely be hooked by group members but also what place they will take in the group dynamic and how they will relate to a group leader. This level of self-awareness of the implications of the therapist's own interpersonal style is essential to FBGT. Without this grounded awareness of the therapist's own hooked state and the feelings that accompany it, they will struggle to notice when invitations are occurring. Equally, without an awareness of their own disowned interpersonal styles and how they pejoratively label that, they will be unaware of the processes of transference and countertransference that occur. The therapist's emotions must be accessible (as opposed to blunted or experienced as overwhelming) for the therapist to be able to practice FBGT.

Consider this example: The therapist who has taken the IIP-32 finds that they have a style Focused on the Needs of Others (Scale 6). They note that this style is warm and encouraging of others and accept the strengths of this approach. However, they also know that the group they are about to begin leading comprises several members who have styles that are high in assertiveness (Scale 1: Highly Assertive) and distance (Scale 3: Distant). They consider that they may experience feelings of wanting to negatively label the group members' style of asserting themselves. Therefore, they make a note to accept the goals of setting boundaries and achieving safety by being in charge because these goals will make these members feel more comfortable. Further, the therapist recognizes that the experience of vulnerability by other group members will provoke anxiety inside the dominant members. The group leader prepares themselves for group by remembering techniques that will facilitate group progress (e.g., blocking, protecting at the start, and then allowing conflict as the group progresses). They also make a note to notice their own feelings as the group progresses and to stay in process regarding what is helpful and unhelpful in terms of choice of intervention.

Third, the therapist must be aware of culture and differences in the way interpersonal invitations and responses are handled. Lack of awareness can act as its own form of transference and countertransference. Therefore, therapists should always be prepared to consider the cultural elements of their interactions with a client and their impact on the client. Working constantly with humility and a willingness to learn about culture is a lifelong pursuit, and empathic or cultural failures should be met with honesty, humility, and a desire to learn and grow.

LEADER EMOTION AND COGNITION IN HARMONY

The FBGT process includes the ability to accept all emotions as a form of data but with a need to then filter them through cognitive models of understanding, including cultural and interpersonal ones. After sorting through emotions to put them in their proper place (e.g., the anger felt toward a client is a hooked response to their behavior and not a displacement from a prior negative interaction with a coworker), they can be used to inform understanding of the interpersonal process in the room. This means accepting and acknowledging all emotions, no matter how unpleasant or unacceptable, without becoming attached to them. For example, feeling angry, inadequate, hopeless, loving, compassionate, distant, jealous, vengeful, or joyous when reacting to group members can all serve as important data about what is happening interpersonally in the room and what the client may be inviting (presupposing that the therapist is not the one bringing the emotions into the room).

The assumption, though, is that the group leader is sufficiently centered to notice, is able to notice without attaching to the emotions, and also understands how their baseline interpersonal style is either being activated or pulled in a different direction by an invitation. The therapist must be self-aware, centered, and able to notice their emotions and be at play with what those emotions might mean. Doing so provides the therapist with an important additional data set from which to draw on during the therapy, pregroup preparation, and screening (TPS) session (see a full discussion of TPS in Chapter 6); group; and debriefing. The therapist needs to work toward the middle ground of mindful noticing of emotions and using it as a data point to understand clients and the group.

LEADER STANCES

As Yalom and Leszcz (2020) stated, perhaps nothing is more important than the group leader's fundamental stance of unconditional positive regard toward each client. Group leaders must always maintain a position of care, compassion, and understanding toward even the most challenging clients. The more challenging the group leader finds a client, the harder the group leader must work to understand their own negative reactions and to maintain empathy. This is no easy feat. At times, clients elicit a wide range of difficult feelings from the leader: inadequacy, shame, anger, self-loathing, jealousy, and desire. These feelings can feel toxic and dystonic to group leaders, and left to fester, these feelings can lead to poor leader performance and resultant negative client outcomes. As Strupp (1993) pointed out in the Vanderbilt psychotherapy studies, "interpretations [that] advanced in a subtly blaming manner or 'supportive' messages that simultaneously conveyed a criticism of the patient" (p. 432) have been linked to negative outcomes. Shaming, blaming, and guilting of clients are antithetical to change and promote poor outcomes. FBGT avoids any interpretations or interventions that promote shame, blame, or attacks on the client, whether overt or covert. However, Strupp's study also noted that the therapists tended not to notice that they had conducted such attacks. Rather, they appeared emotionally activated by hostile and aggressive clients and responded in unconscious ways.

There are solutions to this morass. Person empathy is a core foundation to preventing overfixation on negative reactions to maladaptive interpersonal behaviors (Shafranske & Falender, 2008). While FBGT focuses on the overt behavior related to client functioning, remember and understand that the attachment style and its origins underlie this behavior. For example, a typical Scale 2: Focused on the Needs of the Self behavior might be to berate the leader and other group members when feeling anxious. However, we know from the dismissive attachment style (that correlates with this interpersonal style) that this positive sense of self and negative sense of others comes from experiences of being consistently unable to get time, love, and attention as a child. Clients with this style sometimes reveal histories of parents who berated them for any expressions of warmth; the parents also met the child's tears and upset with disdain and disgust (M. E. Connors, 1997). It is no wonder that clients with the style are wary of showing vulnerability when it was dealt with so severely when they were children.

The Need for Person Empathy

Typically during the TPS sessions but also during the life of the group, the therapist needs to develop empathy and understanding of a client's attachment style. During the initial TPS interview, the therapist should ensure they have compassion and understanding for the client, which, in some cases, may be easy to achieve. For example, a socially inhibited therapist may have little trouble developing empathy for a socially inhibited client. However, for the therapist to develop empathy and compassion for all clients, they should be in progress toward interpersonal self-acceptance. Once the therapist is rooted in self-compassion for their interpersonal style and its strengths and limitations, they are then able to more successfully achieve compassion toward the client, regardless of invitation. The therapist must evaluate and find compassion for clients with every kind of interpersonal style and distress. Whether this comes through person empathy and understanding the client's interpersonal history or by maintaining a deep empathy for each style and its origins, the therapist must find what it is about a client that is worthy of compassion. Unless the therapist fundamentally believes that the client is always doing their best with what they know, then little progress will follow. The therapist must also remember that cultural differences in interpersonal interactions are very real and that the same interactions can have different meanings in different cultures. They should carefully ensure that they are considering cultural factors and that interpersonal disconnects are not related to different cultural ways of relating. The therapist must be in the process of learning and empathizing, both interpersonally and culturally.

The client is always trying their best to manage relationships based on what they have learned. Therapy is a chance for a reparative experience; therefore, the group leader must root themselves in the role of compassionate helper or risk falling into being another person who rejects the client for their maladaptive strategies.

Case Example: Difference Between Hooked and Unhooked Responses

Without the requisite self-awareness, feelings and urges risk becoming the hooked response (Kiesler, 1996) rather than the unhooked, helpful response. The following case example illustrates the difference as two therapists—Rosa, Group Leader 1, and Ronny, Group Leader 2—experience the same events in Session 2. Rosa, who is centered, and Ronny, who is more reactive, respond to an incident involving a group member (client), Wendy.

WENDY (CLIENT): So, listen everyone. I am tired of this group and all your mewing about one problem or another. Frankly, you all make me sick, and you just need to suck it up and get on with things. Rosa and Ronny, you group leaders need to do a better job of telling everyone to just stop acting like babies and toughen up.

ROSA (GROUP LEADER 1): (*Feels both irritated and protective of the group and the work the group members have been doing. She also feels angry with Wendy for calling her and Ronny out in front of the group.*)

RONNY (GROUP LEADER 2): (*Has been feeling inadequate lately after a difficult week during which several clients have gone into crisis. He feels flushed and angry, and he tries to decide what to say next. Ronny's interpersonal style is Highly Assertive [Scale 1; see Figure 1.2 in Chapter 1], and this comment from Wendy feels like a challenge to his and Rosa's authority. He thinks he must quickly counter by putting Wendy in their place.*

Ronny decides to call Wendy out and begins to formulate a response. Ronny prepares to say, "Wendy, that is really unfair to the group, and you really are demeaning them. You need to work harder at understanding and empathy." However, Ronny is so caught up in his own emotions that he freezes and shuts down, afraid of harming the group member and worried how the group will be impacted.)

ROSA: (*Notices that Ronny is having a big reaction to Wendy's statement. Rosa herself notices that she feels flushed and anxious, experiencing a surge of anger and disappointment together with a twinge of inadequacy. She also knows that she tends toward an Uninhibited (Scale 8) style.*

Because Rosa spent a few minutes centering before the group began, she recognizes that she had been feeling frustrated with a coworker earlier in the day and is carrying some residual irritation. So, Rosa takes a moment to breathe and check in with her feelings. She realizes she is being hooked in a predictable way: She is feeling competitive with the client.

Rosa considers how to respond. She notices she is feeling angry and disappointed and is having the urge to both protect the group and defend herself. She breathes into the moment and turns to speak to Wendy.)

Wendy, I wonder what happened just then. I noticed you were trying to be helpful, but I wonder if it got you the opposite of what you intended. Would you like to hear from the group about how they would have liked to hear it and then give it another go? (*Rosa turns to the rest of the group.*) Group members, please let Wendy know what you would have liked to hear and how it would have made you feel different.

The difference between these two stances predicts the effectiveness of leader interventions and the likely pathway of the group. Centered, mindful noticing followed by unhooking is key to leader success.

COUNTERTRANSFERENCE IN FBGT

Yalom (Yalom & Leszcz, 2020) took the position that there are two types of countertransference: (a) objective and (b) subjective. According to Yalom, *objective countertransference* is considered the therapist's objective reaction to a client that any other person might reasonably experience—for example, experiencing a client as dismissive. Yalom described the process of *consensual validation* as aiding in this distinction: If other group members also report the same set of reactions, then there is consensual validation that this reaction is a shared one. *Subjective countertransference* occurs when the therapist is consumed with their own material and is reacting to a client as if they are a figure from the group leader's past, such as a parent or a sibling.

FBGT takes the position that there can be four types of countertransference: (a) objective, (b) subjective, (c) both objective and subjective, and (d) multicultural. In the FBGT model, *objective countertransference* is perceiving the client as they actually are; that is, the therapist is experiencing the client in the same way as other group members. If the group were consulted, all members would report some variation on this retelling of events. FBGT also views *subjective countertransference* as the therapist's not seeing the client clearly because of their own unprocessed childhood material. So, the therapist experiences the client based on their own—and not the client's—early interpersonal experiences. The combination of both objective and subjective countertransference in FBGT refers to the idea that people's early experiences can result in feelings that are subjective to them (e.g., their brother was a bully and left the person feeling victimized). However, when this person meets a person Focused on the Needs of the Self (Scale 2), they both reexperience that person as being like their brother but also experience something objective: that people with this scale score can be very domineering, aggressive, and attacking. Therefore, the distinction between what is subjective and objective can become blurry. Being able to notice that both can be true is an important step in noticing a hooked position and being able to unhook. FBGT categorizes countertransference in three ways. First, it states that the therapist must process their own interpersonal material to avoid being unaware of being hooked. Second, the therapist must understand and accept their own interpersonal style. Third, the therapist must continue to progress their multicultural awareness. These factors must then be within the therapist's awareness before they begin group.

Reactive, Unaware, Hooked Countertransference

This first category involves a failure on the therapist's part to either accept or understand their own interpersonal style. Distress sets the therapist up for misalignment and for a reactive stance to the client's invitations in which they are likely to be hooked. While the therapist may remain functional with respect to some clients and might achieve some degree of empathy, they will be more easily hooked, resulting in unhealthy repetitions of interpersonal patterns, dislike of clients, and ultimately worse leadership that results in poorer client outcomes.

Baseline Awareness and Mindfulness

The second category involves leaders acknowledging their own interpersonal style and culture and rooting themselves in mindful noticing, humility, and self-compassion. Once they have rooted themselves in mindful noticing, they can notice when they are being hooked and then subsequently unhook. The therapist notices their feelings, which, as therapeutic data, can inform interventions when used thoughtfully and mindfully to unhook and be helpful.

This is slightly different than Yalom and Leszcz's (2020) conception of being objective. Rather, this conceptualization rests in the notion that the leader is able to root themselves in the knowledge of their own baseline interpersonal style. For example, a therapist who is normally somewhat socially inhibited notices that they are even quieter than usual, or a therapist who is used to pleasing others is feeling an urge to remain distant. They are mindfully aware of when they are then being pulled off this style by a group member's invitations. In this sense, the leader is not an empty vessel but, rather, is a vessel aware of its own shape and when it is being pulled out of that shape by the invitations of others. Thus, there is no conceptualization of the therapist as a blank slate with "perfect" interpersonal functioning. Instead, there is self-compassion toward one's own interpersonal preferences and a noticing of how those are being engaged. Thus, there is a mindful noticing of the pushes and pulls from the group based on self-knowledge of trait-level interpersonal style.

Multicultural Countertransference

In this third category of countertransference, the therapist must be mindful of the role of culture. Within FBGT, cultural understandings and practices can produce their own form of impediment to empathy. If the leader is unaware of how both the therapist and the client's cultural background informs their interpersonal functioning, then they risk being as ineffective as the leader who is stuck in reactive, hooked countertransference. The notions of multicultural transference and countertransference (Aggarwal, 2011) are that leaders and clients have cultural ways of relating with specific meanings attached that can become a distorted aspect of the relationship. What results are myriad interpersonal implications (see the discussion in TPS session and group process chapters).

The group leader needs to remember that interpersonal behavior is loaded with cultural meanings that may have negative connotations in some cultures and positive connotations in others—whether this behavior is cross-cultural, is within cultures and subcultures, or depends on more microsystemic spaces. For example, in some cultures, people address conflict directly and tell the truth directly with little concern for sugarcoating. In those cultures, giving direct corrective feedback can be a sign of respect, strength, and love. In other cultures, direct expression of disagreement or conflict is considered a taboo and is a sign of rudeness or disrespect.

However, cultural differences are extremely nuanced. Within-group differences can be as great as between-group differences. For example, two people of the same ethnic background may have grown up in an urban and suburban environment, respectively. Each has had a different experience of what is needed to survive and thrive in their respective world. Moreover, the person's interpersonal style also represents a variable that may be syntonic or dystonic with their specific cultural group. The group leader therefore must elicit cultural data from clients to shed light on cultural manifestations of their interpersonal style. By asking group members what cultural norms are informing these styles, the therapist can step outside of their own experience and begin to empathize.

Rather than seeing interpersonal differences as purely trait based, the therapist should view interpersonal differences as a combination of both culture and trait that combine in complex ways and play out in different contexts and in relation to different life roles (e.g., mother, daughter, sports center director, church deacon, friend). This "both" category assumes that people internalize schemas as children that, when added to our basic personality set, form an interpersonal style. This interpersonal style becomes a baseline that we return to under stress. So, if we tend toward warm dominance, then we return to this style even more strongly when experiencing anxiety.

LEADERSHIP WITHIN THE GROUP DYNAMIC

Leadership in FBGT requires that leaders notice their own interpersonal style and recognize the invitations and emotional reactions that occur as they interact with clients and the group. For example, the group leader with a Warm/Self-Sacrificing baseline who works with a group entirely comprising clients on the Unassertive (Scale 5) end of the interpersonal circumplex likely experiences an urge to be even more warm and dominant to fill the space left by the Unassertive group members. The leader likely experiences the anxiety of this interaction as anxiety provoking and may describe feeling as if they are racing or feeling pressured to make things happen. Therefore, the skill set the FBGT therapist requires is to be able to notice the invitations, see when they are being pulled off their baselines, and respond therapeutically. That process involves being hooked by an invitation, noticing it, and then consciously deciding to be unhooked by responding with interventions that do not react to the initial invitation but, rather, promote awareness and understanding through process comments. A comment might be, for example,

> I notice that I am feeling an urge to be really talkative right now, and yet I wonder if that is robbing you of a chance to fill that void. I wonder who is sitting on something they would like to say or struggling to find the right words?

While the therapist's basic stance is to be warm with slight dominance, the leader must also work to match to the interpersonal style of the client by becoming unhooked. This requires the FBGT leader to be able to root them-selves in their baseline interpersonal style and also be flexible when necessary. For example, the client struggling with issues of being overly hostile may well begin the TPS session by making an early claim for dominance. This may take the form of challenging the therapist's skills, credentials, expertise, or knowl-edge base.

The therapist's task is to avoid becoming hooked and either responding with angry submissiveness or returning with more dominance. Instead, the therapist should respond by allowing the client to feel as if they are in charge while the therapist still actively guides the session. For example, by using "disqualifiers" (a technique used in functional family therapy; Sexton, 2012), the therapist allows the client to feel in charge. The therapist, for example, might say, "I could be wrong about this, but I wonder if you have ever con-sidered that some of the aggressive comments you make might be preventing you getting what you want? What do you think?" The use of disqualifiers allows the client to retain feelings of dominance but also allows the therapist to exert influence and direct the session.

PROFESSIONAL DEVELOPMENT, HUMILITY, AND SELF-DOUBT

The therapist's attitude toward therapy and their practice should also balance gaining expertise alongside humility and a willingness to consider that, at any moment, they could be wrong. Collecting data locally, clinicians can see how they are doing with different types of clients and make adjustments accordingly. This effort could be based on interpersonal circumplex scales; for example, the clinician finds that one group leader performs well with people high in warmth but poorly with those high in unassertiveness. Or it could be based on other diversity-based variables; for example, the clinician finds that there are differential outcomes by factors such as age, gender, or ethnicity that require them to examine their skills and build greater effectiveness with cross-cultural techniques. Doing so requires courage on the therapist's part. To be willing to unflinchingly consider the possibility that blind spots exist or that room for improvement is possible requires that the therapist maintains a stance that they are always a work in progress. This attitude of constant willingness to improve is what can differentiate an average therapist from one committed to mastery.

Research on deliberate practice (Clements-Hickman & Reese, 2020) has emphasized that true expertise is only acquired by *reflective practice*—that is, practice around specific skills related to the skill sought that are followed by feedback, supervision, consultation, and learning to improve and enhance areas of weakness while consolidating areas of strength. Regular assessment of outcomes and processes can be a part of this movement toward true expertise. Research also has shown that humility, a willingness to be professionally unsure at times, and the willingness to entertain the possibility of being wrong are also linked to more effective performance on the part of therapists.

Professional self-doubt (as opposed to low self-esteem or constant feelings of inadequacy) is an important predictor of improved performance (Nissen-Lie et al., 2017) and should extend to multicultural humility. Regardless of how accomplished a person may feel in working with diverse groups, blind spots abound. Research has found that therapists are not equally effective with clients based on their racial and ethnic minority background (J. A. Hayes et al., 2016; Pinner & Kivlighan, 2018). The multicultural orientation model (Owen et al., 2011) teaches three core essential practices: (a) multicultural humility, (b) multicultural opportunity, and (c) multicultural comfort. Group leaders should be seeking to remain humble, seek opportunities to learn about other cultures, and work on becoming comfortable in processing and discussing multicultural material.

Whether the therapist is meeting another person from their own ethnic or other diverse group and assuming they understand them completely or is working with someone from an unfamiliar minority group, the potential for assumptions to be made is considerable. The ability to truly listen and to compare and contrast assumptions about that person's identity variables requires considerable humility and internal stability. Therapists prefer to feel competent, and there is nothing wrong with that desire; working toward it is important. However, FBGT practice requires a combination of taking what is "known" (e.g., an interpersonal style profile that seems clear) and being willing to consider that some or all of it may be wrong or that the specific nuances might be complex. Holding a balance between confidence and humility is an ongoing one that keeps the therapy process alive, real, and genuine because it maintains the constant possibility of genuine connection and understanding. This process is not only novel and enjoyable for the client—to be understood—but also creates joy for the therapist who then truly understands another human being more deeply and feels that connection.

SPECIFIC GROUP LEADER INTERVENTIONS

Basic group leadership skills are helpful in running a group and should not be underestimated. Group is a specialty, and the skills and attitudes involved in running groups are enshrined as common factors (Whittingham et al., 2021). Therefore, the core techniques that mobilize those factors are essential.

Basic Group Skills

A multitude of leader interventions exist, and detailing them all is beyond the scope of this book. However, some core skills are important to mention because they have particular relevance to FBGT. This discussion is not exhaustive but may offer guidance that can help FBGT leaders select interventions to match to the needs of each stage and session. These core skills are drawing out, blocking, supporting, protecting, interpreting, framing, reframing, summarizing, modeling, linking, thematizing, and processing (Morran et al., 2004).

Drawing Out
Drawing out involves both structured activity, such as dyads, and unstructured interventions, such as verbally or nonverbally encouraging a member to speak. Nonverbal invitations can be extremely effective with judicious use of eye contact or hand gestures, but they may not be effective in all cultures. A simple glance at a hesitant client and a nodding, silent prompt can sometimes be all that are needed to encourage a reticent group member. In other cases, interventions can be more direct and targeted at individuals or the whole group. Examples of drawing out include asking a client what they think about what another client said, asking the whole group for their reactions to a statement or incident in the group, or inviting people to give feedback to a client.

Blocking
Blocking is a set of techniques designed to protect members from themselves and each other. For example, it is not uncommon for a member with a high distress score on Scale 2: Focused on the Needs of the Self to use a dismissive tone or comment early in the life of the group as a means to self-protect and gain status. With inoculation completed, this member is forewarned to not do either, and they have constructed goals intended to prevent this from happening. However, the temptation to fall back onto known behaviors that serve as self-protection can be overwhelming and can occur almost automatically. Therefore, the leader must carefully block this moment to prevent self-sabotage and potential group breakdown.

Members must know they are protected from attack and that the group is a safe place. However, once the blocking attempt is made, there is now a need to also protect the target of that block to prevent their being shamed or feeling embarrassed. Doing so models that the leader kindly protects people from themselves and that shame, blame, and guilt are not a part of the group milieu.

Supporting

Supporting involves siding with clients in work that they are completing or supporting the whole group in its endeavors. Supporting might involve interventions as simple as smiling and nodding as a client works through a difficult moment or works on a goal or a desired behavior. It can also involve more direct, verbal support, such as congratulating the group on working hard or congratulating a member on accomplishing a goal. Supporting can take other forms, ranging from supporting someone as they assert themselves by giving prompts, offering nonverbal indications to continue, or overtly intervening to help someone when they become stuck.

This core skill can also involve siding with a member who is being scapegoated to help the group and the member make therapeutic sense of what is happening. It can also involve supporting the group as whole through a critical incident or an impasse. Supporting takes many forms, but its role is the same: to provide the facilitative conditions for the work to take place by ensuring the groups and its members that they are not alone in either their struggles or successes.

Protecting

Protecting is a more direct form of support that involves siding with clients who are under attack to allow them a sense of safety and alliance as they work through the process of responding. Therapists can protect clients in many ways, and they should carefully assess the balance between providing a sense of security and safety in the group against needing to allow the group or the person being attacked to respond themselves. Thus, the need to provide a sense of safety must be balanced against giving clients and the group the ability to respond to an attack in a way that feels empowering. This requires a sophisticated analysis of the factors in play, and no easy formulas can explain when and how to do it.

Protecting also varies by culture: Different cultures understand and experience corrective feedback in various ways. The therapist must carefully appraise each situation and decide, based on many factors—ranging from clients' interpersonal styles, the group dynamic, therapeutic opportunities, the strength of the working alliance, and group cohesion and group stage—how to proceed. Sometimes protecting can be as simple as offering an empathic look, giving permission for a client to express themselves, or waiting for the group to step in and help. In other cases, support can be far more direct an intervention, including directly siding with a client and actively supporting them as they are under attack or trying a new behavior.

Interpreting

Interpreting must be conducted carefully and tentatively in FBGT. The therapist must use interpretations carefully and judiciously because the purpose of FBGT is to have members engage with each other rather than rely on the therapist as the font of all knowledge and wisdom. Thus, an interpretation that leads to members' being invited to connect is preferable to one that delivers only an insight as a coup de grâce.

In most cases, interpretations should be delivered in an escalating fashion, ranging from lower levels of inference (e.g., "I wonder what is happening right now?") to moderate levels of inference (e.g., "I wonder if the group tension is relating to what happened a few minutes ago?") to high levels of inference (e.g., "I am wondering if when you all asked if you could go out for dinner together between sessions and I advised against it, was a bigger deal to all of you than you admitted?" The therapist continues: "I noticed that the subject was quickly changed, and we all moved on, but I have noticed the group feeling stuck and preoccupied since. I wonder if those things are connected and whether we can talk about that now?") As can be seen from this example, even at the highest level of inference, the therapist still presents an interpretation as one to consider, not as an absolute truth: "I wonder if . . ." allows the group to consider the interpretation without seeing it as an absolute truth that forces them to accept the therapist as the arbiter of truth.

Framing

Framing occurs when the therapist gives meaning to an activity, group, or incident by front-loading it. For example, the therapist provides a summary of the last group session at the beginning of group and sets up the next session as a continuation:

> Last session, we really underwent a lot of discussion about managing intimacy and feeling close to each other. Several people worked on goals related to connecting with each other, while others worked on support and encouragement. I am mindful that today we have two sessions left, so let's hear everyone's goals before we start and pay particular attention to those who have a need to work on goals but haven't yet had a chance. If you already worked on yours, then perhaps this is a time to let others work.

This framing sets up the following session for success.

Reframing

Reframing is a helpful technique to change meanings around an event that will move the group forward. Sometimes reframing a behavior is needed with respect to intent and impact. It is not uncommon for clients to make maladaptive attempts to relate to others. Sometimes these attempts to manage relationships need to be reframed to allow the group to understand the underlying motivation. Reframing is best used in FBGT to explore intent and not impact—to treat people as if they are always doing their best with what they know. The following example illustrates the use of reframing:

GROUP LEADER (SPEAKS TO GROUP MEMBER): Kara, I can see that you wanted to say something to Taylor [another group member] after they disclosed that they were upset that their cat had died. You looked upset and worried, but when you spoke, you told them to get over it and that they will be fine. I can tell you were trying to help, but I wonder if the impact was what you had intended? Can you check that out with Taylor, and then maybe let's see if the group can help you with that?

This example also combines some protecting (of both group members Taylor and Kara) as well as the opportunity for feedback.

Reframing can also offer the opportunity to maintain realistic hope after a difficult interaction or session. This does not mean creating a fake reality— that a difficult session did not happen. Rather, it means acknowledging reality, offering hope, and providing validation of what did happen. Take this example:

GROUP LEADER (SPEAKS TO GROUP MEMBER): Vik, I think we all felt how upset you were about what was said to you in group just now. We are right at the end of the group, and I wanted to acknowledge that I noticed that you are still having angry and hurt feelings. I am really sorry that we have run out of time in the group today to process it. That feels unfair and not okay, and I want to acknowledge that. It feels really important that we don't shelve this and ignore it, and so I am going to suggest we discuss this next week so we can make sense of what happened and honor the process.

I also want to say to the group that although some of you may be worried about difficult feelings that come up with this kind of discussion, you need to particularly need to come back next week. It is easy to find an excuse to not come and avoid the discomfort, but we are a strong group, and we can tolerate this and learn from it together. I have faith in all of you to have the courage to do that.

This intervention is important on many levels. It validates what happened and does not diminish it. It places the incident into a therapeutic frame. It also anticipates potential dropout because people avoid a conflict (which, for some group members, who are conflict-avoidant at a trait level, is highly likely). And it conveys hope and belief: The leader believes that the group is strong enough to tolerate conflict, and the therapist will contain and help make meaning of the experience.

Summarizing

Summarizing can take place during the session and at the end of the session. When the session is drifting or needs focus, it can be useful for the therapist to summarize what has been happening and to then provide direction. In this example, the therapist talks with the group about two other group members:

> We just spent some time listening to Marcus and Prisha working out how they can better connect with each other. That really took us on some interesting tangents, where different people talked about a desire to connect with each other. I wonder if now is an opportunity to try that out.

Summaries can also be useful to end sessions. Sessions are often complex, and much can happen. Therefore, the therapist should consider a way to summarize, frame, and reframe events to ensure a therapeutic focus is achieved, as in this example:

> Everyone really worked hard today and showed a lot of courage. There were some difficult moments that were resolved and some moments that felt unfinished. It is okay to have unfinished moments even though it feels unsettling. We can tolerate that as a group and as individuals and come back next week and make some sense of it together. That is some of the work here, and this is what makes group worthwhile—that we can deal with challenging things in a way that helps us grow as individuals and as a group.

This kind of summary offers the group both reality and hope. It does not sugarcoat a difficult session or avoid stating that not enough time was available to process some unfinished threads. It does, however, offer hope and a sense that this is what the group can sometimes provide: opportunities to work on difficult things and to learn and grow.

Modeling

Modeling takes place whether the leader wishes it to or not. Group members are aware of the personhood of the therapist and pay attention to how other group members act as well. A well-worn group maxim states that groups take on the personality of the leader. There is likely significant truth in that statement, particularly in longer term groups in which subtle behaviors and overt actions can lead the group to shape their behavior to match. However, even with a brief group, subtle and overt leader behaviors can lead to a degree of group conformity, depending on the group composition. The group leader should be able to demonstrate a degree of self-acceptance, interpersonal awareness, and interpersonal flexibility to model what they want the group members to understand about themselves from the group.

Linking

Linking is a key intervention in group in general and no less so in FBGT. Linking involves connecting members together around common issues, content, themes, and concerns and can take place at the individual, interpersonal, and group-as-a-whole levels. For example, the therapist might say to a group member: "Andrew, I noticed you were nodding and smiling as Nur was talking just then. I wonder if you can share your reaction with her?" Linking can also take place in a more general way: "Kerry, I heard you share that sometimes this group can feel a little avoidant when issues around caring and compassion come up. I wonder if anyone else has noticed that?"

Linking members together is important for cohesion and can also help functional subgrouping occur as members shift in and out of alliances with each other on different topics. In FBGT, linking can also provide a concrete means to connect members around common goals. For example, the therapist notes that two members are working on the same issues and asks what it is like to hear that someone else has the same concern, or ask if group members feel connected to another member around their goals. This type of linking can be a powerful means to create cohesion, unity of task, and goals and to move the work along.

Thematizing

Thematizing can be an important therapeutic device to keep work focused. Therapeutic drift is not helpful if it occurs in every session of a group. In brief groups, time is limited, so the work must be focused. Thematizing involves developing themes from the work that move the group work by summarizing ideas, concepts, and directions that the group is moving in. In FBGT, the helpful themes that organize work can sometimes be to point out that the group is working on issues related to power, boundaries, connection to each other, difference, and similarity—that is, the content of the interpersonal circumplex and its allied constructs, such as thoughts, emotions, and cultural differences and similarities, that accompany and inform these issues.

FBGT themes can also be linked to other aspects of the group and individual process: ambivalence about change, anxiety that comes with approaching change, managing time, working inside the group versus outside the group, understanding each other more deeply, and mentalizing. Themes should be accurate and provide clarity and focus. Therefore, leaders should look for therapeutic threads that thematize and bring to the fore the focus of the work, as in this example of a theme being brought into a here-and-now goal with some urgency: "At different times so far in the group, we have all been struggling with connecting to each other. I wonder if someone who is seeking connection would like to try that now?" Using the theme of connection creates the possibility that a group goal that needs working will take place.

When selecting interventions, this thematizing approach becomes particularly helpful. For example, if late in the group two members have yet to work on their goals, and sessions are running out, bringing a theme that unites those two members in some work can provide a needed impetus for work. For example, one member has yet to work on their goal of asking follow-up questions, and another has yet to work on their goal of asking the group for help. The leader offers, "We were just talking about how we sometimes hide what we are feeling because it is hard to trust we can get help. I wonder if anyone else is struggling with that?" This thematizing carries with it an invitation for those who have yet to work on their goals. If the group leader has successfully used a prior technique—framing—to ask the group to make room for members who have yet to work on goals, then the invitation becomes a therapeutic opportunity.

Processing
Processing in FBGT involves discussing what happened interpersonally during the session. Yalom (Yalom & Leszcz, 2020) called this *process illumination*: drawing attention to what is happening in the room in the present moment. Processing can range in its level of inference from a simple "I wonder what is happening right now?" to a more inferential prompting:

> I wonder if this long silence has to do with the fact that everyone is feeling uncomfortable about discussing the conflict that just happened between Julie and Alex? I wonder if anyone has any reactions to what happened that can help us learn from it?

Processing can also be pointed toward goals. For example, a group member has stated feelings of sadness after the death of a beloved pet. The group, which comprises people high in distance and inhibition, remains silent before subtly changing the topic onto something lighter related to the care of pets in general. The group leader brings the group back to the moment by sharing that something important just happened and asking the group how they felt when the member shared about their loss. One member reports being emotionally impacted by the disclosure and feeling compassionate, and they state that they wanted to say something but were afraid to do so out of fear of saying "the wrong thing." The leader offers them an opportunity to try and say something anyway, knowing that perhaps the intent is all that matters. The client does so, and a feedback exchange ensues.

In this case, the process of the group led to a goal completion because the therapist noticed this group dynamic and used process commentary to enlist members in attaining their goals. In a group comprising many people with inhibition as their area of distress, difficulty with moments requiring compassionate and empathic reflection is to be expected and to be particularly difficult because the precise thing that they are struggling to do is in fact the problem that they need work on the most. Therefore, in this moment, process leads to group leader-initiated goal completion.

Other FBGT Core Techniques

Core techniques common to all group therapies, including FBGT, are important to outline. However, some specific techniques are not always used in every type of group and are also quite nuanced within FBGT. These techniques—feedback, disclosure, and here-and-now activation, are discussed next.

Feedback

Feedback is also a core technique in FBGT. At the beginning of the group, feedback interventions should be kept positive. Research has shown that group members will discount corrective feedback if it is offered too early in the life of the group (Moran et al., 1998). In cases in which this happens, group members tend to discount the messenger rather than absorb the feedback. Some group members discount the positive feedback because they sometimes see it as insincere, and they are seeking corrective feedback. Leaders should resist the temptation to engage in corrective feedback too early, even when members are enthusiastic to do so. My clinical observations from working internationally showed that even in cultures in which direct, immediate feedback is preferred, premature movement into corrective feedback can lead to some members' plunging into an emotional crisis and prematurely terminating. Given the short-term nature of the groups, this can be extremely hard to recover from and can damage both the individuals and the group.

From the beginning, FBGT has used early positive feedback in U.S. university counseling centers both as an example of how to engage in the here and now and also as a buffer against premature group dropout (by increasing feelings of warmth and cohesion between members). In some cultures in which directness is prized, it may be that corrective feedback can be elicited sooner because it may promote more culturally normative bonding and lead to cohesion. However, bearing in mind within-group differences and varying levels of ego strength, the therapist should still exercise caution in encouraging too much early corrective feedback because even if some group members request it, others may not yet be ready and will feel threatened by its early introduction.

Disclosure
Disclosure, that is, self-disclosure by the therapist, has its uses in FBGT, but the therapist should use it very carefully and judiciously because the approach is a brief one and can unnecessarily shift the focus away from the group and onto the therapist if used too often. Interventions that involve use of *self-involving self-disclosure*—for example, "I feel like something important is happening right now"—which has a low level of inference, invites the group to take control of the processing. This is often preferable to *self-revealing self-disclosure* in which the therapist self-discloses personal information about their lives.

Although self-revealing self-disclosure has its uses, particularly in medium- or long-term groups in which the therapist sometimes becomes idealized to an unhealthy level by the group, in a brief group, it is seldom as helpful. By contrast, self-involving self-disclosure can accelerate the work of FBGT groups. The level of inference can also be escalated depending on the timing and need. For example, the therapist's question, "I felt sad and anxious when that last interaction happened, and I wonder if anyone else experienced that?" offers some emotional content to begin to allow others to ascribe meaning.

Leaders can further escalate the level of inference if the group is struggling to express the moment by adding process illumination, as in this example, when the group leaders says, "When I felt sad and anxious, I began to wonder if the way that Erin and Chole [group members] interacted with some tough words for each other had resulted in them both feeling hurt and misunderstood." At this point, an inference is being made that invites direct responses from the group and the individuals named. However, this level of process illumination should be used judiciously because overinterpretation can block the central mechanism of change in the group, namely, members behaviorally activating their goals for themselves.

Here-and-Now Activation
Here-and-now activation is a key skill for FBGT leaders and is crucial to the success of the approach. The notion of the *here and now* is one enshrined by Yalom (Yalom & Leszcz, 2020): It involves members interacting with each other in real time about how they are experiencing each other in the present moment. The *there and then* is when members talk about past events, such as what happened in the prior week. FBGT involves a delicate dance between

the here and now and the there and then. Members begin by talking about their past week or things on their mind, such as relationships with significant people in their lives.

COLEADERSHIP

Individual members benefit from different types of modeling. Coleadership can therefore provide opportunities for vicarious learning for group members because if those coleaders are sufficiently different on variables ranging from interpersonal style to multiple identities (e.g., gender, race, age), then members have more opportunities for social learning and modeling. These opportunities can also arise from leaders' disconfirming stereotypes (e.g., a male leader behaving in ways that are emotionally expressive). Leaders can also consider how to leverage the different kind of bond they have with each client to decide on interventions. For example, if a group is having difficulty confronting a specific member in the group around noncompletion of goals and that member could benefit from confrontation around that issue, then leaders might consider who has the strongest bond with that client and thus is a safe enough person for that client to hear feedback as helpful and not injurious.

Equally, at different times, certain groups that are heterogenous for member interpersonal style may require a considerable rethink of strategy (e.g., including more skills-based training in groups comprising entirely clients with distress around social inhibition [Scale 4: Socially Inhibited]). FBGT assumes each group presents different challenges that a leadership team must meet in different ways. Therefore significant flexibility is required on the part of leaders, who can move to meet the demands of what is needed from each team.

Coleadership is influenced by the interpersonal styles of the group leaders. As can be seen from illustrations of group dynamics, both leaders' interpersonal styles are part of the group dynamic. FBGT theory suggests that two leaders with similar styles need to, at times, be interpersonally flexible so that they can model behaviors for the group, manage critical incidents, or use techniques that move the group forward. For example, if a group could benefit from self-involving self-disclosure from the leaders (e.g., during a prolonged tense moment or when there is an "elephant in the room" that the group is avoiding), but both leaders have styles that are high in distance (i.e., they often struggle with sharing and being open), then some flexibility is needed.

Coleaders must be aware that their baseline interpersonal styles impact their response to the group dynamic. If both have similar styles, then they may have similar reactions to what is happening in the group, feeling validated by each other and feeling that things are progressing as a leadership pair. However, they risk having the same blind spots. For example, two leaders who are high in assertiveness might be similarly preoccupied with dominant group members that they feel challenged by and similarly oblivious to what is happening internally with the members who are socially inhibited and unassertive. They may also be unconsciously modeling lack of warmth and encouragement while providing a united front of authority. A pairing of leaders who are similar on other dimensions—distance, unassertiveness, focused on the needs of others, and so forth—brings the strengths of those styles, but those leaders also may struggle with skill sets that are less well developed but are sometimes vital to group leadership.

Group leaders should therefore carefully assess their own styles and look to work on their flexibility. Leaders' understanding what is at 180 degrees to their own interpersonal style is an important part of understanding what techniques they may be comfortable with and which ones they find more difficult. Techniques ranging from protecting and blocking to using self-involving self-disclosure and modeling all have contained within them a set of matching interpersonal styles that make these interventions either a natural fit for a practitioner or a challenge to work through. No technique is beyond any leader, but each leader must be aware of which techniques they find challenging and work to become more flexible and therefore more skilled in how they implement them. They may also wish to consider coleadership with someone whose skills fill in the gaps.

Another consideration is the role of being hooked and unhooked and the impact on each therapist. This is where the importance of a therapist's baseline style becomes apparent. Therapists have different reactions to each member's invitations based on their own baseline style and also invite different things from group members based on that style. Therefore, a group comprising members who are all unassertive feels more comfortable to a leader who is also unassertive (because they have less internal urges to be in a dominant position and to take charge) than it does to a leader higher in dominance (who feels highly stressed by the level of inactivity and fights the urge to dominate and take control).

When processing together, leaders therefore have to be careful to consider how each of their styles is influencing their perceptions and also their combined choice of strategies. It could easily happen that one member with an opposite interpersonal style feels invalidated by the other group leader who states, "But I don't feel that way" about a group member or the group dynamic. It is important that each coleader understands that the impact of every group member feels different and depends on baseline scores of the leaders and how they impact complementarity and invitations. It is also essential that each group leader shows compassion for their own style as well as empathy and compassion for their coleaders. Understanding and working successfully together should go hand in hand.

Combinations of leadership interpersonal styles can also account for being hooked and unhooked by each other. For example, two leaders high in dominance might feel competitive with each other, subtly undermining each other's ideas, techniques, and interventions. Failing to notice this underlying dynamic is problematic and could result in deleterious results for the group. Consider this clinical example: A group member once approached me to intervene as a supervisor because the competition between the two group leaders—who were negating each other's interventions—had become so problematic that the group felt that the competition was interfering with the group's work. Group leaders must process this feedback honestly and with sensitivity. Their discussion should be ongoing both about how each feels about the group and how the process of coleadership is going. These discussions should take place with nonjudgmental compassion for each other that seeks to empathically understand and listen. Each member of the leadership duo should also remain focused on retaining self-and-other compassion, being careful not to project their own disowned feelings onto the other member. Both members should also be willing to consider what is the most effective combination of strategies that can move the group forward based on an analysis of the group dynamic and the needs of the group.

This process can be challenging but enjoyable. Leaders stay mindfully centered and act as a participant–observer in their own meetings with each other. Coleaders may wish to consider discussing their interpersonal styles before the group begins so they can anticipate not only how they will feel as a part of the group dynamic, but also so they can predict how their own coleadership process will unfold. Being able to predict possible conflicts, resentments, or intervention techniques the deficits and strengths that they both have is an important part of growing together and being able to move the group forward.

It is important, too, to consider the role of planning. Coleadership is a process involving considerable discussion, planning, and comparison of perspectives and impressions of what is occurring. Coleadership effectiveness is predicated on communication that is consistent. In my experience supervising coleaders, the largest predictor of session "drift" is whether the two leaders had met to plan before the group therapy. That planning did not have to be directly before the group, but it had to be close enough so that each leader was on the same page regarding a plan and focus for treatment. When supervising group leaders conducting FBGT, it became clear that even with the most skillful leaders, lack of planning is highly predictive of session drift and failure to accomplish work. Leaders who spent time planning (even sometimes having lunch together to do so) and thoughtfully considering (e.g., sharing their own emotional reactions to clients, talking through how they wanted to improve, talking over each client, and discussing the cotherapy relationship) how they could improve together tended to progress at a faster pace than their colleagues. Doing so required humility, openness, and a willingness to be vulnerable. At times, it also required an open and honest discussion about the coleadership relationship, including sharing feelings about strengths and challenges that each person faced and embracing the journey of growth together.

SUMMARY

FBGT leadership involves maintaining a balance between continually learning and acquiring new knowledge, technical competence, and comfort with working with diversity while maintaining humility and openness to new information. Above all, it requires unconditional positive regard and empathy for clients as well as self-compassion and grounded awareness from the leader.

Leading within FBGT is a process of lifelong learning that requires its practitioners to maintain balance, awareness, and a desire for personal and professional growth. The skills of leadership should emanate from a combination of attitudes, techniques, and a sense of clinical structure that moves clients toward change. Coleadership also needs mindful centeredness when processing events and planning. Leaders should be aware of and be able to process their own leadership strengths and weaknesses based on their own interpersonal styles. They also need to be committed to growing together. Complementary and noncomplementary interactions are part of this process, and denying disowned parts of themselves is important to consider as part of that progress.

PART **II** THE MODEL IN PRACTICE

5 PREPARING FOR FOCUSED BRIEF GROUP THERAPY

Referrals and Assessment Integration

For focused brief group therapy (FBGT) to be successful, it is essential that referral sources are well trained on what is and what is not a successful referral and that the therapist begins the process of integrating measurement-based care. Once the referral has been made, the client is administered three pregroup measures, and the therapist's task is to develop tentative initial hypotheses regarding the potential interpersonal problem the client is bringing. This chapter outlines how these key processes set the stage for the treatment to be successful.

PREPARATION OF REFERRAL SOURCES

Discussions should take place with referral sources on inclusion and exclusion criteria as well as helpful referral techniques. Follow-up on these discussions then occurs to reinforce when referrals are accurate and to discuss thoughtfully and respectfully when referrals are inappropriate. It can take a while for referral sources to understand interpersonal subtype patterns that relate to diagnostic distress. Therefore, the group leader should ask

https://doi.org/10.1037/0000389-006
Focused Brief Group Therapy: An Integrative Approach to Reducing Interpersonal Distress, by M. Whittingham

permission to return and check in to affirm good referrals and also to discuss and brainstorm how to work on increasing accuracy in referrals.

Client and Therapist Reluctance

Clients may not follow through on their appointments, or they may refuse the referral outright for many reasons. They may have formed strong negative impressions of group therapy from the media, may believe they are entitled to individual therapy, may be unaware of the benefits of group therapy, may be unwilling to share time, may see group therapy as inferior to individual therapy, or may have had prior bad experiences with groups (Parcover et al., 2006). Clients' own personality styles also predict reluctance. For example, clients high in distress on Scale 4: Socially Inhibited are very likely to see a referral to group as equivalent to being asked to jump into the ocean after just informing the therapist that they cannot swim. Interpersonal styles present different challenges to the referral process in terms of forming a working alliance from the very beginning. Chapter 3 outlined how each client's interpersonal style predicts their response to an invitation to join the group as well as their contribution to a group dynamic.

Remember that not all referral sources are strong advocates for group therapy (Marmarosh et al., 2006; Parcover et al., 2006). Whether because of a lack of exposure to research on the effectiveness of groups, poor prior experiences with groups, or purely a lack of understanding about what any group can do, referral sources may also have issues with their willingness to refer. For example, research has also shown that therapists who are insecurely attached are less likely to refer clients to group therapy (Marmarosh et al., 2006). If a therapist is afraid of, dismissive of, or anxious about being in a group, they likely will be disinclined to direct a client to what they see as an aversive event. Therefore, helping referral sources understand the benefits to their clients, seeing the results of clients' work, and checking in with them about progress can all help in ensuring clients are well served.

Referrers also initially need help understanding who to refer. In my clinical experience, referral sources are quick to refer anyone with obvious social difficulty, such as people with social anxiety. However, the FBGT leader needs to explain how other interpersonal difficulties can impact presenting problems and diagnoses. A referral source may not realize that a client who is angry and aggressive has an interpersonal distress around that issue or may fail to identify that someone is binge drinking at the weekend because they are lonely or struggling with their relationships. These are important indicators that need discussion and may require an informal, one-on-one explanation, a brown-bag presentation, a more formal presentation as part of an in-service, or combinations of these strategies, depending on the specific organizational structure of the agency. This should include a thorough description of the interpersonal circumplex and exploration of how different scales impact treatment at the level of presenting problem and also process.

The FBGT leader should also discuss with the referrer how to overcome resistance to treatment. Although some research (e.g., Abraham et al., 1995) has suggested that clients prefer to deal with their problems in individual therapy rather than in group therapy, this is not always the case. My clinical findings from FBGT showed varied reactions to a recommendation for group therapy, depending on the client's interpersonal style. These reactions ranged from apprehension (e.g., clients with a Distant or Socially Inhibited style) to excitement (those with styles higher in warmth). However, reluctance can take many forms. The referral source may wish to explore with the client their reasons for reluctance. Doing so allows the referral source to more fully understand the client's reasons before working with them to open to the possibility the group may be effective.

In many cases, referrers take the first answer of *no* from a client as a definitive one. However, the referrer should be encouraged to take at least 7 or 8 minutes to explore the client's reluctance. Carter et al. (2001) showed that following 1 minute to 5 minutes of discussion about groups, only 33% of clients planned to follow up with the group, whereas after 6 to 10 minutes of discussion, 70% of clients planned to join (Parcover et al., 2006). The time spent is worth it. Except in cases in which there is clear contraindication, the referrer should encourage the client to meet for a therapy, pregroup preparation, and screening (TPS) session to find out more about the group.

Successful Referrals

Several components to a referral are suggestive of success, and they follow the lessons learned from primary care integration handoffs (e.g., Horevitz et al., 2015). These components include naming the problem (e.g., depression), clearly explaining how the group may help (e.g., "by helping you find ways to connect to others through asking for help or sharing about yourself"), giving a warm handoff whenever possible, prescribing or strongly recommending the group, and allowing time for discussion. Referrers might also be introduced to techniques related to forming the working alliance with the client based on interpersonal style. For instance, they might discuss when to use direct recommendation and prescription (e.g., "I recommend this strongly") with most clients but use disqualifiers (e.g., "I could be wrong, but I think this might be really helpful for you. Why not meet with the group leader and see what they say?") for clients with styles higher in dominance. Refer to Chapters 5 and 6 to explore how to best tailor referral interventions to each client.

Referrers can also be introduced to the idea that some clients may see completing assessment tools as an opportunity to develop self-awareness, so this can be a means to engage them with the idea of therapy. Online personality tests have become a commonly accepted form of entertainment and self-knowledge, and, for some clients, this will add to the allure of the group. However, for other clients, completion of self-assessment can feel threatening, onerous, or like an invasion of privacy. The referrer needs to assess cultural and personality factors on a case-by-case basis—in discussion with the client—to determine each client's perceptions of assessment and whether the client sees assessment as enhancing therapy or as a potential obstacle to the therapeutic alliance.

The referrer must also determine the suitability of the client for FBGT. A poor referral sets up the client for a painful rejection or to potentially fail in the group. Therefore, inclusion or exclusion criteria must be considered carefully, a topic addressed next in more detail.

PRE-TPS ASSESSMENT INTERPRETATION AND HYPOTHESIS FORMATION

Preassessment of data before meeting the client is an invaluable tool in FBGT. It allows the therapist to form an initial but tentative hypothesis that can set the therapy up for success by anticipating the strengths and challenges of therapy. Comparing and contrasting assessment data beforehand allows the therapist to enter the TPS session with more sophisticated clinical insights and to be better prepared to form the working alliance. This type of prework significantly augments the therapist's clinical judgment, allowing them to be better prepared to cocreate the conditions for change with the client.

Combining the self-reports allows the therapist to begin to simultaneously accelerate the mechanisms of change while also ensuring the guardrails are in place to prevent premature dropout and client worsening. The data from the measures can also be compared and contrasted with intake notes. For example, if the intake therapist or referral source notes that the client has many interpersonal problems and explains what they are, then this information adds data that can be compared and contrasted with the assessment tools that are a part of FBGT.

Instrument Selection

Two of the three instruments used in FBGT are constants: the 32-item Inventory of Interpersonal Problems (IIP-32; Horowitz et al., 2000) and the Group Therapy Questionnaire–Short Form (GTQ-S; MacNair-Semands et al., 2010). The other instrument is an outcome/quality of life measure that should be selected based on being valid, reliable, sensitive to change, and normed against the population being studied. The quality of life measure is important because it lays the foundation for the implications of interpersonal distress and how it plays out in overall life distress.

Quality of Life Measure

Choosing the correct quality of life measure is an important step for a therapist or agency. Examples of quality of life measures that are empirically sound include the 30-item Outcome Questionnaire (OQ-30; Ellsworth et al., 2006) or Outcome Rating Scale (S. D. Miller et al., 2003). Other examples of behavioral health care instruments for the United States are available from The Joint Commission (n.d.). These measures are good examples of reliable, valid, and sensitive-to-change assessment tools that can be used for different populations within the United States.

Therapists should refrain from using their own self-constructed measures because the results are unlikely to be valid, reliable, sensitive to change, or correctly normed; they, therefore, could negatively impact treatment. Whenever possible, therapists should choose instruments with norm groups appropriate to the population being served at the location where they are based. When it is not possible, clinicians should use item analysis to check instruments— to ensure their culture suitability—while also ensuring that any results are then considered with some caution (Whittingham et al., 2023). If the client group is sufficiently different than the norm group, then clinical judgment in interpreting results and listening to the client's interpretation of results should become even more strongly weighted.

The outcome measure serves several purposes. First, it is used to understand the client's level of life distress at the start of treatment. This can then be used later as the pretest paired with a repeated measure of that same test at the end of treatment. Second, it can be used to help the client understand their current level of distress with their life. It also has multiple other uses when combined with the other instruments and explored collaboratively with the client in the TPS session (see more on this topic in Chapter 6). When combining output of this instrument with the other two assessment tools (i.e., the IIP-32 and the GTQ-S), it can also cross-validate assumptions. For example, items on the GTQ-S indicate difficulties with being shy, finding it difficult to be assertive and struggling with socializing. Endorsement of these items would be further evidence that a high score on Scale 4: Socially Inhibited on the IIP-32 represents an underlying interpersonal style. Equally, a high score on a quality of life measure can help the client understand the distress that they are feeling. If, during the TPS session, in collaboration with the therapist, the client is shown the high quality of life score and a high score on a specific scale (e.g., Scale 4), they then can make the connection between how their interpersonal distress is connected to overall feelings of life distress. This connection helps with the working alliance.

IIP-32

The IIP-32 (Horowitz et al., 2000) provides a considerable amount of information that can be helpful in establishing a working hypothesis. It gives a set of scores on the scales. The highest scale distress score is typically considered to be the primary target for change (see Figure 5.1 for an example

FIGURE 5.1. Example of a Highest Scale Score

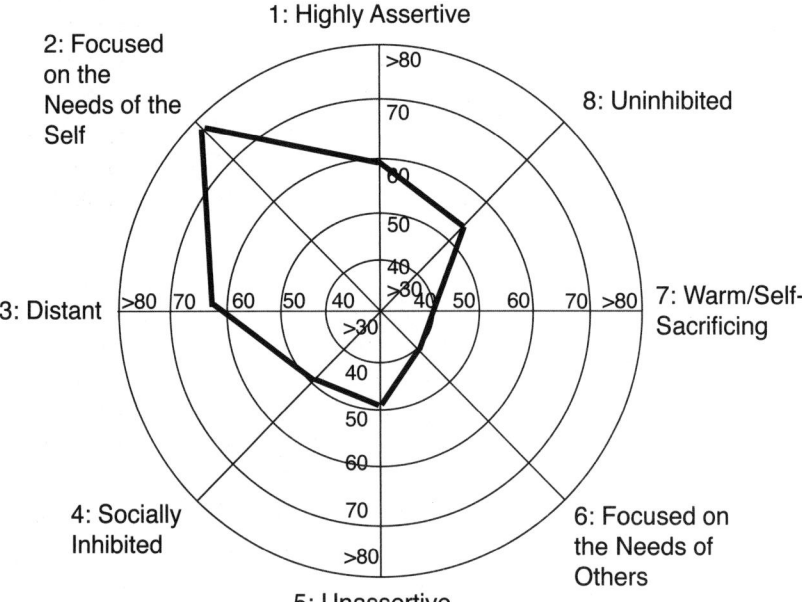

Note. This figure shows a client with the highest level of distress being on Scale 2: Focused on the Needs of the Self. Adapted from the manual for the Inventory of Interpersonal Problems by special permission of the Publisher, Mind Garden, Inc. Further reproduction requires the Publisher's written consent. Copyright © 2000 by Leonard M. Horowitz, Lynn E. Alden, Jerry S. Wiggins, & Aaron L. Pincus. All rights reserved in all media. Published by Mind Garden, Inc., www.mindgarden.com

of a highest score that is on Scale 2: Focused on the Needs of the Self), although this score may be adjusted if the therapist—in collaboration with the client—has a compelling reason to do so (e.g., the client indicates that their highest score may be important but that their second highest score represents a more significant construct that would immediately improve their life). Research on the model has shown that the effects of the therapy may be diffuse; for example, if the client works on Scale 2 distress and also has a high score on Scale 1: Highly Assertive, then Scale 1 may also end up reducing as well (Allison & Whittingham, 2017). The instrument also gives a total distress score that sums all scale distress scores and can be used to compare with the distress score of the quality of life measure as well as used for conducting prepost change measurement. Further, an evaluation of the overall profile is also helpful.

Understanding how the other scale scores impact the client's overall interpersonal style is clinically important. For example, someone with their highest score on Scale 7: Warm/Self-Sacrificing but with other high scores on Scale 8: Uninhibited and Scale 1 would feel very different in the room and the group than someone with their highest scale score on Scale 7 but the next highest scores on Scale 5: Unassertive and Scale 6: Focused on the Needs of Others (see Figure 5.2). In the first instance, the person is likely warm, is outgoing, shows leadership, and is assertive and highly influential over the group. In the second instance, the person is warm but is focused on the needs of others and is unassertive—a far quieter and more gentle presence who would be well liked but would struggle greatly with conflict.

The highest score can also be used to begin mapping out the group dynamic (see Chapters 4 and 8). Assuming the empirical premise explained in prior chapters—that under stress, people go to their highest score—the group dynamic is mapped out using people's highest scores plotted on the interpersonal circumplex. This enables the therapist to begin to predict into the group dynamic and, in some cases (depending on the agency setup), may give them the ability to ensure the group is more heterogenous for interpersonal style. While groups that are homogenous for interpersonal style can be effectively worked with, heterogeneity of style does offer the group the opportunity to work with and better understand people who are like and unlike them.

FBGT uses the IIP-32, an interpersonal circumplex instrument, as its main measure. Because the IIP-32 measures distress and not style, this gives some latitude for the therapist to explore the reasons for this distress and allows for the interaction between interpersonal distress, interpersonal style, and contextual and cultural factors. Typically, the initial data collection focuses on the

FIGURE 5.2. Highest Scale Impacted by Other Peaks

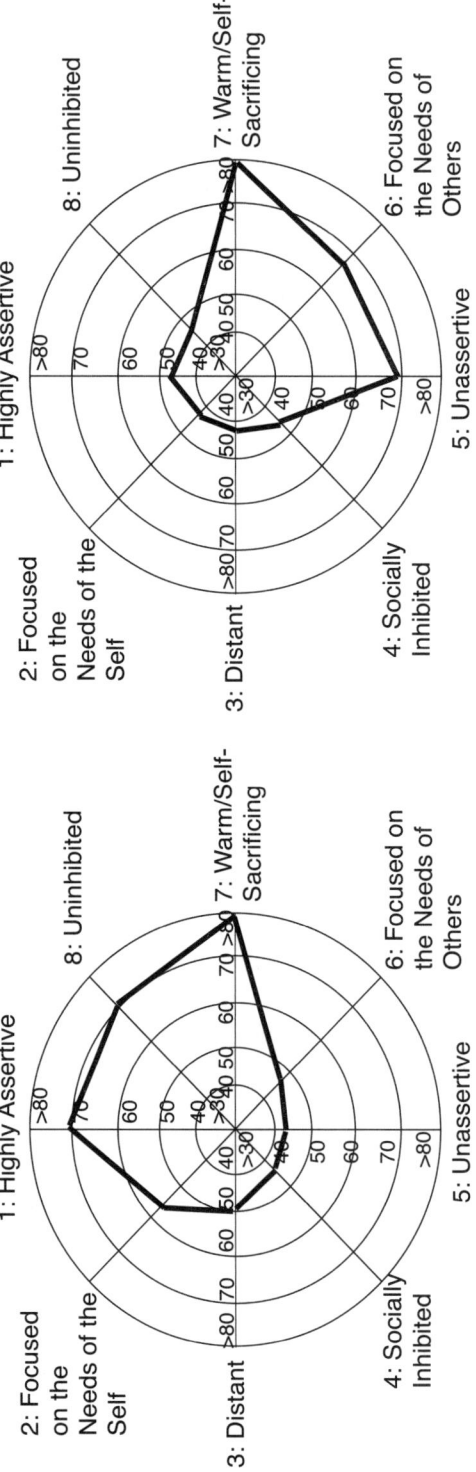

Note. Example of highest scale scores with other scales altering overall profile. The shape on the left shows a highest score as Warm/Self-Sacrificing but with next highest scores being Uninhibited and Highly Assertive, leading to a warm but controlling interpersonal type of distress. The shape on the right shows a highest score as Warm/Self-Sacrificing but with next highest scores being on Focused on the Needs of Others and Unassertive, signifying a warm but less assertive and more compliant interpersonal level of distress. Adapted from the manual for the Inventory of Interpersonal Problems by special permission of the Publisher, Mind Garden, Inc. Further reproduction requires the Publisher's written consent. Copyright © 2000 by Leonard M. Horowitz, Lynn E. Alden, Jerry S. Wiggins, & Aaron L. Pincus. All rights reserved in all media. Published by Mind Garden, Inc., www.mindgarden.com

potential role of interpersonal rigidity and interpersonal style as potentially causal factors, with cultural and contextual data being integrated during the TPS session. Levels of interpersonal distress can therefore be assigned based on client validation—also known as *idiographic validity* (Wright & Zimmerman, 2019). The measure is also sensitive to change (Ruiz et al., 2004), making it ideal as an outcome measure. It has been well validated across multiple cultures and continents (e.g., Clifton, 2018, Martínez-Arias et al.,1999; L. Z. Wu et al., 2015).

Scores on the IIP-32 represent affirmative endorsement of perceived problems. The higher the score on that scale, the more distress a person has for that construct. They are identifying that they are behaving in a way that is too extreme or identifying behaviors that they have a difficult time performing. For example, a high score on Scale 4: Socially Inhibited means that the client is distressed about being too shy and too afraid of social interactions. They are in distress and upset that they are too reticent in their attempts to connect to others. Conversely, a low score means they do not have a worry about that issue. For example, people with low scores on Uninhibited (Scale 8) are not concerned that they come across as too demanding of others or are too intrusive. They do not feel that this is a problem; however, seeing this as not being a problem means that they feel they do not do too much of this. It may mean, though, that they do not do enough of it. For example, a high score on Scale 7: Warmth/Self-Sacrificing and a low score on Scale 3: Distant often means problems setting boundaries. In other words, someone who has a score high on warmth may feel that others take advantage of them and that they can be too self-sacrificing. If they have a very low score on distance, it only means that they feel they are never accused of being too aloof. However, it may mean that they are not sufficiently able to use the strengths of that scale—the ability to set boundaries. Therefore, scale assessment should consider not just what problem is present, but also what strengths may be missing.

GTQ-S

The GTQ-S (MacNair-Semands et al., 2010) is an empirically validated tool to determine readiness and suitability for group (MacNair-Semands & Corazzini, 1998) that has been revalidated (Baker et al., 2013) and updated. It is used primarily to determine potential group dropout but also functions as a cross-validation of answers on the IIP-32, is a place to address multicultural variables, and is a beginning place to discuss goal formation. (The GTQ-S is available as Appendix A online at https://www.apa.org/pubs/books/focused-brief-group-therapy)

The GTQ-S has five major scales: (a) expectations about group, (b) family patterns, (c) drug and alcohol use, (d) interpersonal problems, and (e) somatic concerns. In addition, a question related to identifying salient identity variables is an essential one that should always be addressed in the TPS session.

Expectations about the group. Motivation levels are predictive of the client's likelihood of dropping out and are therefore essential to note and discuss in the TPS session. Low motivation may be expressed as a desire not to attend; ambivalence; or an expression of logistical issues, such as a need to arrive late, leave early, or attend intermittently. None of these options is possible in FBGT, as I discuss in the next chapter.

However, motivation is a malleable concept within FBGT (although not infinitely so). An initial low score is not unusual because it is not uncommon for people to consider group therapy a less effective and desirable treatment than individual therapy. However, interpersonal style is also a factor in motivation. For example, people with a warm or uninhibited style are quite likely to endorse enthusiasm for group work because it fits with their desire to be connected with others. Conversely, people with scores lower in warmth likely endorse lower motivations. For example, those with distant or socially inhibited styles often indicate very low motivation to join therapy groups because connectedness is viewed as either toxic or unwanted.

Chapter 6 on the TPS session explores how to change motivation from low to high by maximizing the working alliance. So, an initial low score on motivation is not necessarily exclusionary for the client. However, if by the end of the TPS session the client is clear that their attendance is uncertain or will be inconsistent, then they should be referred for other treatment. Motivation is therefore an essential construct to assess.

Family patterns. This scale in the GTQ-S can be used to cross-validate against the client's IIP-32 to determine if the two are consistent. For example, if a client reports becoming avoidant of conflict in their family and being afraid of confrontation, then this might add cross-validation to the hypothesis that the client's high score on Scales 5 or 6 (both conflict-avoidant scales) may be an interpersonal style. This item also suggests how the client may react to expressions of anger or conflict in the group.

Drug and alcohol use. Drug and alcohol use in the past is not necessarily exclusionary for FBGT, but considerable clinical judgment should be exercised to determine whether each client is a good referral or not. Severity, chronicity, past treatment, client variables such as comorbid personality disorders, the degree to which other treatment components are compatible with FBGT, and other agency and clinical factors need to be considered. Addictions and attachment style have been clearly linked (Flores, 2004), so it is possible there may be value for a client with addiction issues in taking part in FBGT as part of a wider treatment program. However, research on the efficacy of the approach with this population has yet to take place. Therefore, clinical judgment about and an assessment of the place of FBGT within a carefully thought out treatment package is needed as is careful consideration that FBGT is a brief treatment.

Interpersonal problems. In this scale, interpersonal problems are presented as a series of checkboxes on the GTQ-S and therefore can provide cross-validation of the IIP-32. For example, if a client shows peaks on Scale 2: Focused on the Needs of the Self on the IIP-32 and also indicates on the GTQ-S that they have problems with being in frequent physical and verbal fights with family and others, then there is evidence that the Scale 2 distress may be indicative of an overly aggressive interpersonal style.

Somatic concerns. This is another key construct measured by the GTQ-S. Somatic concerns may seem abstract but reflect another core, exclusionary construct for FBGT. A feature of somatization is *rigid externalization* (Yalom & Leszcz, 2020), the tendency to attribute problems to external events, states, contexts, or outside forces. A high score on this or evidence elsewhere that the client is incapable of insight is a significant factor that the therapist must consider. Because the approach relies on the client's ability to gain insight and understand the role they play in social difficulties, it is of vital importance that the client have some basic level of this quality. If the client rigidly externalizes, then the ability to understand and own one's own contributions to their interpersonal distress is limited, and treatment will be unsuccessful.

Salient diversity variables. These variables are particularly important to FBGT because a discussion about them opens up a deeper, collaborative understanding about the intersection between culture and interpersonal distress that can strengthen the working alliance. The GTQ-S (see Appendix A online at https://www.apa.org/pubs/books/focused-brief-group-therapy) includes a diversity question that states the following:

> Are there any aspects of your identity that you would like to share with the group, or that might be challenging to discuss/explore? Aspects of identity that might be discussed include race, ethnicity, language, nationality, sex, gender identity, sexual orientation, religion, ability, and socioeconomic status. (Question 8 under "Family")

Without this information, a vital aspect of interpersonal functioning can be missed. Behaviors take place within boundaries, contexts, and power structures that are rooted in assumptions about people with different backgrounds, genders, ethnicities, and other diversity variables. The client's sense of identity and their overall identity development are therefore important to establish. Cultural identity and intersectionality of identities offer important information about how clients experience the world and other people (Anders et al., 2021). Having a clear and strong sense of cultural identity can be a powerful protective factor (McIvor et al., 2009). Conversely, the intersectionality of marginalized identities and the frequency of daily experiences of discrimination have been found to impact mental health (Vargas et al., 2020). Understanding the client's experience of these factors gives important information that must be integrated into the TPS session and can help determine the most effective treatment goals for a client.

In some cases, this can involve referral to a group working on identity issues, if one is available, and something that, after discussion, makes more sense to the client and therapist. In some cases, identity variables are more important to work on in a support group for that identity. Careful discussion needs to take place around the impact of identity variables on the presenting problem to collaboratively determine what will offer the most leverage toward change. The concept of client choice is also important. For some clients, a support group can be helpful in working on identity issues and mobilizing support, but other clients will identify the acquisition of social skills as more important and salient to them. Equally, social skills that focus on the interpersonal aspects of identity (e.g., being assertive in the face of microaggressions) can be a focus of treatment in FBGT.

On the last page of the GTQ-S is a question about goals for the group (see Appendix A online at https://www.apa.org/pubs/books/focused-brief-group-therapy). Typically, clients will write goals that are diffuse and difficult to measure. For example, "to feel better" is an oft-stated desire but is challenging to quantify for the therapist and client and therefore too broad and difficult to accomplish. This section of the GTQ-S can be used as a starting point to gently move the client toward more discreet and focused goals. Doing so ultimately helps the client feel more in control of the antecedents of the problem and ultimately less overwhelmed by the scale of the solutions.

Administration Timing

Once the intake and referral have been completed, the client should be administered the three instruments described in this chapter: the IIP-32; an empirically validated outcome measure, such as the OQ-30; and the GTQ-S.

Sufficient time should have been given for the clinician to score and review the instruments and to begin to make a clinical hypothesis. Therefore, it is strongly recommended that clients be asked to stay after the initial intake or to come in several days before the TPS intake and complete the paperwork. Some assessment tools also use computer analytics that render a printout of current progress as well as other helpful highlights regarding clinically important issues.

Review of the Instruments and Formation of a Hypothesis

Reviewing the instruments requires the ability to identify the connections between them and to form a coherent clinical hypothesis. The process for exploring the meaning of measures and preparing a hypothesis involves several stages. First, the therapist should score the IIP-32 and note the highest scale scores and total score while also mapping out the overall profile. The highest scale score becomes the place for the tentative hypothesis to take place. The therapist then reviews the scores from the quality of life measure. They note the total level of distress as well as any other clinically relevant data points that the instrument may provide. Then, the therapist reviews the GTQ-S score and explores this hypothesis with the client in the TPS session. Each assessment tool can add something to the different questions involved in the working alliance.

Exclusion Criteria
First, it is important to determine whether there are any clear exclusionary criteria. For example, a referral source has sent someone who is endorsing low motivation to join and has somatic complaints, serious current addiction issues, and interpersonal distress scores that are high on every scale. In this extreme example, the person is exhibiting low insight, externalizing strategies of using substances to manage their distress, low motivation, and interpersonal distress that is unfocused. In isolation, each factor is a potential issue, but combined, these factors suggest a low likelihood of success for the client. In most cases, the reasons to exclude are more complex and include potential for gain combined with some risk—for example, a client who has previous addiction issues but is now sober, is working on their relationships, and is motivated toward self-improvement.

IIP Profile
Seeking to understand the client's IIP-32 profile is the next step. This step involves looking not just at their highest score, which always remains important

because it is their core interpersonal strategy, but also the balance of the profile. Understanding the balance of the profile both enables the therapist to predict how the working alliance might unfold and presents the therapist with the opportunity to consider how they may need to adjust their own interpersonal style to improve the bond. For example, the therapist who is typically Warm/Self-Sacrificing (Scale 7) notices that the client coming for the TPS session has a score high on Scale 3: Distant. The therapist makes a note to hold back on their natural warmth to prevent anticomplementary impacting the bond.

Group Dynamic Evaluation

Noting how the group is beginning to cluster in terms of interpersonal styles is also important in terms of beginning to understand how the group will begin as well as how it will cohere. For example, the therapist notices that this is the fifth client with a Distant (Scale 3) or Socially Inhibited (Scale 4) scale profile. Realizing that the group would benefit from some warm or dominant members, they make a note to mention that to their referral sources. They also prepare to make adjustments to the group in terms of leadership style in the event that the group entirely comprises members who are high in distance and inhibition. FBGT has also worked on models of predicting group dynamics and conflict in groups. Barry (2011) suggested a model that broke down combinations of interpersonal styles into predicted interactions with each other. This mirrored a similar idea by Markin and Marmarosh (2010). These models predict group-as-a-whole behavior as a function of interpersonal dyads interacting within the larger matrix.

Culture and Context

The complexities of how interpersonal style, culture, and context interact with each other should also be considered. A good example of this is a discussion by Rahmawati and Taylor (2018) in which the first author described how their Javanese and Indonesian culture's emphasis on avoidance of conflict made it difficult for them to deliver needed feedback to the teachers they were training. This author, Rahmawati, described a process of evolution in learning how to deliver feedback in ways that allowed students to be helped while still retaining a sense of cultural pride and identification. This example of how cultural norms, role performance, and interpersonal skills interact illustrates the complexities of interpersonal challenges that life presents us. Interpersonal flexibility involves many layers, and clinicians and clients face the challenge of navigating toward a future that involves recognizing strengths both in personality and culture while embracing flexibility in desired behavioral options.

CASE EXAMPLE: COMBINING DATA AND HYPOTHESIS FORMATION

This case example illustrates how data points from the different instruments may be combined. The client intake report states that the client is a 30-year-old White woman who is working in the entertainment industry as a specialist in set design. The GTQ-S report shows that she wants the therapist to know that she is "Italian American, asexual, Catholic, and has dyslexia." She identifies her personal pronouns as "she/her/hers." She is currently single and lives at home with her parents. The client has received a diagnosis of social anxiety and dysthymia from the intake therapist, who also notes that the client is having problems sleeping and reports being unhappy at work and at home.

The GTQ-S shows low scores for motivation to join group. The client reports growing up in a family in which everyone was extraverted and close to each other, and she felt on the periphery and ignored. The client notes that conflicts in her family were "very loud" and that she felt unable to stand up to her parents or her siblings. She has no endorsement of either problems with alcohol and substances or of somatic complaints. She endorses feeling shy, being unassertive, having difficulty with social relationships, and not enjoying or desiring close relationships. She notes that she is feeling pressured at work to be more social but that she feels uncomfortable going out but is unable to say no. The therapy intake notes also show that she is feeling pressured by her parents to move out of the house and to find a romantic relationship. The client notes that she has no friends.

The OQ-30 shows a score for overall distress in the range of someone who might be in outpatient therapy. The client did not endorse critical items, such as suicidality, alcohol, or substance abuse or any other areas of concern. The IIP-32 profile shows high peaks on Scale 4: Socially Inhibited. The next highest score is on Scale 3: Distant and is in the clinically significant range. No other scores show significance, thus making the profile clear: The highest distress is on social inhibition with the next highest on distance.

Combining Data to Form an Initial Hypothesis

In terms of connecting the dots of all instruments, it appears from the preceding case example that the client is endorsing several indicators of social inhibition that may be tied to feelings of loneliness and disconnection. The client has identified that she has difficulty socializing, so it is quite possible that her distress is linked to loneliness from difficulty in initiating and maintaining friendships. She may also be highly ambivalent about wanting relationships, given her high score on distance. The client's overall distress is fairly high, so it will be important to determine in the TPS session if the loneliness and social inhibition is casual (or at least implicated in a significant way) in terms of her overall distress. The client's identification as asexual has many potential meanings because, as a definition, its etiology is unclear. It has been linked to either sexual behavior, hypoactive sexual desire, self-identification, or combinations of those three; therefore, care must be taken in making assumptions about meaning (Van Houdenhove et al., 2014). The therapist notes to ask the client in the TPS session what her sexual identity means to her and how she felt it emerged.

In terms of identity variables, the therapist also makes a note to ask more about how the client feels she fits into and identifies with her Italian American cultural background. The therapist notes to ask about the interactions between the client's family, her culture, and her interpersonal style to determine how she sees person–environment fit and identity interacting.

The client's identification as a person with dyslexia is also something important to explore in the context of her reported distress. Research has suggested that dyslexia can be integrated the person's identity via either externalization or internalization (Livingston et al., 2018). For example, some people develop compensatory strategies that result in their becoming more verbally skillful and able to work around difficulties in writing or reading. For others, negative internalization may take place and result in an inaccurate, deficit-focused set of cognitions (e.g., "I am not smart") that result in lower self-esteem and lower perceived efficacy in interacting with others. How the client makes sense of their experience with dyslexia therefore is important to investigate with them.

It is essential to explore all aspects of these identities with an open mind and by listening to the client. It is also critical to understand how these factors interact from the client's perspective, thereby allowing for a stronger working alliance between therapist and client, which ultimately enhances the likelihood that the client will feel heard and will select goals that will be meaningful to their life.

Other factors cross-validate the tentative hypothesis that the problem is one of style and is not purely situational. For example, in the case example, the client endorses low motivation to join group therapy, which is characteristic of people with social inhibition (and contrasts with those high in warmth or those who are uninhibited—who eagerly respond to the idea in the affirmative). To a person with social anxiety (which typically correlates with social inhibition), being around other people—particularly in groups in which they must interact—represents a feared stimulus. Therefore, suggesting that a client with this kind of distress join a therapy group represents the same fear as asking someone who is afraid of heights to go rock climbing without a rope. For the client in the case example, her family background in which she reported being the most insignificant member could be related to being someone who is shy at a trait level being in a family in which other members may have less trait-level shyness (as indicated by the client's GTQ-S responses) and in a cultural milieu in which being highly social is valued (which would need verifying with the client to see if that is how she experiences people from her cultural background and her family). The client also endorses feeling lonely but ambivalent.

Exploring Other Factors

Considering the case example, all these factors present the tentative hypothesis that the IIP-32 score represents a person who is distressed by social inhibition and that this may be a style. It is unclear what role the client's diversity variables play in her social inhibition, and the therapist makes a note to listen to the client's account of them. It is possible, given what the client has already written, that her social inhibition is cross situational and rigid. However, because she has identified work and home as the two major places where the distress is activated, the therapist focuses on whether the client wishes to make changes related to those two scenarios.

In terms of work, the therapist notes to ask what the specifics of the recent distress are. For example, it is possible that the client is generally happy at work but has recently become distressed as people have solicited more social involvement from her and she feels both anxious about it and ambiguous about enforcing a boundary by saying no. The therapist needs to explore the specifics of this distress with the client because they could implicate goals. For instance, a goal to set a clear boundary with the group by saying no or retaining distance after an invitation into a discussion could be worth considering if the client identifies boundary setting as an issue. Equally, the client may also wish to work on goals such as asking follow-up questions of others or engaging in brief conversations that she initiates. Doing so then offers her the opportunity to have more choices—to engage or to keep a boundary—and to have more skills in managing whichever alternative she selects. The therapist prepares for this possible set of goals while remaining open to the possibility that the client may provide information that could suggest goals that are very different.

At the TPS session, therefore, the group leader expects someone to present themselves in a shy and withdrawn manner. They might expect to see them avoid eye contact; have difficulty making a warm connection; and struggle at times to manage basic social skills, such as making small talk or going beyond basic responses to questions. The group leader might expect to feel an urge to fill the awkward silences and to feel anxious and faltering themself. Conversely, a highly dominant group leader might find themself overtalking and acting in an even more dominant manner than normal. Either of these reactions represents feeling "hooked" by the client's interpersonal style. The group leader then needs to unhook to be effective. If the client presents in a very different way than this, further exploration is required. Assessing group dynamics is also possible once the interviews have all been completed.

ASSESSMENT OF HOMOGENEITY AND HETEROGENEITY IN GROUP DYNAMICS

Remember that people perceive the group climate in ways that reinforce their interpersonal problems (Kivlighan & Angelone, 1992). This has important implications for group dynamics. Self-fulfilling prophecies operate as mental schemas. For example, someone who is highly assertive perceives a group as more anxious and avoidant, thus giving them license to behave in ways that are more domineering and active in challenging others. This set of cognitions and therefore the behaviors that attach to them can lead to a self-fulfilling prophecy as members react with quietness to the domineering behavior and, in some cases, take a more passive role.

In FBGT, prediction of group dynamics is an important process that can help leaders plan interventions and anticipate possible alliance ruptures, premature termination, conflicts, and impasses. FBGT plots three important dimensions when mapping out a group dynamic: (a) each group member's interpersonal style, (b) who each members feels allied to, and (c) what the group leader's interpersonal style is. This presupposes that the three connecting threads that represent the deep structure of human behavior in groups are affiliation, agency, and alliances. The way these three play out are idiosyncratic and are based on cultural norms; roles (if at work or in a family); and expectations, such as group norms. It also presupposes that the group leader's interpersonal style is an important part of the group dynamic to consider.

Affiliation and Agency

It is important to map out each member onto the interpersonal circumplex using their highest score. In some cases, it is also worth adding an "extender" in the form of a dotted arrow to illustrate where a style has more than one peak or the profile is more complex. One needs to understand alliances and the group leader's interpersonal style.

In the following group dynamic, several patterns can be seen (see Figure 5.3). The group is fairly heterogenous for interpersonal style, which is not always the case. In some groups, members may cluster around certain scales, axes, or hemispheres. For example, a group may comprise members who are all high on distance and low on warmth. Figure 5.3 illustrates that most scale types are represented within the group: Julia's style is represented with the addition of broken arrows to represent that Scale 5: Unassertive and Scale 6:

FIGURE 5.3. Example of a Group Dynamic With Highest Scale Scores of Each Client

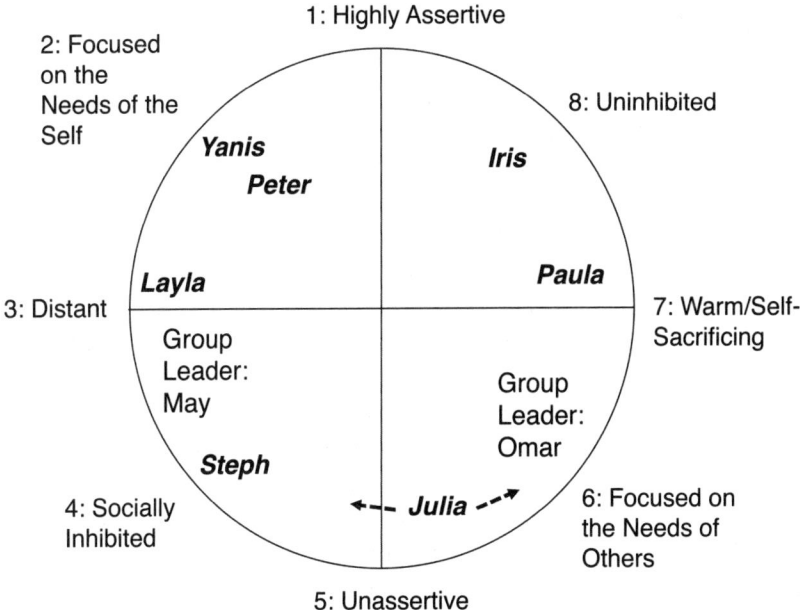

Focused on the Needs of Others are approximately equal in terms of scoring on her IIP-32. This means she may move toward Scale 5 or Scale 6. Notably, this combination of scores also suggests she may exhibit features of dependency. This group looks to have members who can be warm, such as Paula and Iris; members who have boundaries; members who are assertive; and members who are unassertive. There is a good mix of different styles, which can make the work flow more easily. Paula, in particular, will attempt to establish cohesion and warmth in the group. However, she may find some resistance to that effort from the members who are less comfortable with closeness— those with strong boundaries and a preference for autonomy.

The presence of three members—Yanis, Peter, and Iris—with scores high in assertiveness is interesting. If Yanis and Peter form an alliance, then this may or may not be productive, depending on whether they inspire each other to work or collude on defending each other against the work. If they choose to defend and support each other against the work and in ganging up on other members, then this could become what Agazarian (2018) defined as a *functional subgroup*, one in which members are helping each other in their work. However, if the leaders and members can hold them to their work, then they could end up being helpful to each other. Iris is also someone who may be highly active in the group. Therefore, there are three members all high in assertiveness. The two leaders are not high in assertiveness, so they do not feel hooked in wanting to compete for dominance. However, if Yanis and Peter remain stuck in their favored position of hostility and assertiveness and do not engage with their goals, then the leader must find a way to block, protect, and encourage them toward their goals.

Given that Julia represents the disowned, vulnerable parts of the self for Yanis and Peter, it is quite likely they will attack her at some point. The leaders must be ready to use the work the axes technique (discussed further in Chapter 8) to help the members involved to process what is happening. Omar, one of the group leaders, may find this quite challenging because his default style is to be warm and to avoid conflict. May, the other group leader, is able to provide more challenge and has the assertiveness to confront Yanis and Peter but will find it difficult to offer the requisite warmth in doing so. Therefore, both leaders may need to stretch themselves interpersonally and therapeutically to be able to craft the correct interventions. Because the interventions require the ability to simultaneously help protect Julia and correct Yanis and Peter, the group leaders will need to conduct firmly but without shame or judgment. Therefore, wording and tone become important; therapeutic tact when addressing these issues becomes a crucial technique. It is also possible that Iris will defend Julia, particularly if she feels supported by the warmth

Julia offers. May may be able to use her position as a person with a more distant style to support Steph and Layla in activating their goals.

Alliances

The role of alliances is important to consider. While it is possible that Peter and Yanis form an alliance, they may also develop enmity toward each other and compete for control of the group. This would shift the group dynamic considerably. In this instance, Iris might attempt to be a peacemaker between them, and members in the group who are in the bottom hemisphere (i.e., Steph and Julia) may feel silenced and afraid as they experience heightened emotions that come with observing a conflict. In this case, Peter and Yanis may eventually reconcile if they can learn more about each other's life histories or if they dysfunctionally unite against the warm or vulnerable members of the group that they perceive as the disowned part of themselves.

Thus, it can be seen that alliances can also significantly impact the group dynamic. Layla could find themself to be an important source of truth for the group. With a style that is based on analysis of situations and goals to offer advice or listen carefully, it is possible that some keen insights into the group dynamic could be helpful for both Layla and the group. Steph is somewhat at risk in this group if the group do not work on their goals. If Steph's goals that involve assertiveness and asking follow-up questions are successful, then this could both help the group process (e.g., by standing up to Peter or Yanis or by drawing out and helping Julia) and therefore help themselves.

Goals and Group Dynamics

Peter and Yanis's goals are designed to help them try something new. The Scale 2: Focused on the Needs of the Self goals (see Chapter 4) are typically to hold back from domineering, to avoid attacking, and to offer encouragement and support. Therefore, completion of these goals offers them the opportunity to avoid the typical outcomes they normally experience: of being seen as aggressive, domineering, and attacking. With group leader and member encouragement, working on those goals can provide them with an alternate pathway to group participation that can deliver significantly different outcomes than they might normally expect.

Remember, though, that even when they are working on their goals, members' default styles remain. While working on goals, those default styles will be hyperactivated, which sometimes leads to members' bouncing back from a goal completion to a preferred, familiar, and more comfortable state so that they can regain a sense of safety. It is important that they then get feedback on goal completion both during and after the group in the debriefing (see Chapter 10). Moving out of their typical comfort zone involves considerable risk that they may become vulnerable and exploitable, so metaphorically laying down their (verbal) means to defend themselves represents a considerable risk.

Group Leaders' Interpersonal Styles

Leaders' styles affect both the group dynamic and their own ability to use their interpersonal flexibility to apply certain interventions. It is possible that group leader Omar (see Figure 5.3) may become the subject of attack from the dominant group members because Omar's style is also one that represents the disowned part of the self of the Scale 2 members. Group leaders Omar and May must prepare to process this with the group and to consider using a modification of the work the axes technique explained in Chapter 8 (but with the group leader as the example).

In this case, Omar would model being at peace with their own style and acknowledge that being warm and comforting represents a risk of being exploited and attacked. However, Omar could then act as a model for other group members by inviting those with Scale 6 (Focused on the Needs of Others) scores to consider what aspects of the style they might find helpful in their lives if they were to take a small part of them. This requires Omar to have previously become comfortable with the strengths and limitations of their own style so that they can both explain it, defend it, and acknowledge when they need to work on interpersonally flexible (e.g., during conflicts). This can be helpful for multiple members in the group and can model both feeling comfortable with one's own style and being able to acknowledge the feelings that go with being flexible when moving outside of a preferred interpersonal style.

It is important that Omar conducts this discussion while being rooted in their own mindfulness and centeredness. This is not a place for Omar to work on themselves but rather a place to demonstrate what work that is ongoing looks like. Omar should first internally notice the hooked state: feeling afraid and taken advantage of for being kind, which translates into an internalized unassertive, upset position of feeling disempowered and removed from the leadership role. Rather than accepting this position, Omar must unhook and take a position of assertive distance: explaining calmly and collectedly what is happening and offering analysis and interpersonal solutions to the group members.

SUMMARY

Accurate referrals from skilled referrers provide a solid foundation for the next phases of FBGT: administration of instruments, hypothesis formation, and the TPS. However, referrals should not be left to chance; rather, they require an ongoing discussion between referrers to strengthen the working alliance and promote successful client progress. Clinical judgment is key in this process, and careful case conceptualization combined with conducting analysis of risks and rewards possible for the client and the group is essential in cases that meet one or more exclusion criteria.

Using the IIP-32 (Horowitz et al., 2000), GTQ-S (MacNair-Semands et al., 2010), and a quality of life measure together provides a rich vein of information that can help the group leader generate important data about the client's presenting problem, interpersonal style, overall functioning, and likelihood of dropping out. By reviewing the instruments together and using them to cross-check each other, the therapist can prepare for the TPS session with a working hypothesis that is ready to be checked with the client. And by including information about salient cultural and diversity variables, the therapist is also prepared to integrate this information into the case formulation.

With these data gathered, the therapist must then hold lightly onto the hypothesis and prepare for confirmatory and disconfirmatory information to arise, allowing their clinical judgment to be guided by, and responsive to, new information and client preferences. Thus, the working alliance, an evidence-based construct, can be refined and strengthened such that the bond to the therapist, goals for treatment, and task agreement are foundational to successful outcomes.

6

THERAPY, PREGROUP PREPARATION, AND SCREENING

The Importance of the TPS Session

The hypotheses generated in the pregroup assessment are an important component of the process of focused brief group therapy (FBGT). However, they should always be held lightly because meeting with the client in person can yield crucial information that may lead to validation, modification, or, in some cases, rejection of these hypotheses. The individual meeting with the client, called the *therapy, pregroup preparation, and screening (TPS) session*, is where the hypotheses can be explored collaboratively with the client and refined with the client's input.

FROM HYPOTHESIS TO TREATMENT

The TPS session—named after its three core functions—therapy, pregroup preparation, and screening—is one of the defining and essential features of FBGT. It is core to the approach because it sets the conditions and focus for all other phases. It is a highly rigorous session that demands a great deal of the therapist. When the TPS session is well conducted, though, it creates ideal facilitative conditions for the client and group to achieve successful

https://doi.org/10.1037/0000389-007
Focused Brief Group Therapy: An Integrative Approach to Reducing Interpersonal Distress, by M. Whittingham

outcomes. When the session performs poorly, however, the working alliance fails, insight fails to materialize, and the group struggles with therapeutic drift and has a higher potential for premature dropout and poor outcomes.

The TPS session is where the "focus" is put into FBGT in terms of correct goal selection and calibration. It is also where group dropout and client worsening are predicted into and prevented via inoculation. However, each of these is interlinked with the goal of developing a strong working alliance that is based around rapid movement to insight. This rapid movement to insight within the TPS session is what makes the session "therapy."

ESTABLISHMENT OF A WORKING ALLIANCE

The key task of the TPS session—what the whole session is geared toward—is to establish a strong working alliance. The working alliance is key not only to positive outcomes, but also to reductions in group dropout. The alliance has three components that must be attended to during the TPS session: bond, goal agreement, and task agreement (Horvath & Greenberg, 1989). *Bond* takes place by several methods: matching to the client's interpersonal style in acomplementary ways that leave the client feeling comfortable but challenged; being culturally sensitive and thoughtful when working on multicultural listening with the client; having an attitude of empathy and unconditional positive regard; and using therapeutic tact that avoids shame, blame, and guilt. *Goal agreement* involves linking the client's overall life distress to a specific interpersonal problem that, if solved, leads to greater feelings of self-efficacy, reduced interpersonal distress, and an increased likelihood of their needs being met. *Task agreement* involves helping the client understand what they will be doing in group, namely, working on goals in the here and now that directly relate to the interpersonal area that they are most distressed about.

The working alliance is woven throughout the session, and it needs establishing and monitoring throughout the session and as the group progresses. Developing skills in the art and science of the TPS session is an essential part of FBGT.

WHO CONDUCTS THE TPS?

One of the group leaders who is leading the group that the member will be joining should always be responsible for the TPS session. This task should never be completed by a separate therapist. The formation of the working alliance, a construct related to reduced dropout and improved outcomes, entails that the therapist develop a bond with the client. The client must like and feel connected to a therapist; they must feel that the therapist understands their issues and will have their best interests at heart. The client can also anticipate the group while being safe in the knowledge that, even though they know the group will be full of anxiety-provoking unknowns—that is, the other group members—the group leader is someone they know, trust, and feel connected to.

The therapist acts as the container for the work and remains the "therapeutic drumbeat" throughout the rest of the therapy as the group begins to take center stage. Therefore, this bond is crucial as a bridge before the working alliance with the therapist is transferred into cohesion with the therapy group. Equally, if the group takes a week or two to form, it is important for the therapist to make weekly contact to maintain that bond by phone (with the client's prior permission). It does not need a long conversation but, rather, a quick update to let the client know that they are still being thought of and cared for, thus maintaining the bond.

TASKS OF THE TPS SESSION

The TPS session comprises several interrelated and overlapping tasks:

- Move the problem definition from a diffuse concept (e.g., "I feel bad") to one with a clear interpersonal focus (e.g., "I think my shyness is impacting my ability to form relationships").

- Determine the validity of the hypothesis that was formed (see Chapter 7) by adding therapist countertransferential reactions and contextual and cultural data.

- Present the quality of life measure and the 32-item Inventory of Interpersonal Problems (IIP-32; Horowitz et al., 2000) to the client as a potential etiology.

- Generate group MATH goals (i.e., goals that are measurable, achievable, time limited, and based in the here and now; discussed later in this chapter) related to a specific interpersonal distress on the interpersonal circumplex.

- Inoculate, if necessary.

The order in which these tasks are carried out varies by individual client, and all are vital parts of the TPS session.

Task: Move Diffuse Problems Into Specific Interpersonal Problem Identification

Clients typically enter therapy with an unclear and often diffuse idea of what they want from therapy. The Group Therapy Questionnaire–Short Form (GTQ-S; MacNair-Semands et al., 2010) has a section on goals for group, and it is fairly typical for potential group members to write, "To feel better" as a main and sometimes the only goal.

This lack of goal clarity is a vital element of progress in brief group therapy. A main task of the group leader in FBGT is to turn a vague goal into one that with a clear focus that is amenable to the mechanisms of change that the group has to offer. This assumes that the referral has been conducted thoughtfully. The client sitting in the waiting room should have been evaluated by the intake therapist as having an interpersonal issue underlying their presenting problem and diagnosis. If the referral has been incorrectly made, such as when someone has no clear interpersonal difficulties, then the therapist may wish to redirect the person to other services and then revisit with the referring therapist to explore the inclusion and exclusion criteria.

Task: Determine Hypothesis Validity

Before the therapist has even considered beginning FBGT, they should have determined what their own interpersonal style is. Establishing their own baselines style is a vital prerequisite in understanding hooked and unhooked states that occur between therapist and client.

Recognize Hooked and Unhooked Reactions

The therapist's emotions and thoughts are a vital part of validating a client's interpersonal style. For example, a therapist with an assertive interpersonal style expects to feel competitive and irritated with a client with a highly assertive style because that response represents the feelings that accompany noncomplementary on that scale. Equally, a therapist who is focused on the needs of others might feel intimidated, emotionally upset, inadequate, and resentful of that same client. The therapist's baseline style determines their typical reaction. They must also check in with any potential for cultural bias with respect to negative labeling of interpersonal behaviors that are outside of their own cultural experience. Therefore, the therapist must be able to mindfully notice their own feelings and understand them in terms of complementarity and being hooked. They must then decide how to best respond therapeutically by unhooking to establish a strong bond based on the client's interpersonal style.

Every client who arrives for the TPS sessions offers invitations to the therapist based on their interpersonal style. This opportunity allows the therapist to confirm whether distress seen on the IIP-32 is in line with the client's interpersonal presentation. Given that, for the client, the TPS session is likely anxiety provoking, research has suggested that the client will move farther toward their typical interpersonal style (Van Denburg & Kiesler, 1993). So, a typically uninhibited person becomes even more unboundaried and intrusive. The person typically focused on the needs of self may attempt to assert themselves as more intelligent than the therapist to gain a sense of safety, and the client with an unassertive style becomes even more quiet, indecisive, and unresponsive.

Thus, in the TPS sessions, the therapist has considerable opportunities to notice the invitations and see if their clinical impressions match what the assessment tool suggests. This impression can sometimes appear in the first few minutes (e.g., when a client does not give eye contact initially or makes a rude statement about the therapist's office on walking in) or evolve more slowly over the sessions. However, observing initial first impressions and noticing feelings that come up in the presence of the client are important aspects of corroborating clinical judgment. For example, feeling liked or being entertained by the client, feeling bored or distracted in the client's presence, or feeling humiliated or inadequate are all data points that should be compared and contrasted with the formal assessment.

A prerequisite of this centered noticing, however, is to actually be centered. The therapist must take a few moments before meeting with the client to take some deep breaths and center. The therapist should then notice their feelings and remind themselves of their preferred interpersonal style. It is vital to center in this reality. For example, they might observe the following:

> I am feeling a little tired today and somewhat anxious. My typical style is Scale 6: Focused on the Needs of Others, which means I have a tendency to be warm and allow others to lead. I am going to keep breathing and notice what I am feeling as I meet the client. This will give me information on whether this IIP-32 matches to what I am feeling as I am with them. Their IIP-32 has a high score on Scale 2: Focused on the Needs of the Self. This means they may try and dominate me and see my warmth and quietness as weaknesses. I may need to be a little more distant and cooler initially and show a quiet strength.

This centeredness is vital. The therapist must notice their feelings and see them as information, not as something to be reactive to. For example, the therapist may notice feeling put down, inadequate, and belittled in the first 5 minutes. Working from a noncentered stance, the therapist may be tempted to refer the client on or offer no resistance when the client suggests the therapy will be ineffective. This kind of response to client hostility is all too common.

As von der Lippe et al. (2008) pointed out, therapists often belittle and ignore hostile clients in subtle ways, leading to a hostile therapeutic climate. The authors described a typical pattern of clients' overt hostility being met with the hooked response of hostile submission. Because therapists are trained to avoid overt hostility, they respond, unless unhooked, with the hostile submission of ignoring and subtly scorning that eventually provides a toxic climate for the whole group.

By labeling the feelings as an invitation and a hooked state, though, the therapist now has verification of the client's style and the choice to give the client an unhooked response, thereby becoming more therapeutically responsive and effective. Alliance rupture can occur even before the therapy is fully underway. Without full knowledge of what is occurring and why, the rupture risks turning into the therapist's disliking the client and the client's feeling uncontained and unconnected.

Conduct an Interpersonal Interview

Yalom and Leszcz (2020) described the *interpersonal interview* as involving taking a history of a client's interpersonal relationships. Its purpose is to establish how pervasive across time and situations interpersonal behaviors are. In FBGT, this interview also involves integrating the interpersonal circumplex and diversity variables. The therapist first looks at the interpersonal circumplex to establish a possible hypothesis and makes the assumption that the distress may or may not be a result of an inflexible style. The therapist then explores with the client how long they have felt interpersonal distress and in what venues. If it has been long lasting and pervasive across all times and contexts, then there is support for the possibility of a restricted style of relating. However, it is also possible that contextual issues may have been involved at all ages and levels of development; therefore, context should not be ruled out as being the most salient issue.

Assess Diversity and Identity Variables and Integrate

The therapist also checks to see if cultural differences are involved—specifically, if the client's self-identified diversity variables impact their interpersonal world. For example, a client from a minority group might indicate feeling interpersonally at ease in groups that share that same minority status but in distress once they join majority groups. Equally, they may identify as feeling distressed in all the groups they take part in, regardless of culture. They may also identify as being more comfortable in majority culture groups than in groups mirroring their own salient identity variables.

The therapist also should carefully consider context. For example, someone may report being seen as interpersonally skilled and likeable in every context in which they have functioned—either in the past or in the present. However, currently, they are being labeled as vindictive and unlikeable at work. It is also possible that a context may be so mandating and strong in its effect that it warps a person's self-image or ability to cope, such as in a workplace with a dog-eat-dog mentality that encourages competition and ruthlessness and, thus, affects employees' self-image and distress. Exploring contexts is important because they may lead to a misreading of the level of distress on the interpersonal circumplex as representing style rather than inaccurate feedback from a particular context.

The possible combinations of factors are complex. The therapist must work out with the client which factors are the most important ones and come to a shared understanding of what is causing the distress and what might solve it. Remember that regardless of the causes of distress, the client still has opportunities to grow—perhaps becoming more assertive, leaving a toxic context altogether, learning to convey to others how cultural differences impact their interactions, being able to connect in more meaningful ways across situations, or numerous other possibilities. The opportunity always exists within FBGT to find new ways of relating that are more adaptive and functional. Although some more functional ways of relating involve learning how to connect and establish better, closer, and more satisfying relationships, they may also involve findings ways to be more assertive, boundaried, and honoring of one's identity.

The key to identifying goals should relate to collaboratively identifying what it is the client wishes to work on, which can be narrow or broad. For example, a client may be highly assertive in advocating for themselves at work but feel disconnected and rejected at home when trying to achieve closeness. The client may also identify identity variables that seem highly salient to the therapist. Remember, however, that the key mechanism of change in FBGT is achieving interpersonal flexibility, so goals should emerge from the client's interpersonal distress that they have identified as a particular problem for them. If the problem is entirely created by a toxic environment, then the client may also choose to find ways to be flexible in dealing with that environment if they do not wish to leave it. They may also identify that their lack of flexibility is causing some of the problems. The link between internalization and externalization is complex and requires careful thought from the clinician in collaboration with the client.

Task: Present Quality of Life Measure and IIP-32

In the TPS session, the therapist shows the client two main instruments: the IIP-32 and quality of life measure. FBGT is transparent and collaborative in its use of assessment, taking a nonjudgmental, nonshaming, and strengths-based approach to how it is presented. The model helps the client understand what is happening and provide a bridge between therapist hypotheses and client reality. This is a mutually influencing process.

The therapist begins by listening to the client and asking them about how their interpersonal life and general life distress interact. The therapist completes an iterative process, going back and forth between the formal data and client descriptions to determine the root causes and to formulate goals. The therapist is asking questions, integrating data, and presenting those data to the client as tentative hypotheses. The client then responds, and the two develop a working alliance around what the problem is and around possible solutions.

Remember that this collaborative process depends on the client's interpersonal style. For example, clients with distant styles may be hesitant, slow to disclose, distancing from a warm therapist, and reluctant to join a group. A client with a more highly assertive style might be reluctant to accept the possibility of anything being an area of vulnerability in their life, whereas someone with a style focused on the needs of others may say yes to the group while feeling highly ambivalent and wishing they said no. The trajectory of each TPS is determined by the client's interpersonal style and the therapist's ability to be flexible in response to it.

Task: Generate MATH Goals

Goals in FBGT must meet the following MATH goals criteria: They must be measurable, achievable, time limited, and implementable in the here and now of the group. Goals clients bring tend to be based on abstract, diffuse notions of "feeling better." FBGT goals sharpen the focus.

Measurable Goals

Measurable goals mean that both the therapist and the client keep track of their progress. By making transparently measurable goals based on behaviors enacted in the group and kept track of by client, therapist, and group, progress is made accountable. Equally, because goals are based on visible behaviors, therapists can track overt processes rather than make assumptions about internal changes.

Achievable Goals

Achievable is an important criterion with two major component parts. First is the quarter turn (Kiesler, 1996), which is discussed in Chapter 2. To keep anxiety at optimal levels, the quarter turn change has proven to be a key strategy but is perhaps the most counterintuitive to how some therapists consider what is a face-valid way of developing goals. Clients attempting 180-degree goals can either become highly avoidant of the goal or become overwhelmed by the goal and emotionally decompensate. The second component, polyvagal theory, tells us that social learning takes place when we are in "rest-and-digest" states, so creating goals that are a logical next step and not an overreach is essential for progress. Ninety-degree goals are sufficiently challenging that no stretch beyond this goal is necessary in eight sessions.

Time-Limited Goals

Time-limited goals are an important criterion because they allow clients to accomplish something achievable in a realistic time frame. Clients fit the work into the available time as long as they know what the work is, believe it is achievable in that time, and consider the outcome to be worthwhile. Providing that the goals are well calibrated, meaningful to the client, and time limited, they should be met in the time available. Clients may even accomplish some of their goals by the end of Session 1. It is quite common for sudden gains to accrue for some clients because they are so well prepared in the TPS session. In this case, they can solidify the gains, get feedback, and help others. Repeated attempts to meet goals over and above what were originally set are not a bad thing because they allow for habituation to take place, which can solidify gains in even a brief group.

Here-and-Now–Based Goals

Here-and-now–based goals must also be based in the here and now and not the there and then; that is, enactment of the goals must take place within the here and now of the group in the course of the interactions taking place. This enables the client to work though their feelings and polyvagal reactions in real time, thereby gaining greater understanding and feelings of control over their own schemas and responses. This idea of interpersonal flexibility is not only behavioral but involves a whole-system response—emotional, polyvagal, cognitive, and interpersonal—as homeostatic reactions occur both within the person and in terms of the group's reactions.

Sample MATH Goal

A full goal that incorporates all MATH goal criteria would be: "To ask follow up questions at least twice during the life of the group." This goal is measurable (asks questions that can be seen and counted), achievable (assumes that the client agrees to it but, in general, is a realistic goal), time limited (is within the life of the group as opposed to after it has finished or at some indeterminate time), and based in the here and now (the questions pre-suppose that they will be acted on as the group is in progress). Note how different this goal is from the client's initial formulation, which is typically "to feel better" or "to be happy"—what they often write in the GTQ-S goals section. Those initial formulations set the client up for failure: Because they rely on subjective noticing of internal states, such formulations are not mea-surable, they rely on fleeting emotions in response to specific situations, and they are based on indistinct periods. MATH goals, however, represent concrete, realistic achievements and, as such, allow for increased locus of control by the client.

Goal Calibration: "Going for Goldilocks"

The test of whether a goal is appropriate is tested by the level of anxiety the client expresses toward the goal. Theories linking anxiety to learning, such as flow theory (Csikszentmihalyi et al., 2018) and polyvagal theory (Porges & Dana, 2018), have come to the same conclusion: that there is an optimal level of anxiety required for learning. Too little challenge, and a goal does not provoke any anticipatory anxiety. Some degree of anxiety is produced by a sense of challenge and is necessary for any goal and treatment itself to feel meaningful. However, too much anxiety pushes people into fight, flight, or freeze mode, and social learning does not take place because the sympathetic nervous system is activated. Therefore, an optimal level needs to be set.

Nonverbal cues can give significant information on the degree to which a client is emotionally activated (Kinner et al., 2017). When discussing goals with clients, the therapist should watch clients' nonverbal cues to begin to understand what level of anxiety comes with what goals. For example, when the therapist suggests a goal, if the client sits up, has dilated pupils, and looks physiologically activated, then the goal has provoked an anxiety reaction. Some degree of this reaction is positive. To name the search for the optimal level, the FBGT team coined the term *Going for Goldilocks* after the Western nursery rhyme that makes repeated allusion to the idea of being too hot, too cold, and *just right*. In the aforementioned example, some pupil dilation is preferable to none, with low arousal and bored appearance, or massive "big as plates" eye dilation with accompanying expressions of alarm.

Group leaders should watch nonverbal cues and ask the client to rate their anxiety about a goal on a scale of 1 (*lowest anxiety possible*) to 10 (*highest anxiety possible*). Goals should be somewhere in the 6-to-9 range to be considered worthwhile. If goals fall below or above that range, they should be altered to place them in this range. When evaluating to ensure data are accurate, therapists should be mindful that cultural variations may exist in expressiveness and scaling.

Task: Inoculate

Inoculation (Whittingham, 2015) is a technique specific to FBGT that involves prophylactically predicting into and preventing group member self-sabotage based on the challenges of each particular interpersonal style. It is a specific technique within goal formulation that cuts across all the working alliance categories because it involves using the working alliance to develop a matched bond while developing goal agreement and task agreement on how to prevent self-sabotage. After the self-sabotage has been predicted, the therapist alerts the client—in a nonshaming way—to the typical pathway of self-sabotage. They then offer that group member an opportunity to practice entering the group in a different way that may provide a more successful strategy to prevent rejection. By forming goals that both prevent the self-sabotage—for example, suggesting holding back from criticizing others and also suggesting different, more adaptive behaviors, such as encouraging others—the client has the incentive to move toward a different way of relating.

Based on my clinical observations, early FBGT findings and cases showed a pattern related to two specific scales: that clients who are initially overly aggressive or overly self-disclosing sabotage themselves and frequently the whole group. This pattern is consistent with the literature that stated that clients who are early provocateurs or highly aggressive tend to have poorer outcomes; thus, the therapist must carefully consider how to manage these potential problems using the FBGT inoculation technique when preparing the client for group therapy (Baker et al., 2013).

Consider the following two examples: A client with a style high on Scale 2: Focused on the Needs of the Self is asked to introduce themselves at the beginning of Session 1. They listen to the other introductions before announcing that they are not sure they want to "hang out with such a bunch of losers and pathetic weaklings" and are considering leaving the group. They fold their arms and watch as other group members react in stunned silence.

A client with a style high on Scale 8: Uninhibited watches two members introduce themselves for 2 minutes each, give their names, describe where they work, and state how they are feeling about starting group. They begin their introduction by taking 15 minutes, rapidly shifting from topic to topic, including graphic details about their sex life, mentioning that they used to self-harm and once tried to kill themselves, and telling the group they want to become close friends with everyone after the group is over. They finish by asking the group leader if it is okay for group members to date.

As can be seen from these two disguised case examples, clients with these styles often launch into their scale distress immediately. Remember the maxim that people go their highest score of interpersonal style under stress.

The beginning of a group is a highly activating and anxiety-provoking situation, and, under these circumstances, clients act in ways that are a heightened version of their interpersonal style. To achieve a feeling of safety, the client with the Focused on the Needs of Self style (Scale 2) attempts to assert control by doing what they know how to do very well: Denigrate others. The client with distress related to the Uninhibited (Scale 8) style attempts to manage their anxiety about rejection by overdisclosing and being overly intrusive of others. Clients with distress on Scales 1 (Highly Assertive), 2 (Focused on the Needs of the Self), and 8 (Uninhibited) typically need some form of inoculation; otherwise, they self-sabotage and can also cause other group members to leave, which is highly impactful on the group.

In the example involving the client with a style high on Scale 2 who made their announcement, the members were shocked, saddened, angry, and hurt within the first 20 minutes of group. Unless the group leader manages that situation well, the group may devolve into either sullen silence (the complementary stance) or angry retribution. However, because that announcement occurred so early in the life of the group without an opportunity for group members to have cohered, the impact on overall feelings of cohesion can be profound. The client may choose to leave and not return, which affects the entire group, and, when that group member returns, they experience the group as having rejected them—providing them with further evidence that the world is rejecting and is not to be trusted. Similarly, group members may flee from the client in the second example who overdisclosed and was unboundaried. The nature of that client's sharing can frighten and overwhelm the new group members. The expectation that other group members may have to disclose at a similar level may serve to overwhelm new group members, and the fear that the group boundaries may not be clear and might involve dating may lead them to leave. The result is a breakdown in the group. And, when the group reconvenes, the client lapses into shame because they realize they have again been rejected despite their best efforts to connect.

An inoculation occurs when the therapist shows the client their IIP-32 profile and describes how a typical social interaction might unfold for someone with this profile. Care must be taken by the therapist throughout the inoculation to emphasize the strengths of the interpersonal style and its overall benefits. The message should always be that the client's personality has strengths and that every strategy they have tried up until now made sense. The therapist then discusses with the client how others with this profile sometimes self-sabotage. They invite the client to consider if this is also something they may do. Next, the therapist presents the client with a chance to adjust their approach for this group and to have a different and more successful experience entering the group.

Given that clients with styles as described in the preceding two examples are most likely to self-sabotage immediately, waiting for the event to occur and then processing can place too much stress on groups that have not yet cohered. Regardless of how the group leader intervenes, the damage has often been done. Clients who are inoculated eventually show those same behaviors, but by the time they do, group cohesion has sufficiently occurred that members can tolerate the invitations and are more helpful to the client, albeit often with the group leader's help.

CASE EXAMPLE: INOCULATION OF CLIENT WITH DISTRESS (SCALE 8)

Consider this case example that shows an inoculation of a person with distress related to being Scale 8: Uninhibited:

The group leader (i.e., the therapist) has already been in the group meeting for 5 minutes and has been asked about their marital status and where they like to go for coffee after work. The leader deflects both comments. The client doing the asking has behaved in an overly disclosing way by using humor and storytelling to hook the therapist into feeling entertained but somewhat wary about boundaries. The leader notes feeling hooked and uses this as concurring evidence when combined with the client's high Scale 8: Uninhibited profile to strengthen belief that the initial hypothesis is correct.

The client notes being an "Irish American" as a diversity variable that is salient, but when the group leader asks the client for more information, the client reports it does not really impact their life except "on St. Patrick's Day, when I dress up as a sexy green leprechaun!" The leader notices their own emotional reactions to this statement as being a mixture of a desire to laugh and a sense of discomfort that the client has been so overtly sexual in their reply. They also note that their feeling a lack of boundaries and being entertained lends support to the idea that the client's Uninhibited distress score may be a style.

The group leader decides to inquire more about the client's interpersonal history and discovers a long history of problems in relationships. The client reports feeling lonely and depressed but with intermittent intense but short-lived relationships. The client states this has happened across time and contexts and is consistent in their life. A discussion continues:

GROUP LEADER: So, it seems like you have been pretty lonely, and I can see that these intense relationships forming and then ending quickly are leaving you feeling really worried about the future.

CLIENT: Yes, it just keeps happening. I can't figure it out.

GROUP LEADER: Well, how about we look at this assessment tool, and let's see if it helps shed any light. (*Leader shows client the IIP-32 interpersonal circumplex shape with scores mapped out.*) People with this high 8 profile can be described as "Uninhibited." They are often described as leaders and as warm, friendly people. They tend to be curious about others and love closeness and feeling connected. (*Leader then focuses on strengths.*) They are also often quite charismatic. (*Leader checks in to confirm.*) Does that sound like you?

CLIENT: Yes, I love to be around people, and I like to lead. I think I am really fun and good to know, but things always start well and then just blow up, and I never hear from people again. I have had so many relationships that start with blazing passion, and it's like our souls were meant to be together. For 2 weeks, we are together night and day. Then they just drop me. It is so disheartening.

GROUP LEADER: Hmm, that sounds familiar. People with scores high on this scale are really great people to know. They have qualities like you and really enjoy closeness and intimacy. However, sometimes that desire for closeness can really build up, and so when they finally meet people, they can want to get close really quickly.

CLIENT: So, you are saying that they want to dive into the deep end straight away. That sounds like me. But what is wrong with that?

GROUP LEADER: Yes. Because they want to feel connected, they sometimes rush things a little. It is like they want to start the book at the last chapter and get to that good ending, where everything feels complete. However, this is sometimes a little too quick for other people, and it can have the opposite reaction than what is intended. Sometimes people feel overwhelmed and run away. Is it possible that sometimes this is what happens to you? [Here, the therapist offers a hypothesis based on typical elements of Scale 8 distress while leaving an option for the client to disagree.]

CLIENT: Wow! Maybe that is true. . . . (*Pauses to think.*) Maybe I do push too hard! Wait, though. Does that mean this is all my fault? [Client has rapid movement to insight followed by immediate worries about self-blame.]

GROUP LEADER: No, you were just doing your best to develop close relationships. You have always done your best to connect as best you know how. The intent was great. You just might be going a little too fast too soon. This is just about tweaking some behavior to get what you want, not changing who you are. Who you are is great! I wonder if we can slow you down a little, though, so you give a relationship room to develop. [Here, the therapist reframes self-blame and moves conceptualization toward behavior. Intent and personality are separated from behaviors.]

CLIENT: Like starting at Chapter 1? [Client begins to understand the task.]

GROUP LEADER: Yes. Let's try it with this group. Maybe we can make some goals. How about if you only disclosed about as much as the middle most disclosing person in the group? Only speak as long as they do and only go as deep in terms of content as they do. [The therapist now connects goal agreement and task agreement.]

CLIENT: That will be hard! [Here, the client correctly identifies anxiety that accompanies this change.]

GROUP LEADER: Yes, it will. You will feel anxious and uncomfortable. However, I think you will get to experience a group differently. You will have the opportunity to build relationships where people don't feel overwhelmed at the beginning and eventually get to know the deeper parts of you at a pace they can handle. On a scale of 1 to 10, where 1 is *easy* and 10 is *impossible*, how would you rank the anxiety that goes with this? [Here, the therapist validates anxiety and reframes, then checks scaling of anxiety.]

CLIENT: It sounds tough, but I do want to connect better. It will probably be an 8 at least. I want to give it a try, though.

GROUP LEADER: So, that is a good goal. If it were too easy, it wouldn't be meaningful to you. Anxiety normally accompanies any change we try. I think this really is a chance to let people get to know you so you can get what you deserve: meaningful relationships and connection. You have a lot to offer people as a friend, and I think this will help others have a chance to get to know and appreciate how much you have to give. [The therapist validates the anxiety and reframes as functional to change and returns to strengths and validation of the client's core self.]

In this case example, the group leader is always strengths based. The client is moving through awareness to insight rapidly, and the potential for shame and guilt is considerable. The therapist also maintains awareness of client anxiety and addresses each concern. The therapist avoids blame, shame, and guilt but, rather, moves toward solutions that are based on maintaining the ability to stay rooted in preexisting strengths and only adding behaviors as options to use.

The focus on strengths and validation of the person's core personality is an essential component of the approach and should not be underestimated. The consistent focus on strengths throughout the therapy, but particularly during the bookends—TPS and debriefing—is essential in keeping a client adhered to a stable sense of identity that is consistent with who they are. The behavioral change they are attempting is merely a means to be flexible around that central theme so they have more choice. It is not the intent of the therapy for the client to become a different person or for them to twist themself into a knot to appease other people. Rather, FBGT is a method to help a client meet their own life goals and needs by having a greater range of choices in how they want to act in any given situation. In many cases, they hold on to strategies that were previously working. However, if the client perceives that they are not getting the outcomes they are seeking—for example, connection to a loved one or the ability to assert themselves at work—then FBGT offers a new range of behavioral options.

As illustrated in this case example, inoculation should not be underestimated as a strategy. If clients with a high Scale 2 or Scale 8 score in particular are left to their own devices, they often self-sabotage, and the group sometimes collapses around them. This intervention was a key development in the evolution of FBGT and, in my clinical observations, has resulted in reduced dropout and improved outcomes. The next case example describes how the therapist assesses the client's motivation for treatment.

CASE EXAMPLE: ASSESSMENT OF CLIENT MOTIVATION FOR TREATMENT

When formulating treatment approaches, motivation for treatment is a key variable for the therapist to consider because it is highly predictive of poor outcomes. Therefore, as this case example illustrates, the therapist must carefully assess the client's motivation by paying attention to their scores on the GTQ-S:

> The therapist reviews the case formulation and tentative hypothesis (see Figure 6.1). They notice that the client is someone whom they are hypothesizing is high on Scale 4: Socially Inhibited. The therapist makes note that if this is the case, then they may have feelings of wanting to dominate and be warm because this would be the hooked response to that style. The therapist also notes that because the client is high in social inhibition, their natural response to someone else's quietness and distance is to sit in silence and wait. Given the amount of work necessary in the session, the therapist decides that this stance would be unhelpful. They instead decide to unhook and become slightly more directive while exhibiting warmth—the acomplementary stance.

FIGURE 6.1. Case Example: The Interpersonal Circumplex Showing High Distress on Scale 4

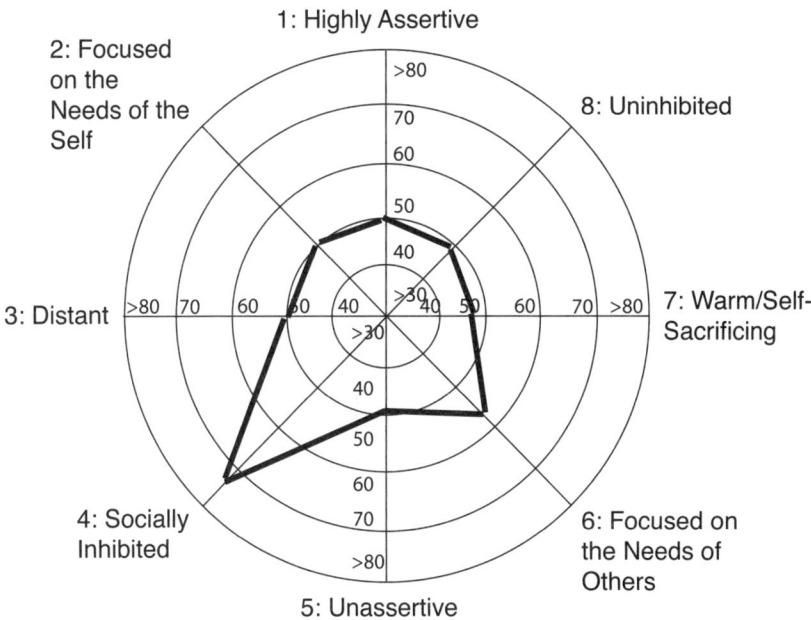

Note. Adapted from the manual for the Inventory of Interpersonal Problems by special permission of the Publisher, Mind Garden, Inc. Further reproduction requires the Publisher's written consent. Copyright © 2000 by Leonard M. Horowitz, Lynn E. Alden, Jerry S. Wiggins, & Aaron L. Pincus. All rights reserved in all media. Published by Mind Garden, Inc., www.mindgarden.com

Although this is an interpersonal stretch for the therapist, they work on remaining directive and warm throughout the session.

The therapist also notes that the client is low in motivation on their GTQ-S. This is common with people with high scores on Scale 4 because the group represents an aversive stimuli: Being judged and rejected by people is a major source of their anxiety. The therapist notes that they expect the client will be hesitant about joining group, so the therapist may need to move toward warm assertiveness when recommending group therapy.

Failure to pay attention to this score can lead to group member attrition at any stage of the group, and, in brief groups, member premature dropout can be devastating to group morale. However, motivation is a malleable construct within FBGT. Many clients enter the TPS session with low motivation, and some scales in particular, such as Scale 4: Socially Inhibited, commonly report low motivation. Clients may be low in motivation for many reasons. Few clients have good information about group therapy before joining groups. They may perceive it as seen on television: as a group of people shouting at each other or as a source of comedy with few good outcomes. Equally, some clients' interpersonal styles may be antithetical to a desire to join groups. Clients with high 4 social inhibition experience increases in anxiety around groups of people, so they typically want to avoid exposure to this feared stimulus. Clients with scores high on Scale 3: Distant experience closeness as toxic and threatening, so they find the notion of group equally concerning, albeit for different reasons.

Further, some clients may seem motivated but are quite ambivalent. For example, clients with scores high on Scale 6: Focused on the Needs of Others may want to please the therapist by expressing enthusiasm, but they retain considerable concern that this may be another group of people they look after without receiving reciprocal help from them. Therefore, they may be highly conflicted about joining but hide this concern from the therapist.

Motivation may also be linked to myths about group therapy. These myths include that group is not as effective as individual therapy; joining a group means having to share one's deepest fears, feelings, and memories; group members gang up on and attack each other; and there is not enough time to get one's own needs met. These fears and concerns need addressing. Research has shown that group therapy is, on aggregate, as effective as individual therapy (Burlingame & Strauss, 2021). Group members need reassuring that they only have to share what they are comfortable with and at their own pace; that conflict may be present, but the group leader helps manage and make sense of it so that the group is productive; that the leader does not allow scapegoating to take place; and that time is available to work on issues—but within a set of realistic parameters. As clients identify worries, the therapist should take time to reassure and counter those worries. The therapist can direct clients to view online videos that show examples of members enjoying group (e.g., CAPSBoulder, 2012), can provide positive images of group therapy, and can also explain how to make groups work for the client.

Motivation can also be impacted by outside, logistical issues. To be clear, therapists should not allow clients into the group who plan to arrive late or leave early for sessions, nor should they allow clients to attend intermittently. Clients who do so create a problematic and fractured group dynamic that can significantly interfere with process in this short-term format. In some cases, logistical concerns can signal a deeper process taking place, and clinicians should be aware of possible secondary motivations—for example, fear of the group or desire for more attention from the therapist—as possible reasons for stating logistical roadblocks.

Motivation also can be affected by the successful application of skills in this chapter and those discussed in Chapter 4. However, if motivation was low at the beginning of the session, it is vital to reassess if it has changed at the end. If not, and the client insists they "may come to a few sessions but likely will not stay for long," then the therapist should consider referral elsewhere. Motivation to join an FBGT group can be improved by strengthening the working alliance. Work on improving the factors involved in that alliance—bond, goal agreement, and task agreement—can result in increased expectancy of improvement, a factor also linked to outcome (Abouguendia et al., 2004).

CASE EXAMPLE: FORMATION OF THE WORKING ALLIANCE

As explained in this chapter, the various strands of the TPS session coalesce to form the working alliance. This case example illustrates how these strands come together:

> The client enters, and the therapist immediately feels the client bringing a quiet, humble energy into the room. The therapist notices that the client is not making eye contact and is looking anxious and somewhat embarrassed. The therapist feels an urge to reassure them. Remembering that a warm and directive stance is helpful and acomplementary, the therapist smiles and invites the client to sit down.

As can be seen from this example, the therapist has first noticed their own interpersonal style and then calculated what the hooked and unhooked positions are. The therapist is then ready for the client's arrival and also moves to a *beginner's mind*, which, in FBGT, involves being in a place in which they let go of the hypothesis and notice how they are feeling as a way to understand the client's impact on them that might confirm or disconfirm on the hypothesis. If the client arrives in a flurry of drama, compliments, and warmth, leaving the therapist overwhelmed, then the therapist may decide to seriously question their hypothesis because that style is far more characteristic of being hooked by the high 8 profile. Cases like that are rare in which a client incorrectly fills out a form, or the therapist discovers that the hypothesis needs significant revision and that the causes of the client's distress emanate from a different source, such as a highly mandating context (e.g., working in a toxic work environment where coworkers with an agenda are seeking to discredit the client with falsehoods). When that happens, the therapist meets the unhooked stance in subtle ways. They smile and are somewhat directive, inviting the client to have a seat. This sets the tone for the energy and feel of the session: that it will be warm but purposeful and have elements of directiveness.

The TPS session continues:

> The therapist begins by asking the client what brings them into therapy. The client mentions feeling unhappy and depressed but is vague and does not specify the reasons. The therapist leads the conversation into what areas of the client's life are causing them the most problems. The therapist shows the client the GTQ-S in which the client has indicated problems with their work and home life relationships. The therapist asks them to explain how this is causing them distress. The client says they are unhappy at work and at home, reporting that they feel pressured at work to socialize, which is making them feel uncomfortable, and they want to leave. They also report that someone at work has been asking them to go on a romantic date, and they are having difficulty saying no, even though they are not entirely interested. They also state that their parents are putting pressure on them to go on dates and to leave home. The client reports feeling angry and upset with their parents.

As can be seen, the client is validating some of what the assessments have already revealed. The therapist is finding information that confirms the working hypothesis.

The therapist then considers how the assessment findings tie together with the diversity information:

> The therapist asks about the client's diversity variables in reference to the dating: "Tell me a little more about the identity variables you wrote down in the GTQ-S. You mentioned that your identity as asexual is important. Can you tell me more about how?" The client responds that they have never had interest in anyone romantically and seldom, if ever, feel attracted to anyone. They also state that they are very shy and are worried about getting into a relationship, which they find to be very anxiety provoking. They share that it is possible they may want a romantic relationship one day but feel ambivalent about the romantic interest. They note that they have a very low libido and no interest in sex, and so they are worried about disappointing the person who is interested in them.
>
> The therapist and client discuss this further, and the client notes that they feel "fluid" in terms of their romantic and sexual interest. They state they would like to see if they feel different once they work on their social inhibition. The therapist affirms the validity and value of all identities and possible outcomes and agrees to go on that journey with the client.

As illustrated here, the therapist is open to the client's explanation of their identity and is listening to how this client defines it. This client has indicated a slight interest in a romantic relationship but has real fears that their lack of libido will disappoint the potential romantic partner sexually. The therapist remains open to what feels right for the client in terms of their definition of themselves. The therapist also notes that once the course of FBGT is over, they might discuss with the client whether the client would be open to following up with a clinician who can work with the client individually on issues that address sexuality identity more directly and in more depth.

Remember: FBGT is not a panacea. For some identity issues, a more in-depth approach is needed, either instead of, or adjunctively to, FBGT. Therapists should discuss this topic carefully with each client, listening to their wishes and preferences, as this therapist does in this case example:

> The therapist invites the client to share about their family. The client describes that life is very unhappy at home. The client notes that everyone in the family is very "typically Latinx—real, expressive, loving, connected, and fun." They note that they feel proud of their heritage and love their identity, but, at times, they feel disconnected from their family because they are very shy. The client reports good relationships with the family individually; however, when in a group, they find the family overwhelming. The client also notes that their mother and father have been pressuring them to leave and also to go on dates and eventually get married.

Here, the therapist listens carefully and notes that the client is proud of their ethnic heritage and that this is an important part of their identity. The therapist also notes their own ethnic identity—as an Asian American—means that the client may or may not feel connected to them. The therapist also notes that their own interpersonal style—as someone who prefers to be warm—means that maintaining that warm style is a good acomplementary fit to the client's inhibition style. The therapist observes that although they identify as heterosexual, they feel comfortable discussing issues around fluid identities because they spent time exploring this topic professionally via workshops and reading and spending considerable time working as an ally and advocate to clients with similar identities.

The therapist also notes a disconnect in terms of the client's trait-level personality style and what the client has reported is culturally normative for their Latinx family. Thus, within-group and between-group interactions are important to consider. The therapist then presents data to the client, showing the client the IIP-32 and indicating the peaks on Scales 3 and 4:

> Listening to you telling me about your relationships, I heard you say several times that you were shy and anxious. (*The therapist points to the IIP-32 profile.*) This profile we made from the form you filled out before really shows that. People who are high on Scale 4 sometimes call themselves socially inhibited or shy. People who are shy are often thoughtful, analyze what goes on around them very well, and think deeply about the world. They tend to be people who prefer one-on-one interactions rather than big groups but can be great friends if they can take time to step back and recharge after intense interactions. Does that sound like you?

In FBGT, the collaborative discussion always begins with strengths and validation. This approach allows the client to reflect on their strengths, keep the problems in perspective, and to see that the therapist views them as more than the sum of their problems, thus strengthening the trust and bond. Continuing with the TPS session,

> the client replies to the therapist's question ("Does that sound like you?") that this is true. The therapist then takes an interpersonal inventory—asks about the client's past and current history of relationships in different contexts, such as romantic, work, and family—to check in to see if this has always been the case across the client's life (trait) and across situations and contexts in the present (trait plus person–environment fit). The client replies that they have always struggled with shyness in all contexts in their life and across their lifetime, but that recently, the demands to go out more in a group have meant that they are feeling more upset and worried.
>
> When shown the 30-item Outcome Questionnaire (Ellsworth et al., 2006) score and asked if the client feels that the interpersonal problems and the overall life distress are connected, they reply that, yes, they are. They look thoughtful and state that this has been a worry for a long time. The therapist considers the nuances between identity and interpersonal style and notes that the interplay between identity and interpersonal style is complex and nuanced.

Here, the therapist uses the interpersonal inventory to determine collaboratively with the client that social inhibition is a style that is rigid and somewhat extreme for them. The therapist notes that the client's cultural identity as Latinx is important to them and that their sexual identity is asexual but possibly fluid. The therapist works to respect the client's culture and identity while working on developing a formulation that will be helpful to the client.

The therapist then narrows the focus to establish appropriate goals:

> They show the IIP-32 to the client again and say, "There are lots of strengths to people high on social inhibition, but some people also report that they find it difficult to form close relationships. Some people say it is tricky initiating relationships, while others say it is hard deepening them. Some have trouble with both. Does that apply to you, and if so, how?
>
> The client replies that they are okay with initiating relationships but have the most problems with maintaining or deepening conversations, which leaves them feeling awkward and boring. The therapist asks whether being able to perform this skill would make a difference to their lives. The client replies that it would make a "huge difference" because they are struggling to form the kind of connections that they want.

This is a key question in FBGT—whether a goal would make a difference—because the question and goal are narrowed sufficiently to be operationalizable, and the client is able to determine whether the goal is worthwhile. This goal agreement is crucial to the success of the group. To quote Yalom (Yalom & Leszcz, 2020) in describing brief group therapy, "Nothing will so inevitably ensure failure as inappropriate goals" (p. 477). This is certainly the case with FBGT. Accurate goal selection in FBGT makes the difference between a successful and unsuccessful experience. Incorrectly selected or incorrectly calibrated goals can set clients up for failure, fail to challenge them, or push them into fight, flight, or freeze mode as they overreach.

The therapist now works with the client on MATH goals:

The client settles on several goals in collaboration with the therapist. They choose these:

- asking follow-up questions to other group members at least three times during the life of the group

- coming to every session, even if feeling anxious or disinclined to do so (the inoculation)

- sharing personal information about themselves at least twice during the group

- nodding and giving nonverbal affirmations to others when they need support at least three times

Each component must be present for the goal to be successful. Calibration of goals can be altered by the number of times a goal should be attempted or by redesigning the goal to be more meaningful. Adjusting the number of times a goal should be attempted needs to be conducted thoughtfully to make sure that committed clients do not overcommit to unrealistic numbers in attempting to accomplish goals. Setting a goal as being at most three times during the life of the group is sufficient. If the client attempts a goal five times a session, doing so overtakes the natural flow of the group because people are forcing issues that can happen more organically. If the client succeeds in more than three attempts, that may be helpful, but success should not be predicated on accomplishment of excessive goals.

Even for the most committed person to grow, the life of the group may overtake their ambitions. They may well accomplish their goals twice and meaningfully, but if the events in the group call for different responses, and the person does not manage the five attempts they set, then they may experience what they did as failure rather than as the success that it was.

Calibration of goals should also be thoughtful in terms of breaking down components of behavior. For example, as in the prior case example, is a client skilled at deepening relationships or initiating them? Clinical observations have shown that some clients can be highly skilled in one but not in the other. Both social skills can lead to dissatisfaction with relationships, but each is a different skill set and has different consequences. It is interesting that sometimes even highly socially skilled people can have difficulty with an aspect of social skills. In a sense, it could be argued that people have social skills that resemble Swiss cheese: Even though they may be highly skilled in certain areas, the holes sometimes appear in unexpected places. These holes need careful consideration and exploration because understanding the exact issue can make a difference between a goal rated as boring and easy or as highly challenging. For example, a client may be highly effective at deepening relationships one-on-one but completely lost as to how to initiate new friendships. This reliance on others to initiate contact may leave the person struggling in situations in which superficial social fluency is required when moving to a new workplace or living place.

OTHER IMPORTANT TPS TASKS

The prior TPS tasks are highly specific to FBGT. However, some other, less model-specific but nevertheless important tasks also need to take place in FBGT. These are discussions based on ethical imperatives (i.e., confidentiality and informed consent), the need to sometimes address myths about group, and important practical discussions about group scheduling (i.e., management of logistics).

Task: Explain Confidentiality

Clients should sign a form explaining confidentiality and be able to discuss it in session. In the United States, confidentiality laws vary by state. For example, at the time of this writing, in the District of Columbia (which contains the city of Washington), the laws state that both therapists *and* clients may not breach confidentiality of any group member. In other states, therapists legally must protect confidentiality, but clients are not breaking any laws if they breach the confidentiality of other group members.

Clients should understand state laws as they apply. However, even in the absence of laws regulating clients who breach the confidentiality of other members, a discussion should still take place, outlining that this action is prohibited and spelling out the consequences of doing so (up to and including possible expulsion from the group).

Task: Obtain Informed Consent

Informed consent should also be discussed in the TPS session. This means the client should be made aware of possible gains and potential harm that could be involved. This discussion is a key part of how FBGT differs from some group models. It foreshadows the idea that when developing goals, growth is possible. FBGT also explains that growth is uncomfortable and that feelings of discomfort when attempting new things can often be a sign of growth. However, FBGT does not shy away from the possibility that some changes may bring about difficulty in a person's life. For example, if someone becomes more assertive with a friend, there are no guarantees that the friendship will survive. Equally, if someone becomes more friendly at work, there is no guarantee that they will not be taken advantage of.

The concept of choice in making changes and consideration of the contexts and places in which change will be most effective are important parts of FBGT. Client autonomy is key in decision making, but it must be informed decision making. FBGT therapists must, for example, point out that once someone with a high score on Scale 6: Focused on the Needs of Others begins to ask for help from others or refuses to offer help when it does not suit them, there is a possibility that some people in their social sphere may be so shocked and upset by the change that the friendship is ended. If the relationship is entirely one way, then this may not be a bad thing, but this is for the client to decide on an individual basis. They must weigh the possible good—feeling less resentful, being able to advocate for themselves, and being able to seek out new relationships with new ground rules related to reciprocity—against the consequences of possible loneliness or negative feedback from existing people in their life who do not want an equal relationship.

Systems are homeostatic, and although, in some cases, change may be positive and also maintain existing relationships, there is no guarantee that this will be the case. The client must understand that sometimes achieving gains on one side of the equation can involve losses on the other. The therapist should also emphasize the importance of selecting the places where change should take place. In some places, existing strategies are left intact (e.g., when they are already working, or when the client is unwilling to accept the consequences of change). However, the client and therapist should also work on selecting places where the new techniques might be successful and ensure that they are well practiced in this environment.

Task: Deconstruct Myths

Whether from watching television comedies that parody group therapy as people mocking each other or constantly engaging in conflict or just from imagining what a group might be like, people often engage in fantasies about group therapy that involve their worst imaginings. Dispelling or reframing these myths can be important. Group leaders should ask group members if they have any concerns or worries when they think about a group. For example, some may have concerns about the presence of uncontrolled and extreme conflict. The therapist can share that although conflict may take place, they will not allow it to devolve into a shouting match or insults, a message that can be important for some clients to hear. The therapist should be ready to explain that some difficult moments may arise, but those moments can be productive, and the group leader will help contain them and help the group work through them.

Other group members may have concerns related to feeling that others will like or not like them based on identity variables, concerns that they will be the only ones who are suffering and who have "problems," or concerns that the group will reject them. A powerful salve is reassuring the client that group therapy is a place in which people come with strengths and struggles and that finding connections is one of the most enjoyable and surprising things about group therapy. The therapist also should carefully discuss the presence of diversity variables in the group. Although they cannot share diversity information about other group members (unless a member has expressly given their consent to do so), the group leader can reassure the client that diversity and identity discussions are important to the work of the group. In some cases, the client may also choose to work identity into a goal, should they desire to do so. For example, sharing about themselves and their identity and asserting themselves if they feel that a microaggression has taken place are just two examples of how to weave identity into interpersonal goals.

Task: Engage in Logistics Discussions

Other clients may have concerns about logistics, including time, date, when to arrive, when and what (and importantly why) assessments are to be completed, and what happens if a session needs to be missed (e.g., because of a medical appointment or wedding). The therapist should spell these logistics out clearly so that the client understands the boundaries of the group. Typically, clients are encouraged to let the therapist know ahead of time if they have an emergency or anticipate a single event (e.g., a wedding) that will result in a missed session. Longer discussions, though, are needed if the client is unable to consistently arrive and leave at the required time, or if they plan on missing multiple sessions.

Equally, given the group's brief duration, it is advised that members begin and end together rather than enter in a "rolling" fashion, which entails a constant reset of the group dynamic. Consequently, cohesion needs to be reestablished, and content that is the proviso of veteran members is unknown to the new member, leading to them feeling left out or unsure of how to move among a preformed cohesive group. Introducing new members can be a significant benefit of long-term groups; however, doing so in a brief group is generally not advised unless there is a compelling reason to do so. For example, introducing someone with a very different interpersonal style into a group that is interpersonally homogenous can, in some cases, offer new energy and modeling of behaviors that otherwise were missing.

REFERRING ELSEWHERE

In the event that the client is not an appropriate referral, it is important to ensure the therapist handles this situation carefully, keeping the client's well-being upmost in mind. Inappropriate referrals may involve different combinations of client and therapist willingness—for example, the client's refusal to join when the therapist thinks it is a good referral or the therapist's deeming that FBGT is not a good fit, but the client wishes to join the group. The TPS session often resolves disagreement because it is designed to anticipate resistance to treatment and to work on motivation. However, in some cases, the differences are not resolved, and referral elsewhere becomes an important consideration based on the therapist's clinical judgment that is informed by the client's preferences.

When the client is unwilling to join and the therapist's attempts to build a working alliance are unsuccessful, then the decision is clearer. Without some degree of goal and task agreement, treatment is unlikely to be successful. Referral in this case should encompass client preferences for treatment. Take this example: A client is unmotivated to join a group, and despite the therapist's best efforts to develop a working alliance during a lengthy TPS session, the client insists they would prefer cognitive behavior therapy on an individual basis. The therapist assesses that their own style, Distant (Scale 3), is one that may respond well to less interpersonally activating approaches, so the therapist agrees.

If the client wants to join, but the therapist has a strong reason for exclusion, then framing of the referral is crucial. Consider this example: The therapist listens to the client discussing a history of being racist and engaging in conflict with people from minority groups. The client has little insight that this behavior is problematic. The group comprises members from minority groups, some of whom have expressed considerable anxiety around feeling safe in the group. The therapist gauges that the client is not sufficiently aware to manage their feelings and is also unlikely to respond to leader interventions. The therapist also considers that the damage to the group may be considerable and likely will result in member dropout and client worsening. So, discussion needs to take place around the need for the therapist to provide the best possible care to the client. For example, framing it as caring enough about the client's well-being to make sure they get the exact treatment they need can be helpful in mitigating feelings of rejection. A metaphor often used in this discussion is that the doctor initially needs to assess which medication is the correct one, and, as new information arises, the doctor may switch treatment to ensure the patient is really getting well. The focus is looking after the client's welfare. In many cases, with sufficient discussion between client and therapist, they will mutually agree on the realization that another form of treatment is preferable.

In other cases, a client may be motivated to join group but is unlikely to succeed in the group. Take this example: A client explains that they are excited for group and wants to join, but they state they can only attend every other session for logistical reasons. Because the infrequent attendance impacts the group dynamic and its stages of development, the therapist should refer the client elsewhere and explain the reasons. Clients who are referred elsewhere often experience this referral as a rejection and may experience deleterious consequences to their self-esteem and sense of self-worth. For those with anxious attachment styles, this referral elsewhere is felt keenly because rejection sensitivity is already heightened (Set, 2019).

The experience of rejection is why preparing referral sources correctly is vital. Ideally, incorrect referrals are not made in the first place because managing them in the TPS session becomes a fraught process for clients. However, when referral elsewhere is in the best interest of the client and the group, the therapist should do it only after careful consideration. The therapist must consider whether the client can be successful in the group but must also balance harm to the other group members. In most cases, the therapist should seek to include rather than exclude; however, when it is clear that the client is either being set up to fail or will prove damaging to the group, referral out is necessary. For example, while clients with scores high on Scale 2: Focused on the Needs of the Self can be appropriate referrals, those with that score and who also diagnosed with antisocial personality disorder in the severe range need referral elsewhere. They may well use the group to manipulate others to meet their own needs and either carelessly or intentionally inflict harm and distress. The therapist should consider that a client with this profile is unlikely to achieve anything from the group and also has a strong likelihood of causing distress and damage to other group members. The therapist must therefore judge whether the client can be successful and whether the group will be harmed.

SUMMARY

The TPS session involves building a strong working alliance. Bond, task, and goal agreement are essential components of treatment. Goals should follow the MATH format and involve movement on the quarter turn on the interpersonal circumplex. Multicultural data should be woven into conceptualizations of interpersonal distress, and goals should be adapted while bearing in mind salient data. Careful calibration of goals is also needed to maintain optimal levels of anxiety that promote social learning.

Inoculation, a key technique, is used to prevent client self-sabotage and is particularly important for clients with distress on Scales 1, 2, and 8 because they have a higher likelihood of dropping out of therapy or having poor outcomes. Therapists must retain a flexible interpersonal stance and use assessment data and self-monitoring of internal reactions to client interpersonal invitations to notice if they are being hooked before they unhook to respond effectively.

Therapists need to handle client exclusion from group therapy in a way that communicates the need for the client to have the best treatment that is tailored to them. Initial reading of assessments before the TPS session can provide a preview that some clients may not be suitable for group therapy. Therefore, that initial reading allows therapist to frame from the beginning of the TPS session that the session is to assess what the best treatment is for the client.

7 LEADING THE FIRST TWO SESSIONS

The focused brief group therapy (FBGT) approach is designed to reduce inter-personal distress in eight or more sessions. This chapter describes Sessions 1 and 2. The first of the eight group therapy sessions is complex and requires a great deal of activity from the therapist to manage the many tasks involved. It is highly structured and uses several activities with specific therapeutic pur-poses, unlike later sessions during which the structure is kept fluid and min-imal. Session 1 also sets up the group for success by setting the therapeutic conditions, providing clear expectations, setting the tone, and providing norms. It is significantly different from all other sessions in terms of structure and level of activity.

Session 2 bridges between the highly structured nature of Session 1 and the move toward clients' working in a more organic way in the middle and later sessions. The purpose of Session 2 is to shape the group toward that work by both training them in techniques, such as feedback delivery, while also introducing and implementing here-and-now intervention.

https://doi.org/10.1037/0000389-008
Focused Brief Group Therapy: An Integrative Approach to Reducing Interpersonal Distress, by M. Whittingham

TURNING BOND INTO COHESION

The central, specific mechanism of change within the first two group sessions is to move the bond with the group leader—established during the therapy, pregroup preparation, and screening (TPS) session—into cohesion with the whole group. This is an evidence-based shift, and research has shown that the working alliance is an important prerequisite to group cohesion (Arnold, 2021) while also being predictive of outcome. The therapist must continue the alliance that was built during the TPS session by keeping a posture of unconditional positive regard and holding the boundaries and norms of the group while simultaneously beginning to build connections between group members.

Although the working alliance with the therapist remains a foundation throughout the life of the group, over time, group cohesion becomes the central vehicle for change. This is analogous to a band's beginning with a drumbeat, and then a bass guitar is added in as the song progresses. The drums remain ever present and can take over if the song falters. Gradually, though, the bass provides the energy for the song to move forward. Other instruments then add to the song, but the structure is still held by the drum and the bass. And so it is with FBGT. The working alliance should always be present—with the group leader maintaining positive regard and keeping the group aligned with the purpose of the group.

As discussed in the next chapter on leading the middle and later sessions, the therapist must also attend to alliance ruptures and other potentially harmful critical incidents that risk premature dropout or poor outcomes. Group members must trust the group leader and also the group to be helpful while seeing the group as the main place to practice change and receive feedback. Thus, the processes run parallel to each other and act synergistically.

GROUP COHESION AS A FOUNDATION FOR CHANGE

Cohesion in groups has been found to be particularly important to outcome in brief groups (Lorentzen et al., 2018). Remember that brief groups have little room for treatment failure. If someone drops out, not only do they experience a sense of demoralization and failure, but the group can become demoralized as well. In a long-term group, members have sufficient cohesion to absorb the occasional premature dropout, particularly if they are introduced on a rolling basis. However, brief groups can fall apart quickly if one or two members drop out in the early stages.

Cohesion is also a multilayered construct. Forsyth (2021) described several strands to cohesion, including attractiveness (i.e., Do members like each other, and are they friendly toward each other?); task commitment (i.e., Is the group unified around the task or tasks?); group structure (i.e., Do the group members understand and buy into the norms, procedures, and boundaries of the group, and is membership stable?); entitativity (i.e., Does the group sees itself as a unit with its own identity rather than as a set of individuals?), group affect (i.e., Does the group enjoy being with each other?), and social categorization (i.e., Do the members identify with the group?). These categories are salient and to be targeted in Session 1. Attractiveness is developed via dyads, human treasure hunt, and a reporting of interest in getting to know each other. Task commitment is engendered by commitment to goals and explanations about here-and-now process and feedback. Group structure is developed through discussion of group norms (e.g., attendance, timeliness, respect, listening). Group affect typically occurs during dyads, the human treasure hunt, and discussions following both. In a slower process that occurs over the life of the group, group categorization and entitativity tend to take place as a group member perceives universality and realize they are working together on accomplishing goals. Therefore, each task in FBGT is purposeful, no matter how trivial or playful it may appear to an uninformed viewer of the process.

Part of reinforcing the task agreement in the group is also letting the members know that Session 1 is more structured and less emotionally intense than the other sessions. Those group members who are eager to plunge into the depth of the work need this framing to understand the process. Remember that each interpersonal style carries with it a preference for how Session 1 will go. People with social inhibition prefer to be passive, people high in warmth want to immediately achieve liking and closeness, and those high in focus on the self want to find comfort and self-protection in asserting their dominance by attacking other members. Therefore, the structure of Session 1 becomes important. With careful structuring of the session, each member is placed in a position of optimal anxiety. Those high in assertiveness are not able to attack at will, those who are highly inhibited cannot hide because of the dyads and activities, and those seeking to focus only on others must also talk about themselves. The group is also placed in a position in which they must connect and cohere but cannot entirely rely on their preferred strategy. This structure provides the opportunity for both comfort and growth to occur simultaneously.

As the group leader nears achievement of group cohesion, their key goal is this: By the end of the first group, each member should be connected to at least one other member. This is the foundation of cohesion within FBGT. To track this goal, a group leader in FBGT may find it helpful to write down on a piece of paper the name of the group members in the order in which those members are seated. As the group progresses, the group leader can draw lines between the names of members, thus indicating cohesive connection (the leader can also draw these lines later if circumstances during the session make doing it then difficult).

The working alliance with the therapist should already be present because it was created during the TPS session. Further, the bond to the therapist should be strong, and goal agreement needs to be clear. The task agreement is slightly less clear to clients during the first two sessions, so the group leader must shape the group toward the task by using a combination of direct explanation of and redirection toward the work in addition to interventions that create the conditions for the work to take place.

TECHNIQUES FOR PROMOTING COHESION

In Session 1, the process of transitioning the bond with the therapist to cohesion with the group begins. It is a crucial shift. Throughout this session, the group leader is preparing the group to see itself—and not the therapist—as the main agent of change. Initial interventions are closely augmented by the therapist's nonverbal and verbal indications for members to look at and address each other rather than talk one-on-one only with the group leader. It is quite common in the first few moments of the group for the group members to address all their comments to the group leader and to ignore the other group members. Because the bond is with the leader, members fall into what Yalom and Leszcz (2020) described as a *spokes-in-wheel model* in which all activity takes place through the therapist. The therapist's role is to redirect activity toward the group. From the very beginning of the group, it is crucial that the leader encourage members to talk to and give eye contact to each other. Doing so sets the conditions and expectations for the group.

Observing members connecting over shared identity variables, common goals, shared personal information, or other perceived similarities are all significant indicators. However, the presence of a similarity is insufficient to be able to assume a connection; it is important to use nonverbal indicators of interest and warmth, verbal indicators of connection, or both, as well as clinical judgment. For example, someone may state that it is nice to see another person of the same ethnic identity in the group and looks at that person approvingly. However, it is a mistake to assume this feeling of connection is always reciprocated. Although in some cases, group members report a similar sense of relief, I have observed clinical examples in which members later stated that they felt concerned about being judged by someone from their same ethnic group or were concerned that a regional or other difference in identity (e.g., sexuality) might make them incompatible. Their identity variables were sources of both connection and potential disconnection.

Interpersonal connection and cohesion therefore need to be considered from the perspective of group identity memberships and also from the point of view of each individual and their multiple identities. This consideration allows the therapist to anticipate which members are disconnected and are therefore at greater risk of dropout. It is also vital that the therapist consider that members with different interpersonal styles have different ways of feeling connected to each other. For example, someone with a distant interpersonal style likely prefers dyads as a way of connecting and may find expressions of warmth from multiple members or the whole group as aversive. People with interpersonal styles that are warmer may prefer a strong, intimate, and expressive connection between members, whereas those with a more distant style may prefer relationships in which connection is unexpressed but is nevertheless present and "understood."

Equally, the therapist should carefully track whether the alliances that emerge are likely to become therapeutic or countertherapeutic. In many cases, alliances emerge that are helpful, such as when two group members work on goals together and engage in feedback loops (discussed further in Chapter 8). However, in some cases, members or even the whole group may also reactively protect each other from change. For example, groups comprising people with scores high in unassertiveness (Scale 5: Unassertive; see Figure 1.2 in Chapter 1) can sometimes covertly band together around small talk that is superficial and lacking depth. Alternatively, two members might form an alliance around resisting their goals of offering encouragement by disparaging the need for enacting the goal. Rather than work on the behavioral activation around that goal, which is likely to prove anxiety provoking and to risk being exploited for their vulnerability (which may have happened in their childhood), they instead band together to claim the goal was poorly selected or irrelevant. Attacking the goal (and therefore indirectly attacking the group leader) is a more comfortable position interpersonally because it is a familiar interpersonal strategy based on their typical style. It is, however, a defense against the work.

This kind of alliance is one that systems-centered group therapy (Agazarian, 2018) describes as *nonfunctional subgrouping*, which is when the subgroup stabilizes itself at the expense of change processes (Agazarian, 2011). The therapist must challenge this alliance carefully and also thoughtfully consider the timing of when to do so. In some cases, this alliance may require an immediate challenge, whereas in others, it may require the therapist to note it out loud while stating it is something to discuss as the group progresses. For example, the therapist might say,

> I can see that goal is challenging right now, and you are feeling ambivalent about it. Maybe that is something we can talk about more as the group continues. It could be a really helpful thing to explore why completing that goal might be challenging.

Thus, an understanding of cohesion requires not just a superficial read on the situation but also a nuanced analysis of the links among interpersonal style, multiple identities, and how alliances are formed.

CONFLICT AND EARLY CORRECTIVE FEEDBACK

As part of Session 1, the role of conflict and corrective feedback in FBGT also needs to be considered. Group therapy has been defined as progressing through group stages: Tuckman's model (Tuckman & Jensen, 2010) suggests that groups begin by forming (i.e., coming together and trying to understand each other and the work), storming (i.e., a period of conflict in which members establish status hierarchies), norming (i.e., group members agree on an established way of working), performing (i.e., members engage in change), and adjourning (i.e., members work through feelings around ending the group). Commentators and researchers on group stages have often bemoaned the lack of linear progression of these stages or that they do not follow the same pattern in every group (e.g., Brossart, 1996; Hurt, 2012). For example, some groups immediately move into storming and remain there, whereas others skip stages or move immediately into working.

Within FBGT, this variability is conceptualized as expected because the interpersonal dynamic of the group influences the progression through stages. For example, a group comprising people with scores high on assertiveness (Scale 1: Highly Assertive) and focused on self needs (Scale 2: Focused on the Needs of the Self) could fall into a group pattern of immediate conflict and may well remain there, alternating between attacking each other and sometimes the group leader. That level of conflict is actually a comfortable place for them to be. It is what they know how to do and perform well at. For another group with a large number of people who have problems around being too warm, the conflict stages may be skipped altogether, and they may move quickly to norming. In both cases, the group stage becomes locked into a place of comfort based on the homogeneity of the group and their preferred complementary interactions. In heterogenous groups, individuals or coalitions of individuals exert a similar influence. Session 1, which is marked by heightened anxiety for all, elicits people's highest interpersonal style, a place from which they derive comfort by virtue of its familiarity. Therefore, once the group leader understands the interpersonal styles, they can anticipate the group dynamics.

Therefore, the group leader's role in Session 1 is to provide structure and expectations around desired behaviors while promoting group cohesion. To promote cohesion, FBGT leaders do work to contain and manage early conflicts by using techniques to block and protect (Morran et al., 2004; Yalom & Leszcz, 2020). Brief groups work when members feel they can manage their anxiety to get the work done. Although members high in assertiveness (Scale 1: Highly Assertive and Scale 2: Focused on the Needs of the Self) might find comfort in early conflicts, those conflicts are overwhelming to other group members, particularly those with styles that find conflict difficult. Remember that polyvagal theory suggests that there is an optimal level of anxiety, which, if exceeded, pushes people into fight, flight, or freeze mode. Given that in Session 1, clients are already highly anxious because of the unfamiliarity of the situation, adding intense conflicts to it often pushes those who find conflict challenging into a level of distress such that they may contemplate not returning the next week.

The position of FBGT is that conflict is typically more helpful when trust has been established (Burlingame et al., 2018; Morran et al., 1998). An outcome of trust is the belief that people are giving you corrective feedback not to destroy or achieve power over you, but because they care about you and are trying to help you improve. Without the presence of cohesion, that trust is not present, and corrective feedback and intense conflicts can feel injurious to people's self-esteem. However, in some cases, local cultures may value intense corrective feedback.

Group leaders should be careful to assess how much conflict to allow. They also need to bear in mind that even if many group members favor conflict and pressure a group leader for more opportunities to engage in it, the leader must keep in mind the timing of that conflict, the impact of the conflict on all members (not just the majority), and that the purpose of early conflict is so important it cannot wait. Even in cultures that prize intense conflict and direct disagreement, the group leader should carefully consider the timing of that feedback and conflict. In running groups in cultures that strongly value corrective feedback, it is important for the group leader to note that there are still within-group differences. A culture that prizes corrective feedback still contains within it people who find too much conflict aversive or may leave the group if distress levels become too high.

Group leaders should also consider their own interpersonal and cultural preferences with respect to conflict. Their own interpersonal style may lead them to accept either higher or lower levels of conflict than are helpful to the group. For example, if the group leader enjoys intense conflict, then they may allow more of that conflict early in the life of the group, potentially creating a cohesion and working alliance issue with group members who find conflict aversive. Therefore, group leaders should consider a variety of factors when assessing intervening, including cultural norms, group membership goals, and their own interpersonal preferences around conflict and corrective feedback. Leaders may also find it helpful to use process measures, such as the Group Questionnaire (Krogel et al., 2013), to assess members' reactions to critical incidents, such as conflicts. Such measures enable the leader to assess the impact of conflicts with the group in real time while also being able to predict whether members are at risk of dropping out.

SESSION 1: KEY PROCESSES

Session 1 has several key processes that differentiate it from other sessions. Because it is far more structured, it demands that the group leader take control of pacing and tone. It is vital for the leader to explain this to the group and frame this session as an important introduction and as a "getting to know you" and "establishing norms" before the group becomes more free flowing. Several important tasks need to take place during Session 1.

Logistics

At the beginning of the first session, the group leader hands out cards (typically note cards) with preformed goals from the TPS session written on them. At the end of the session, the leader collects the note cards. This collection of cards is necessary because it is not uncommon for clients to forget their cards either because they are disorganized or because of unconscious resistance. The leader may also choose to let members keep the note cards or allow members to choose whether to keep them or hand them in. However, leaders should always have spare cards just in case.

For Session 1, as with any group, the group leader should first cover informed consent with confidentiality. Confidentiality discussions should include reference to state laws regarding whether only group leader or both group leaders and members are legally required to maintain confidentiality. The discussion should then move into talking about how to manage confidentiality within the group (including issues such as what to do when seeing another member in public or refraining from social media contacts). Then the leader needs to outline group norms and rules, which typically include emphasizing attendance and arriving on time and not leaving early. For this first session, the leader also should have members introduce themselves.

Norm Creation

Norms should include articulation by the group leader of the idea of using "I" rather than "you" statements. For example, rather than say, "You are an idiot" in response to something another group member says, the client should state, "When you said . . . I felt. . . ." This is an important idea for clients—an idea that is commonly used in process groups of putting thoughts and feelings into words and not actions. Norms can also involve general ideas of "respect," but this needs some operationalization: Discussion should take place in terms of refraining from name-calling, taking care with respecting each other's identities, and addressing other issues related to feeling respected. The leader should state norms around turning off any electronic devices and admonish members about contacting each other using social media or looking each other up online. They also should remind group members of confidentiality.

Rules and Structure

From the outset, it is essential to set norms around lateness and absences, something the therapist should already have addressed during the TPS session but is worth repeating at the beginning of the group. As mentioned in Chapter 6, a group member can never join a group with the expectation of arriving late every session or leaving early. The group leader needs to let clients know that the expectation is that clients will arrive on time and leave at the same time as other group members. They also need to state the rule that people must attend every session except under exceptional circumstances and with advanced warning. Group members should call ahead if they need to miss a group session—and it should only be for extreme situations, such as a personal emergency. If the expectation is too loose at the beginning, then groups can quickly devolve into members' arriving and leaving at different times, which results in increasing group dysfunction. Holding the group boundary is important.

Group Member Introductions

Next, the group leader asks members to introduce themselves. Typically, this involves an instruction to state their name, where they are from, and what their favorite dessert is. The leader also typically instructs them to keep this information to under a minute and that the leader may interrupt to allow others to be heard. The brevity allows people to hear themselves speak early on but also prevents any members from derailing the group with anxiety-driven overdisclosure, attacks on other members, or other acts of self-sabotage. The question about dessert is designed to increase the sense that this first session is fairly emotionally light and to encourage group positive affect by discussing something pleasurable.

Key Moments

Bear in mind that as soon as clients are invited to speak, they behave in a way that is consistent with their interpersonal style. This is the moment of peak anxiety; therefore, it triggers each person's highest interpersonal style. The only thing holding them back might be inoculation goals that were set in the TPS session related to group and self-sabotaging behaviors, such as attacking another member immediately or overdisclosing provocative material. For example, someone with a style that is high on Scale 8: Uninhibited will likely overshare during this introduction, whereas someone with a socially anxious style will tend toward freezing and the minimum possible disclosure.

The Setting of Time and Depth Boundaries

When explaining the task of introducing themselves to group members, the group leader needs to set time and depth boundaries around this introduction. It is crucial to keep the initial introduction brief and to avoid initial deeper dives into material that could be emotionally activating. For example, in addition to asking clients to share their names and where they grew up, it can be helpful for them to share their university major (if at a university counseling center) or career and a "fun fact." Typically, the fun fact might be sharing what their favorite dessert is, but fun facts vary by culture. For example, while working in China, I observed that desserts are not a common part of a meal, so naming a favorite movie or book might be more appropriate. The point of the exercise is to merely give people an easy way to make a quick, positive impression.

The group leader needs to ensure that members stick to the time limit. Because there are only eight sessions, time is at a premium, so the leader should keep Session 1 moving along. Gentle corrections such as "Mark, I am really enjoying listening to you, but is it okay if we keep it to 1 minute? We will have a chance to get to know each other better with some activities in a second" provide a nonshaming means to keep the group focused. This then allows the group to move onto the next activity: dyads. Therapeutic tact is key because it allows the client to retain a sense of connection to the therapist while also understanding the parameters of the exercise.

Dyads

Dyads are an important icebreaker because they provide an opportunity for the one-on-one connection that promotes cohesion. People with styles that are high in distance (Scale 3: Distant) and social inhibition (Scale 4: Socially Inhibited) also find the dyads a significantly easier way to begin to talk than talking to the whole group. Dyads also allow members with a warmer style a moment to connect so they can reduce their anxiety about the lack of intimacy. For clients high in distance, this activity also provides a one-on-one moment that allows them to feel close without being overwhelmed by the warmth of a cohesive group. Overall, this activity can provide a significant reduction in anxiety that promotes group cohesion while allowing members a chance to feel connected to at least one other group member.

The group leader breaks the group into dyads or threes if there is an uneven number. Typically, the leader does not join a dyad, depending on the cultural meanings behind the leader's joining in. In most cases, members should be given the chance to connect with another member because the goal of the activity is beginning cohesion with the group rather than continuing a bond with the leader.

The leader asks the dyads to quiz each other on where they live; where they grew up; what pets they had, if any; and about details of their current occupations. Leaders carefully note the time and announce when 5 minutes has passed and that it is time for the other person to talk. The members then report to whole group about what the other person told them. In the event that someone forgets their partner's name or misses details, the leader may want to normalize it by saying that is normal and is a product of this being an anxiety-provoking moment.

Dyads are an invaluable tool, and despite their seeming simplicity, they are not to be underestimated. During groups, clients sometimes refer back to moments in those dyads. Sometimes surprising connections between members can emerge.

Human Treasure Hunt

Following the dyads activity is another structured activity: a *human treasure hunt*, an activity based on finding others in the group who share commonalities. Examples of a human treasure hunt are available online, or a group leader may wish to create or modify one to make it their own. The group leader provides each member with a list of topics that a client might connect with someone else on (e.g., "favorite movie," "has a pet," "born outside of this state"). Members must then stand and mingle to find at least one group member who shares a commonality with them for each item on their list. They need to move from person to person to do so. The leader then debriefs the event. This icebreaker can be useful and enjoyable and is designed to promote group cohesion and a sense of shared communality. In most cases, this is the sole purpose of the activity, and for many groups, it fits into the goal of working on group attraction.

However, in some, but not all, cases, members have profound experiences during this activity, and it can be worthwhile processing those experiences. In one notable example, a group member had expressed some doubts about their ability to relate to any other group member because of their self-identification as both a Black woman and as pansexual. During the activity, she discovered that another group member also enjoyed a television show that she considered a "guilty pleasure" and had doubted anyone else would enjoy. The person she connected to was someone she had earlier dismissed as being a person she would unlikely feel connected to: a White man whom she had assumed was cisgender and heterosexual. This finding—that someone she had dismissed might be someone she had important things in common with—was something she continued to remark on throughout the life of the group. It opened something up inside of her about resisting the urge to label and dismiss people that she found life changing. While this example is more extreme than most, the process is a universal one. Finding rapid connections around common interests provides an important shortcut to cohesion that can prepare the group for the more challenging work ahead.

After the mingling, the group leader debriefs the group, asking questions, such as "What was that like?" "Was anything surprising?" "Did you feel connected to anyone?" Allowing members freedom to reflect can result in superficial comments, and it then may be time to move on. However, in some cases, more involved discussions can ensue and need processing. During this time, the leader should look for opportunities to link people or themes together.

Feedback Training

Another important part of Session 1 (or sometimes Session 2, depending on time) is feedback training. Research on feedback (Morran et al., 1998) has shown that early corrective feedback leads the receiver of that feedback to dismiss it and think less well of the person who delivered it. Equally, that same research also has shown that corrective feedback needs to be preceded by at least two positive statements about the person. Early corrective feedback, if delivered in the first two sessions of the group, should typically be blocked by the leader, who should encourage members to reword their statements. Over time, members can deliver corrective feedback and often find doing so valuable. However, remember that while some people have a stronger memory for positive feedback, others have a stronger memory for negative feedback (Sedikides, & Skowronski, 2020). Interpersonal style, levels of perfectionism, and culture, can all be factors in how feedback is received and processed. For example, clients with styles that are unassertive are particularly anxious about negative feedback and are likely to react to it with shame and vulnerability. Equally, perfectionism can predict poor responses to negative feedback, leading to depression (Nepon et al., 2011).

Culture can be highly impactful on how feedback is interpreted and integrated. In its early years of development in the Midwest, FBGT tended toward avoidance of corrective feedback early in groups (because of the previously cited research on this topic; see, e.g., Kivlighan, Ali, & Garrison, 2020; Morran et al., 1998), but did not discourage it in later sessions when cohesion was established. However, the group was always ended with no new corrective feedback in the last session.

My time spent teaching FBGT in China resulted in an awareness that corrective feedback had a different meaning there. Instead of seeming wary of it, group members invited it and seemed honored by receiving it from other group members. Members would sometimes share that they felt ending the group with only positives was inauthentic. This became a significant evolution of FBGT over time. It became clear that factors, such as culture, were clear mediators in how feedback was delivered and internalized. However, it also became important not to "pendulum" and assume that, moving forward, corrective feedback was a free-for-all. Rather, the therapist should be sensitive to both within- and between-group differences when considering culture and diversity. The group leader must weigh the cultural meanings behind corrective feedback against the personal ego strength of each member and their interpersonal styles. Interpersonal style is worthy of consideration in this equation. The aforementioned unassertive style is the most obvious case of style predicting response to corrective feedback, but other styles also absorb information based on their idiosyncratic combinations of personality and cultural variables.

Despite this assertion, in the first two sessions, leaders should look for an opportunity to invite here-and-now feedback that is positive. Positive feedback allows the group to develop trust that other members are working in their best interests and not seeking to destroy them or gain power over them. For example, asking group members to mention who they have felt helped by already or someone they want to get to know better can enable processes that lead members to feel connected and have a sense of belonging. These moments can prove powerful because members learn that they are visible to others and "seen," providing a strong sense of belonging. At the end of the group, the leader typically expresses positive statements about the work of the group that day and about looking forward to seeing people the next week.

If the group has been challenging with more conflict or difficult moments than expected, then the group leader should focus on the positives, acknowledge the challenges, and state optimism about the next session. The leader should reaffirm that it is important to come back especially when members are worried about the next session. In some cases, leaders may choose to make a note to phone a group member if they believe that a member is at risk of dropping out. However, in such cases, the group member should be encouraged to take their worries and concerns back to the group so they can be dealt with there. Therapists should use their clinical judgment to decide on the suitability of this intervention based on a thoughtful case conceptualization. This option is always available during the life of the group and should be considered on a case-by-case basis. Group leaders may want to explain to the whole group that sometimes they will call between sessions to quickly touch base, depending on the need and that it would be on a case-by-case basis.

Use of Lap Sheet Guides

Each group leader should have two main worksheets on their lap during the group. Both require only one blank sheet of paper that the leader fills out. The first of these, the cohesion lap sheet, is used in Session 1. The second, which is addressed in Chapter 8, is used in the middle stages.

At Session 1, the cohesion lap sheet (see Figure 7.1) should involve a clean piece of paper with group members' names written in the order in which they are sitting (including group leaders' positions). The group leader should then draw lines showing connections between members as they emerge. By the end of Session 1, ideally all group members should be connected to at least one other person. If one person makes multiple connections to other members, then all well and good. However, it is more important to note if anyone has not connected to another member because this indicates higher potential for dropout. Some connections are easy to see and may well be clearly articulated by group members. For example, a member may report feeling closer to someone or wanting to know another member better. It may also be noticeable that two members share a common issue or seem to be emotionally connected as they speak. However, others are more subtle and internal. These are connections that the leader should track and spend time considering whether they are meaningful but internal or peripheral and nonmeaningful. The leader must consider each member's typical interpersonal style when making these determinations. For example, someone who is highly socially inhibited may display connection with slightly more eye contact than normal or by smiling during a dyad.

FIGURE 7.1. Lap Note for Cohesion

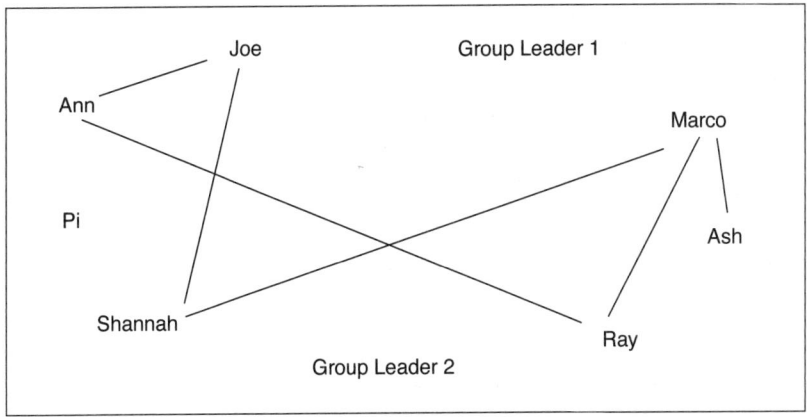

The lap sheet (see Figure 7.1) shows that Marco is a point of cohesion for a few members. Joe and Shannah are also connected to at least two others, as are Ray and Ann. Ash is connected to one other member, Marco, so their connectedness is established but would benefit from more links to other members as the group progresses. However, it is notable that Pi does not seem well connected to another group member and is therefore someone the group leader should attempt to link to at least one other group member as soon as possible. Other key processes that facilitate cohesion include basic group leadership skills, such as linking.

Linking Technique

A key, basic technique in the group is linking. Linking member concerns is essential, particularly early in the group when the group leader is attempting to draw out members and generate group cohesion by establishing connections. This skill can be accomplished in a variety of ways. It can be as simple as nonverbally gesturing for one member to talk directly to another. It can also be asking if a group member has felt impacted by something another member has said. More directly, it can be inviting two members who seem to have connected on an issue to share with each other. Therefore, the interventions can range from the indirect and open to the direct and focused.

These interventions are particularly important at the beginning of the group as members begin the process of group cohesion. It is common for group members to direct their initial comments toward the group leader because that is the person with whom they have the bond. To transfer the therapist bond into group cohesion, it is crucial that members learn to talk directly to each other. Here is an example of this move:

CLIENT: (*Looks at therapist*) When Johnny said that just now, I felt really connected to him. I was surprised he felt that way.

GROUP LEADER: Why not tell him (*gestures at Johnny*) that?

CLIENT: (*Looks at Johnny*) I felt really connected to you just now. I didn't realize you were worried about me and I felt really cared for.

Checking Out

Another technique is to check out. Depending on what has happened in the group and how much time is left, *checking out* can take several forms: It may include a one-word feeling check-in in which members are asked to give one word that states how they are feeling at the end of the group. This can serve to take the emotional temperature in the room and for the group leader to begin to understand how the group members are feeling. Depending on time, the group leader may also choose to ask who has either felt helped by someone in the group or who in the group they are looking forward to getting to know more. This prompt can sometimes serve as a helpful introduction to the here and now in a nonthreatening way that promotes group cohesion. The leader typically summarizes the group, often in the form of thanking everyone for attending, noticing the hard work that was accomplished, and expressing positivity about the next session, as in this example:

> We are at the end of the session, and I just want to say thank you for all your hard work today. It takes courage to join a group, and I want to thank all of you for taking risks. We will meet at the same time next week, and we will spend more time exploring goals together and working out how we can help each other. Thank you all, and see you next week!

Leader summarizing can also help members make sense of difficult moments that were either resolved or unresolved. It also can build trust in the group leader—that they noticed and that building trust is part of the process. Consider this example: At the end of the group, group member Lana expressed frustration at not being able to express themselves more. The leader took note and included the following in their closing statement:

> Unfortunately, we are out of time today. Thank you all for coming. There was a lot of hard work and risk-taking, and I appreciate the courage you all showed. I want to say that I know that not everyone felt heard today. Lana, I am sorry we ran out of time. However, I am looking forward to hearing you share more next week so we can get to know you better.

This statement reflects the reality while also acknowledging feelings. It also presents the group as a place in which repairs can happen the next week, thus providing a model for clients that feelings can be hurt, but the possibility of repair happening later also offers hope for the future.

Administration of Instruments

Instruments such as the Working Alliance Inventory (Horvath & Greenberg, 1989), Group Climate Questionnaire (MacKenzie, 1983), or the Group Questionnaire (Krogel et al., 2013) can provide important group and individual-level data on factors related to climate and cohesion. These assessment tools can add considerable value to clinical judgment, allowing the group leader to make more informed decisions on how to intervene and facilitate evidence-based relationship factors in the following sessions. They also allow for the possibility that a member is at risk of not returning for Session 2. Therefore, the leader can opt to call the client to check in between sessions and to discuss what happened and ensure that the client returns to work through the issues.

SESSION 2: KEY PROCESSES

Session 2 is less structured than Session 1 and involves introducing members to the format of the group as well as shaping the group members toward desirable behaviors. It therefore involves several key processes: introducing goals, clarifying how feedback should be delivered, and bringing the group into the here and now. Thus, it provides a bridge between Session 1, which is highly structured, and the rest of the sessions, which are more based in the here and now, by shaping the group members toward the tasks of the group (which is a key part of the working alliance). Put simply, it involves clarifying what work will happen every week by beginning the work and helping the group understand how to conduct the work so it will be most therapeutic.

Task Agreement Revisited

The session begins by summarizing the previous session, as in this example:

> Last week, we completed a lot of activities and got to know each other a little. I appreciate you all taking the risk to come back this week and to continue that work. This week, we will be really beginning to explore the work and talking about goals and sharing them with each other. We will also be talking about how to deliver feedback so others can hear it and how to ask for help.

Orienting the group to what will be happening in session is important in settling the group down and continuing the working alliance. While the group should be more cohesive after Session 1, they are now going to be unsure as to the actual task of the group, so Session 2 provides valuable orientation.

It is useful to talk about feedback first. Feedback in FBGT is based on Stockton's research (Moran et al., 1998) on feedback delivery that is still considered the gold standard in the field (Burlingame & Jensen, 2017). That research showed that for groups in the United States, participants tended to dismiss corrective feedback if it was delivered too early in the life of the group. The research also found that corrective feedback needed to be delivered as a "sandwich" in that it was surrounded by positive feedback or had two positives preceding the corrective. Further, it suggested that early feedback exchanges would be positive, later ones would involve some correction, and the leader would model feedback. It also indicated that group leaders should be aware of the recipient's readiness for change; that is, if the client can tolerate corrective feedback at that exact moment. The research stressed the importance that feedback focus on behaviors that were observable.

FBGT adheres to these principles in how it considers leaders should facilitate feedback delivery. Gently correcting, blocking, and protecting members when they immediately lead off with corrective feedback are essential parts of FBGT. However, it is also crucial to not invalidate people's feelings or identity variables, and blocking corrective feedback is not always desirable, even early in the group, if doing so invalidates a client and leads them to feel unsafe (Miles et al., 2021). Chapter 8 addresses this topic in more depth.

Cultural Differences in Feedback

Not every culture gives and receives feedback the same way. In some cultures, corrective feedback is delivered early and often and is received as a "gift." Thus, what is experienced by one person's culture as harsh criticism is a "loving truth" in another person's culture. Therefore, in adapting the FBGT approach to different cultures, the role of the meaning of feedback in a culture needs consideration. For example, as previously mentioned, when running experiential groups in China with therapists, it became clear to me that corrective feedback, when delivered with care, was highly valued, whereas positive feedback was sometimes seen as disingenuous. Therefore, the group leaders gave more latitude to corrective feedback, providing it was well intentioned and well received.

However, regardless of culture, there are limits. Within each culture, group leaders should be careful to ensure the feedback is well intended and is delivered in a way that is intended to help and not just to hurt or scapegoat.

Even in cultures that value corrective feedback, group forces and individual differences can still lead to hurt and countertherapeutic outcomes. Therefore, titration of feedback (Yalom & Leszcz, 2020), although needing adjustment across cultures, is still an important consideration (Kivlighan, Ali, & Garrison, 2020). Leaders should be thoughtful in how they consider and evaluate the potential impact of feedback in terms of factors such as intent, severity, timing, and amount.

Group Goals Readout

Group members next need to read their goals. The group first places limits around this task so that each member is heard by asking everyone to read their goals to the group in turn and to hold onto their questions and comments until everyone has been heard. Once everyone has read their goals, the group leader can invite questions, comments, and follow-up.

In some cases, members meet their goals quickly. For example, someone may have a goal of asking a follow-up question of another group member. If they ask someone else to explain their goal a little more, this then meets that goal. Therefore, a feedback process should be engaged by the group leader, who invites the group member to get feedback on how activating their goal went.

Here-and-Now Activation

In some groups, the here-and-now activation occurs quickly and spontaneously. Some groups automatically address each other directly and give each other feedback. However, in many groups, members look to the group leader as a conduit between themselves and the group. For example, they look at the leader and say, "When they [Paolo] said that, I felt sad." The leader can then redirect that comment toward a one-on-one interaction nonverbally, verbally, or both. For example, the group leader, gesturing toward Paolo with an open hand, says, "Why don't you tell Paolo that?" This type of redirection is typical in many groups and is part of conveying expectations about here-and-now interactions between group members.

Shaping the group toward desired behaviors is an important part of group leadership. After a few rounds of redirecting, simple gestures can be enough to convey the same message of talking directly to each other. The session can be continued by asking members for reactions to each other's goals, eliciting here-and-now interactions (see more in the next chapter), and by capitalizing on the content that occurs to eventually focus again on process.

End of the Session

Sessions 1 and 2 typically end with check-ins about feelings and the therapist's summary. Both tasks provide the sense of continuity for future sessions and keep the group aware of how the group is impacting them.

These tasks also allow group members who felt ignored, left out, or impacted by something in the group to leave "breadcrumbs" for the group to follow in the next session. For example, someone who states they feel "empty" when the rest of the group has reported having positive feelings suggests that this group member wants and needs attention in the next group session. Such breadcrumbs also allow the therapist to note in their closing remarks that not everyone has the same feelings about the same events and that this can add richness to the group experience to discover, in the next session, why.

SUMMARY

Session 1 of FBGT is highly structured—more so than subsequent sessions. Such structure provides the basis for cohesion and serves as the container for the later work. The therapist actively encourages member-to-member interaction to move the working alliance toward group cohesion. In Session 2, the therapist should move the group into the here and now as the session progresses and should also provide instructions for how to deliver feedback. In addition, the therapist needs to consider cultural differences in structuring feedback but take care to ensure that the working alliance and cohesion remain central to the group process.

8 LEADING THE MIDDLE AND LATER SESSIONS

Sessions 1 and 2 of the group therapy, as discussed in the preceding chapter, are intended to set the stage for the middle and later sessions during which work continues and deepens. In these sessions, the art and science of the therapy combine, and the group leader's interventions become less structured but no less impactful. The group leader must attend to the deep structure of the sessions, keeping members focused on the work and maintaining a time focus while also managing alliance ruptures and providing a facilitative environment. In addition, the leader must manage the complexities of the final session and confront group members' ambivalence about leaving while ensuring that termination provides a platform for modeling endings. Focused brief group therapy (FBGT) middle sessions are defined by working toward behavioral activation of goals within the here and now and integrating feedback immediately afterward. This chapter addresses the tasks and skills related to these processes.

https://doi.org/10.1037/0000389-009
Focused Brief Group Therapy: An Integrative Approach to Reducing Interpersonal Distress, by M. Whittingham

STRUCTURE OF EACH SESSION

The basic structure of each session should be consistent and needs to include these tasks:

- Hand out the goal note cards at the beginning of each session. Collect them again at the end (clients tend to forget to bring goal note cards, so this is an easier path to successful goal focus using the cards).

- Maintain a time focus by reminding members how many sessions they have left to work on a goal.

- Begin with a summary of the previous session.

- Ask members to read their goals and comment on their progress so far.

- Invite members to work on their goals in the here and now.

- Provide feedback as soon as a goal is worked on.

- Finish the session with a summary and collect the goal note cards.

A consistent structure ensures the group is maintaining its focus on the work. On occasion, an issue may have surfaced during the prior group session that the group leader stated would be addressed in the next session. In this case, when summarizing that previous session, the leader should indicate that the group will begin with this issue after everyone has gone over their goals.

KEY GROUP LEADER TASKS

The group leader performs a number of key tasks during the middle session of group therapy to set the container and facilitative conditions for the members to engage in their work (Moss, 2008). These tasks are (a) working on goals in the here and now as well as illuminating process; (b) keeping a goal focus on behavioral activation; (c) engaging feedback and feedback loops; (d) ensuring that cohesion and the working alliance are maintained; and (e) helping group members work through rupture and repair in the group using techniques, such as *working the axes*, which involves reconciling each person in the interaction with a disowned part of themselves by helping members see the positives in those whom they see as unlike them (the technique is discussed in more detail later).

The group leader should also keep a balance between forces that drive the work forward and maintain progress—the up-regulating processes—and the forces that threaten progress and premature dropout or client worsening. The up-regulating processes include placing the group in the here and now and having members work on goals and feedback.

Working on Goals in the Here and Now

The *here and now* as defined by Yalom and Leszcz (2020) is the shared interactional space in which members' behaviors emerge. In Yalom groups, members are encouraged to share reactions to each other in real time, and this activity is used to uncover maladaptive relational patterns and provide the basis for behavior change. The concept of the *social microcosm*, an empirically validated concept (Kivlighan, Gullo, et al., 2021), is important to understand. It states that given enough time, people inevitably replicate during the group process the behaviors that they exhibit in the real world.

FBGT similarly assumes that the social microcosm is a real phenomenon and that members enact their maladaptive interactional strategies during the life of the group. However, because FBGT has already moved individual members to insight using the 32-item Inventory of Interpersonal Problems (IIP-32; Horowitz et al., 2000) in the therapy, pregroup preparation, and screening (TPS) session, this shared space instead becomes a place in which members enact their behavioral goals. Thus, the here and now is used to work on behavioral activation and to manage the emotions, cognitions, and polyvagal responses around that. People in FBGT groups still feel the urge to behave as they always have done. Indeed, they still play out their interpersonal styles during the group. However, because FBGT works on either inhibiting the extremes of some styles or having group members work on growth into a more flexible style, these behaviors sometimes exhibit less frequently than usual. Moving the group into interacting with each other in real time, discussing issues that are real to them, and delivering feedback to each other constitute the space in which the work takes place.

As mentioned in Chapter 7, FBGT interventions during group are predominately horizontal (i.e., into the here and now of the group) rather than vertical (i.e., into the client's past). They are also directed at group members' exploration of their reactions to and with each other rather than being focused on their reactions to the group leader. Thus, the leader's main task is to model and facilitate the climate that fosters exploration of new behaviors and encourages safe feedback from members.

Group most frequently begin with the group leader's inviting group members to read their goals. The leader then either waits for a spontaneous discussion to emerge or asks who wishes to work on a goal. As the group progresses, the leader also asks members to report on their progress toward their goals so far. These two strategies usually lead to some combination of task and process emerging organically. Sometimes the group immediately begins working on goals; in other cases, the members ask for support around a there-and-then issue that occurred in the past week or two.

Invitations to the Here and Now

Initial invitations to the here and now take place as early as Session 1 but are kept positive. At the end of sessions, it is sometimes helpful to leave time for members to give each other positive feedback. Typical questions might be: "Who have you felt connected to today?" "Who are you looking forward to getting to know more?" "Who did you feel helped by today?" The group leader needs to monitor time and ensure members have an opportunity to briefly speak but still allow brief mentions of positive connections to each other. Doing so models here-and-now interaction, which the leader and group build on in the middle sessions.

Levels of Inference

These interventions to the here and now can range from the simple and non-inferential to the fully inferential interpretation as the group progresses. For example, a noninferential invitation to process might be: "I wonder what is happening right now?" or "Something just happened." This type of invitation allows the group space and time to consider their feelings and readings of the situation without the group leader's overly prescribing the problem. A more fully inferential process might be this: "There was a real moment of tension and anxiety just then as we had our first disagreement in the group. I wonder what is happening right now as we all sit with that?"

Another level of inference might be the group leader's using self-involving self-disclosure. For example, the leader may say this after a powerful interaction between group members has taken place: "I noticed that I am feeling a mixture of things right now: sad, worried, deeply moved, and grateful. I wonder if anyone else is having similar or different feelings to what was just said?" This intervention performs two tasks: It promotes emotional awareness in the group about something happening in the here and now and also opens a window for awareness about process. The last level is one of more inferential interpretation; for example: "Jeff, I saw you looking at Sam like she had really injured you. I wonder if her comments that you were behaving like a baby really felt wounding to you."

Other interpretations can be highly inferential. Take this example: A group member named Chantelle reported that they had been attacked in the street the previous week and had to run away to escape. After a long delay and pause, a group member with a Distant (Scale 3) style stated, "I like to go running on the weekends. It keeps me energized!" Another group member with a similar style stated, "I like to go running too! I bought a new pair of running shoes last week!" The group discussed running shoes for some time, avoiding the major disclosure from the group member. After multiple attempts to elicit from the group that a major event had happened, the group was still silent. The group leader noted that all the members have a similar style—distant or socially inhibited—and were clearly struggling with how to respond to the disclosure of a very important and traumatic event. So, the group leader stopped the group by asking, "Can I just stop everyone and ask a question? What just happened?" The group was silent.

So, the group leader increased the levels of inference: "Chantelle just told us all about a really traumatic event that happened to her, and all of a sudden, we were talking about running shoes. I wonder what was happening inside you all in that moment?" A group member responded, looking ashamed of themselves: "I really did feel awful for Chantelle, but I was scared of saying the wrong thing and making it worse, so I kind of changed the subject." Others in the group nodded. "Would you like to try again?" the group leader asked that member. The person nodded: "I felt horrible when I heard you talk about being attacked and chased. Are you okay? That must have been terrifying" Chantelle responded that it was nice that the group member cared. The other group members now take took this opportunity to state how they were feeling; they had similarly been afraid of saying the wrong thing. The group then moved into the work of trying new things while also receiving feedback from the recipient.

As this previous example illustrates, although motivation and insight are important, the therapist is also looking to prompt the behavioral activation and engage feedback loops. The FBGT therapist is less interested in deep exploration of the "why" of an event (e.g., "I remember saying the wrong thing once to my parents, and they shouted at me") than in ensuring that the person understands the pattern and expands their behavioral repertoire, and then receives feedback. The two processes do not have to be mutually exclusive. There are times in FBGT when exploration of the past can be useful; however, typically, attention needs to shift toward insight about present moment behavior and behavioral activation of a new behavior.

Interpretations should be used judiciously in FBGT. The key intent of FBGT is not that the group learn to rely on the group leader as a fountain of wisdom but, rather, that they have time to practice new skills in a safe environment and to get feedback from each other. In FBGT, the group member making the changes is the main focus, and group leaders should avoid overreliance on interpretations that may cloud their view of what constitutes success in the group.

Illumination of Process

Process illumination is described by Yalom and Leszcz (2020) as a multistep process involving factors such as recognizing and interpreting what is happening in the present moment and using this as a force for change. In FBGT, this process is used similarly—to step back from the content of a discussion (e.g., a member sharing about a conflict at work) and to shift focus onto a process happening in the group (e.g., that the member sharing about the conflict is also sharing for the first time with the group about something important to them). Remember that although the group process involves some fascinating and sometimes powerful content, the central task is to attend to attend to the content but then move into process. Specifically, this means working on goal completion by individual members during the here and now of the group. The here and now does not refer to recent events that happened outside of the group; instead, the here and now comprises interactions between members in the group in the present moment—that is, how members react to each other's interpersonal invitations and behaviors in the present moment. For example, a group member states that they have recently struggled with the fact that their life partner left them for another person. The content is compelling and important. Members likely offer support, ask questions about the client's emotional well-being, and express concern as to that person's future and also reflect on their own relationships. This content can provide an important function for the group.

Once the content has been processed, though, the group leader then directs the group toward the process. During this discussion, group members may have acted on their goals, such as asking follow-up questions, expressing concerns and encouragement, or offering advice. Therefore, although the content is compelling and helpful to process—and it should be validated—following this up by drawing attention to the processes is the primary mechanism of change. Having members discuss what it was like to offer support or advice and then receiving feedback from the group on how they came across are the central tasks of the group and what the leader should be facilitating.

Focusing on What Generates Behavioral Activation: From Organic Processes to Targeted Interventions

The group almost always starts with a brief summary of the preceding session and a reading of group goals. Afterward, the group often takes on a life of its own: Members either launch into goal work immediately (e.g., someone who has a goal of asking for time from the group makes a direct appeal to talk about their issues), or the group may become preoccupied with something that happened inside or outside of the group. For example, a group member may be concerned about something that felt unresolved with another member during the previous week's session, perhaps an unresolved conflict or a reaction to an unexpected disclosure. Equally, a member may have arrived following a difficult moment outside the group, such as a conflict with a coworker, and is in distress. On other occasions, the group may feel flat and be silent as members struggle with what to do next.

The group leader's task is therefore varied. Once the group understands the work—to focus on goals in the here and now and to give each other feedback about those goals—then, at times, the leader can choose to be passive if that work is taking place. In that case, the leader may sometimes direct traffic by occasionally prompting or redirecting work toward themes or interpersonal interactions that enable members who have been unable to work on goals to do so. In other cases, the group leader may need to let the group play out an issue and find ways to work in a goal over time. That issue may begin as here and now (e.g., feeling hurt about something another group member said and wishing to process it) or may be there and then related (e.g., telling the group how they felt injured after a microaggression at work). The issue, though, should always end up being related back to the here and now and ultimately to the interpersonal goals being worked on in the present moment. For example, as a person processes feeling hurt by someone in the group, the leader eventually turns the process back into what it feels like to express a need, assert oneself, or continue with whatever goal or goals were worked on during that here-and-now work on the in-group conflict.

Illumination of process by the group leader—who may ask, for example, "We all just had a conflict play out, so what was that like, how did it go for you, and what feedback would you like?"—is the core work of the group. While simultaneously expressing that the content is also important (e.g., the content of the conflict is about feeling disregarded and dismissed), the *process of the conflict*—that is, how the conflict occurred and what interpersonal behaviors took place—is the main therapeutic work. A key skill of the therapist is to treat the content of the conflict as important but to ultimately move the work toward goal completion.

Addressing Microaggressions

In the earlier example of the group member who had experienced microaggression at their workplace, important work is to be completed that can aid in terms of goal completion. While the person is expressing the manifest content—that they felt angry and upset in how they were treated related to an important diversity variable—a second, highly valuable process also is taking place: how interpersonal behaviors are playing out in the group in relation to that issue. Group members need time to air issues of identity (Miles et al., 2021), and the process of group members' listening and validating experiences is important in and of itself. A process of sharing should not be cut short by shifting too quickly into process. It the shift is too fast, it can feel like a minimization and invalidation of an important issue, so the group leader should ensure that the discussion is given time to air and not foreshortened because of another member's discomfort with confronting difficult work. Without this adequate time, a second, in-group microaggression takes place: a minimization of the content and the feelings involved, which leads to a second injury. However, once the process has been discussed thoroughly and the person feels heard and understood, issues of process can then also be worked on. For example, if the member who brought the issue up also completed their goal of going first in the group or asking for time, then this can become a time for the group leader to mention that the goal was completed and to check in with the member's feelings about the issue. Group leaders must ensure that they maintain a high level of cultural comfort in group by modeling open and humble attitudes toward members' cultural identities. Making room for discussions around diversity, identity, and how those play out in the life of the group is a key part of group process (Kivlighan, Swancy, et al., 2021; Miles et al., 2021).

Remember that although the manifest content is important, the process can also be highly activating, particularly if this is a new behavior. For example, the group member may report that this was the first time they had ever spontaneously asked for group time to listen. Now, they are worried that they were too demanding of the group and may be rejected. Hearing reactions from the group can provide a powerful disconfirmation that their interpersonal behavior did not result in the expected disaster. Identity variables and interpersonal traits are important, and how they combine requires considerable finesse to both understand and therapeutically work with. Discussions of how interpersonal behaviors and identity issues combine and the resulting interpersonal interactions are a powerful source of growth for both individuals and the group.

Simultaneous Goal Work

Often in FBGT groups, people are working on goals simultaneously. By inhibiting their response, the second member is now both helping the first member to meet their goals and simultaneously working on their own goal. Thus, there are now two members working on their goals simultaneously. What may end up happening is that the second member takes the spotlight away from that first member or works on a goal of asking follow-up questions. Each moment in the group has therapeutic potential and can be the source of work and growth for multiple participants simultaneously. This is part of what makes FBGT so exciting for both its members and group leaders. The synergies involved allow for what some group members have described as the "magic to happen" as members find the space to work on powerful content and powerful processes at the same moment.

Engaging Feedback and Feedback Loops

These simultaneous moments require the therapist to notice what is occurring and thus begin the process of feedback. Multiple types of feedback might be occurring that call for the therapist to keep track of the different types of goals that were enacted. Each of these goal completions then requires, in turn, implementation of feedback. For example, as one person completes their goal of going first, the group leader asks them how that felt and whether they wish to check in with the group about how it went. The leader can then shift focus to how it was for another member to ask follow-up questions. These follow the same intervention process (i.e., asking how that felt and inviting the member to check in with the group on their reactions).

Feedback loops (Yalom & Leszcz, 2020) occur when group members give each other feedback during the group and goals are enacted within that loop, providing a recursive process. For example, one member asks for feedback about how the other members felt about their asking for time and then use that feedback to discuss a personal problem (a goal on Scale 6: Focused on the Needs of Others; see Figure 1.2 in Chapter 1). The member receives feedback from a second group member who has been working on improving their ability to offer encouragement to others (a Scale 1: Highly Assertive goal). Because the second group member had the individual goal of "offering encouragement to another group member," they therefore also completed their goal during this feedback sequence. The group leader then turns the feedback back onto that person (the one who had provided feedback to the first member), asking them how they felt having completed the goal of offering encouragement.

These feedback loops can be powerful. Members feel the energy of working together on issues, which provides a sense of communal belonging and esprit de corps that they are working purposefully together to help each other. The group provides individual growth and an increased sense of altruism.

Ensuring Cohesion and Working Alliance Are Maintained

The energy of FBGT comes from being in the here and now and illuminating process. This is what differentiates it from a psychoeducational social skills group: Behavioral activation take places organically in the here and now of the group, and all the risks involved in attempting new behaviors are in the flow of a set of group interactions. These attempts also come with stakes:

The member risks being disliked and rejected for their behavioral change. Role plays do not provide as great a sense of risk because they sometimes involve mechanical enacting of specific techniques. Yet, they are still highly valuable, and some more unstructured group therapies underestimate the importance of social skills as technique.

FBGT, however, blends the need to implement technique with the risk of actual rejection. The space is therefore inherently a higher stakes one, contains more potential for members' sympathetic nervous systems to become activated, and allows for fight, flight, or freeze behaviors to emerge. This process involves setting and retaining the facilitative conditions for the group to take place, so members sometimes need guidance on tasks. Although this guidance should have been provided in Sessions 1 and 2, it should also be provided in the middle sessions. Holding the group in the therapeutic space to complete the work is an ongoing task. This means building on the work of Session 1 by continuing to maintain cohesion and bond while keeping a focus on the task and goals, that is, using the working alliance and group bonds to move the work forward as it becomes more challenging and stress inducing. Keeping a focus on the task and goals might involve working through problems with task agreement, goal agreement, and bond as well as group cohesion. Typically, goal agreement problems are caused by issues in the TPS session; however, task agreement needs clarifying and facilitating as the group progresses, as does the form and nature of group cohesion.

Conflict and Cohesion

Consider, for example, that conflict can be extremely helpful in the middle to late sessions of group if the group leader provides the container for it to happen (Flores & Porges, 2017). For some group members, standing up for themselves and holding their own in a conflict and then later getting group feedback on that is a stated goal for the group. If the conflict is well titrated by the group leader, then it can be a force that promotes group cohesion via more authentic reactions between members.

The group leader, however, must be aware of the differential impact of the conflict on the whole group and notice that while, for some members (e.g., those high on Scale 2: Focused on the Needs of the Self), conflict is a safe, happy, and comfortable skill set, for others (e.g., those on more unassertive or warm scales), conflict can present significant discomfort and anxiety. Therefore, the group leader should be mindful to maintain that cohesion by ensuring members can engage in productive conflict, which will be discussed later in this chapter.

Structure

Within FBGT, though, remember that these forces take place not only for the group as a whole but also on an individual basis. Therefore, the tension between the structure of task completion and allowance of the process to emerge organically is where the art and science of the process meet. Too much structure, and the group becomes forced and psychoeducational; too little focus on the goals, and the group risks drifting into a general therapy group.

Although there are strengths to both general therapy groups and psychoeducational groups, the art of FBGT involves skilled therapists working with process and the here and now to allow goals to emerge either organically or with some prompting. In FBGT, both occur. The use of note cards and the reminding of members that the purpose of the therapy is to activate those behaviors can result in members' plunging into the work without further prompting. In these cases, it is the therapist's job to notice this has happened and to facilitate feedback loops.

Equifinality

The lines among organic emergence of goals, members driving the work, leaders driving the work, and group-as-a-whole progress depend on the group. Remember that "all roads can lead to Rome": Some groups need more group leader activity and prompting to get there, whereas others can leave the leader feeling that they are just along for the ride. For example, a group that is homogenous for distance or unassertiveness requires far more leader activity than a group that is more heterogenous for interpersonal style and is ready to work.

The routes to get to behavioral activation are varied. What works in one group—for example, members freely interact with each other, and the leader sits back and makes the occasional intervention—does not work in another. Some groups may require more direction and skillful intervention, ranging from interpretations, to prompting, to managing alliance ruptures and conflicts that may need some group leader facilitation.

Leader as Facilitator

As Yalom (Yalom & Leszcz, 2020) described, the group leader is a facilitator of the process. Although in some groups, the leader may be highly active and, in others, may be able to more passively watch as the growth unfolds more organically, the type of activity is important. The group leader plays the role of conductor, not lead soloist. Therefore, their interventions should be directed at setting the facilitative conditions and ensuring the group stays on track in working with each other.

In FBGT, the group leader sometimes uses interpretations; however, this is not their main mechanism of change. Rather, the leader should spend more of their time prompting members to work with each other instead of being the fount of all wisdom for the group and providing individual therapy in the group. As discussed in Chapter 7, Yalom and Leszcz (2020) described this as the spokes-in-wheel model: The therapist looks to help the group make connections to each other by setting the facilitative conditions—unconditional positive regard, empathy, and cohesion via linking—and container for the work to take place. The group leader therefore needs to set clear norms about what the work of the group looks like and thus should step in to help the group do that work whenever the group gets off track.

Working Through Conflicts and Ruptures

Of course, not every group moment provides a sense of joy and shared purpose. Change can also come about through conflict, resolution of difficult moments, and by working through emotionally activating material. Managing these alliance ruptures and repairing them are important parts of evidence-based practice (Marmarosh, 2021). The job of the therapist in these instances is to provide a calm, supportive container for these experiences to take place in. It is essential that the therapist remain centered and thoughtful about what is occurring.

There is a place for conflict in FBGT. Although the early session or two of FBGT is where conflict is highly contained, once cohesion has been established and the rules for giving feedback made clear, corrective feedback and conflict can be given room to breathe. Polyvagal theory suggests that working through a conflict should involve allowing clients to experience up-regulation and then a sense of control as they down-regulate as the conflict eases (Flores & Porges, 2017). The group leader's role is to titrate the conflict so that as issues emerge, they are discussed using "I" statements (to help others understand the impact of their conflict strategies). The leader then makes meaning of the event. For example, the leader may choose to open the group up to discussion of what having a conflict is like for everyone. Whether the group then processes this event effectively or needs guidance to do so, the leader must ensure that group as a whole and its members make sense of the event. By validating the groups and its members' ability to tolerate and process a conflict, there is much to be learned by each member. However, remember that conflict for some members (depending on their interpersonal style) is either very easy and energizing or deeply upsetting and pushes people into fight, flight, or freeze mode. Understanding the different reactions each member is likely to have during a conflict is an important part of reducing premature termination.

This does not mean that the conflict should go unmanaged. Conflicts can arise for a variety of reasons: power struggles and fights for dominance; micro-aggressions; feelings of hurt or injury; feelings of being belittled, ignored, or silenced; scapegoating; or group anger at member deviance. Deciding on a therapeutic strategy requires the ability to first determine the reason for the conflict (Kellermann, 1996).

The following case examples describe different reasons conflicts ensued. They also demonstrate three different solutions to address these conflicts.

CASE EXAMPLE 1: PLANNING AHEAD

The FBGT therapist notices that the group comprises seven members who are very high in warmth and one member who is high in distance. The therapist anticipates that at some point in the group, the other members will attack the member who prefers more distance for not being sufficiently warm or for not participating in emotional connections in the same way as the other members.

Planning ahead, the therapist intends to side with the client who prefers distance for support and to process this with the whole group using the working the axes technique. The therapist intends to work on having the warm group members understand the need for boundaries and distance and to begin to empathize with the person who is more distant by considering how they each could integrate boundary management into their own lives.

CASE EXAMPLE 2: USING THE WORKING THE AXES TECHNIQUE

A group member called Dev with a score high on Scale 4: Socially Inhibited has a group goal of being able to assert themselves around issues important to their identity. Dev identifies as Indian American and pansexual. At one point in the group, another group member states that they have always wanted to date an Indian American person because they are "super sexy." Dev states that this feels like they are being objectified and fetishized. They add that the person has turned people of their ethnicity into something that is less than a real person.

The group member is initially offended and disputes this statement. The group leader invites Dev to share how they feel by using "I" statements. Dev then states that what the group member said impacts them because it makes them feel that someone might only be dating them for their ethnicity—as an "exotic" person rather than for who they truly are inside. The other group member realizes the impact of their statement on Dev and looks tearful and sad. The group member thanks Dev and says that they have been given a lot to think about.

The group leader, noting that this is an instance not only of a microaggression that needed addressing but also an example of Dev's completing a goal, moves to the next intervention. The leader turns to Dev: "Dev, that was really powerful. You really spoke from the heart and expressed yourself. I wonder how that was for you and also what it was like to complete your goal." Dev replies that they feel a mixture of emotions: pride that they could state how they felt and own their own identity but sadness and pain that the conflict may have injured the other group member.

The group leader invites Dev to seek feedback. Dev does, and the other group member states that it was hard at first, but that after they heard how it impacted Dev, they felt they had learned something. They stated that although they now felt guilty and slightly ashamed, they felt glad Dev had said something. Other group members expressed their support of Dev for standing up for themself and also gave appreciation to the other group member for being open to learning.

The leader then directs a discussion on how some goal completion comes with mixed feelings afterward. The group considers what it is like to embrace the need to sometimes experience discomfort when in relationships.

CASE EXAMPLE 3: PUTTING POLYVAGAL THEORY INTO ACTION

The group, which predominately comprises members with scores high on warmth and focused on the needs of others, is struggling with a member, Luna, who is high on Scale 2: Focused on the Needs of the Self. Luna has been harshly critical of several members for being "overly sensitive to every little thing that happens to you." The members express a mixture of sadness and hurt that Luna is being too judgmental.

The group leader notes that this is a difficult situation because for several members in the group, being assertive and engaging in conflict is a 180-degree goal and is therefore highly activating for them. The leader mediates. First, the leader invites Luna to consider how their perception of the rest of the group may be shaped by Luna's own difficulty in owning their own vulnerability. The leader initiates a working the axes intervention (discussed in more detail later in the Working the Axes to Handle Tension and Conflict section) by asking each side to consider what aspect of the other might be helpful to integrate into themselves. The leader also invites Luna to consider how their goal of asking follow-up questions can be used to better understand the role feelings of vulnerability that can be helpful for the rest of the group.

After the intervention has finished, the group leader invites the group members who are less comfortable with conflict to reflect on the process. While several group members express pride that they could share their feelings, one member becomes tearful and expresses that they are feeling "very shaky" after the conflict. Luna shares with the tearful member that although it was hard, that person did survive the experience and that perhaps this was a template for being able to survive other experiences with conflict. The group shares that they like the way Luna expresses this far better and also provides comfort to the upset member. The therapist encourages the upset group member to see that they were successful in managing a conflict and that, over time, they may find that holding steady in the middle of a conflict, while uncomfortable and upsetting, can sometimes lead to positive outcomes. The group discusses this process.

Here are the takeaways from these three examples. The posture of the therapist depends on their identification for the constructs involved and the reasons for the attack as well as their consideration of what interpersonal forces are involved. In Case Example 1, the group leader notes that the group should expect to have a significantly different experience of closeness based on their interpersonal styles. The leader also notes that the person with a distant style may end up being scapegoated by the rest of the group for representing the boundaries and distance that they find so difficult to enact. The leader therefore makes a conscious choice to ally with the isolated member and protect them against the scapegoating while also helping the group understand the process that is happening. In this example, the opposing interpersonal forces have generated a group-as-a-whole phenomenon: scapegoating.

In Case Example 2, a macroaggression has occurred that also allows a group member to work on a goal. The therapist's stance can therefore be supportive while acting to contain the conflict and ultimately provide the facilitative conditions to work through. Feedback can also take place that allows the member who asserted themselves to understand the impact of their actions and allow for the fact that change is not always accompanied by universally positive emotions.

Case Example 3 shows how a group conflict represents an opportunity for members to become more adept at managing their feelings and tolerating conflict while also working on their goals. This is an example of polyvagal theory in action. As Flores and Porges (2017) indicated, an effective pathway for becoming more able to manage conflicts is to be exposed to them and become up-regulated but then to experience them as safe and manageable. In this case, the group leader manages not just the conflict but also helps the group find meaning in what was a challenging experience, strengthening their ability to see future conflicts as manageable and survivable.

WORKING THE AXES TO HANDLE TENSION AND CONFLICT

Many moments of tension, conflict, and sometimes serious rupture need repair when a member externalizes parts of their disowned self. Once such moment often occurs when an individual with a high score on Scale 2: Focused on the Needs of the Self (or with that as a secondary peak) experiences the internal tension of encountering the vulnerability of the other group members, and that individual begins to externalize. Remember that each style contains within it a set of behaviors that are considered acceptable and unacceptable. Sullivan (1947) mentioned the idea of the me, bad me, and not me as representing parts of the self that are either owned, labeled negatively, or completely disowned based on parental reactions at childhood (p. 10). The "not me" represents the aspects of the interpersonal self that were treated so severely in childhood that they became completely disowned. For example, a child who was treated with disdain or punishment every time they failed or showed vulnerability may learn to dismiss that part of themselves as "weak and pathetic," internalizing the words of their parent as a truth that they needed to organize themselves around. Because part of the trait-level style of Scale 2 is to externalize, that disowned part of themselves is externalized onto others. Therefore, when someone in the group acts in a way that is vulnerable, such as by crying or exhibiting other forms of emotional release, the person is immediately and sometimes vocally and harshly dismissed as "weak." In this moment, the person with a high score on Scale 2 is externalizing that part of themselves they have dismissed. It is "not me"—it is "you."

There are many ways to deal with moments of tension and conflict in group therapy. One such intervention within FBGT is the technique called *working the axes:* After the initial aggressive attack, the group leader intervenes. Their job at this point is to help frame the interaction as relating to disowning parts of themselves. While it is easy to see the disowned vulnerability, it is also worth remembering that the person who is being attacked also has a disowned side. For example, someone with a Scale 6: Focused on the Needs of Others style will find it difficult to argue, defend themselves, and externalize. The therapist typically begins with reframing the attack by defining the problem as one of polarities—that each person in the interaction is in conflict with a part of themselves that they have disowned.

A brief explanation of how we sometimes label things as bad when we cannot accept them in ourselves also provides a frame that the attack is as much a personal one against ourselves as it is against the other person.

The therapist then invites each person to consider what small part of the other person they would wish to have a part of. This has proven a useful intervention as members begin to own aspects of themselves that they had previously disowned. In one clinical example, the client with a high Scale 2 score stated, "The ability to monitor what I say and be careful of others' feelings is something you do really well and I wish I had," while the member who had been under attack acknowledged, "I wish I could be more spontaneous like you and not always overthink everything." The intent of this intervention is to help each member begin to see the disowned part of themselves—their 180-degree side, or what Jung might have considered part of the "shadow self" (Jung, 1959/1968, p. 20).

In some cases, the rest of the group intervenes and defends the person under attack. Some learning may come from this set of responses from the group, and it can be helpful to let it play out—but with some parameters, such as using "I" statements and refraining from using insults. In these instances, it remains important for the group leader to monitor what kind of learning takes place that relates to the skill building or insight of the group in general—which depends on the group dynamic and the mix of interpersonal styles. For example, a group of people with high scores in warmth respond very differently than a group comprising people high in unassertiveness. Each group needs a different level and type of intervention from the leader to ensure that meaningful learning takes place. Thus, the leader must frame these events thoughtfully, taking into consideration the critical incident, the group dynamic, and the interpersonal styles of the members involved. Ultimately, there may be some gains to the group from a variety of responses to this moment, but remember that addressing the underlying interpersonal circumplex issues should always remain front of mind for the group leader. While managing conflicts and ruptures in any group is crucial to its success, a leader task in FBGT that is just as important is maintaining a focus on time (Piper & Ogrodniczuk, 2004): a process named "holding feet to the fire."

HOLDING FEET TO THE FIRE

For any brief group, while managing alliance ruptures and providing a facilitative environment, a main task of the group leader is *holding feet to the fire*, that is, maintaining a focus on time (Piper & Ogrodniczuk, 2004). FBGT is no different. Clients tend to fit the work into the available time but only if they are made aware of the parameters and reminded of them. The therapist should bring attention to these parameters at the beginning of each session, noting the number of sessions left to complete the work.

The group leader must treat the penultimate group as the last chance for group members to work on their goals. Because the last session is devoted to ending, group members should be clear that this is their final opportunity (see The Final Session section later for further discussion). Group leaders are wise to check their notes to ensure that members who have already worked well on goals are not taking up more of the group's time. Therefore, the final session should involve inviting members to report if they feel all their goals are completed or not and to ask for time if they have not been previously completed. The leader's statement at the beginning of this session should be clear and unequivocal in noting that this is the last chance to do so. Equally, the therapist and the group should be working to help those who have not yet completed a goal. The therapist should be active as they need to be inviting and making this happen.

GROUP WRAP-UP

Wrapping up the group at the end of sessions typically entails a range of options, depending on time. In most cases, it may entail a summary of the session and a prediction about the next session. For example, the therapist might say,

> Today was a good session where you all really worked hard on your goals. Pat and Ira, you really got a lot accomplished today. Ki, you really were taking it all in, and I know you got a lot of good feedback from the group about your goal. Marsha, I know you wanted to say more and asked for help, so I wonder if we can start off with you next week?

Interventions can also address a group-as-whole issue, such as a difficult conflict that happened too near the end to effectively process. The therapist might say something like this:

> We had a good session today, and lots of work got accomplished. I know this session ended in a tough place, and we didn't have time to really see it through. That happens sometimes. Sometimes conflict can seem frightening, and some of you might be tempted to stay away next week. However, in my experience, working it through in a safe environment can really add a lot of depth to the group, and there can be a lot of learning for everyone. So next week, it is more important than ever to turn up. I look forward to seeing you all next week. We will work it through and see what we can all learn from it.

Summaries after sessions end in this way need to predict into a hopeful outcome. Members who are conflict averse may feel frightened by the affect and be worried that it will be uncontained. The group leader therefore must put things into perspective so that the conflict is not the only work being identified as important. Equally, the leader predicts into members' desire to flee. This prediction is important because members are now alerted that they may be tempted to not return. By identifying the impulse, the member can no longer engage in the pretense that missing the next session is for another reason, such as an urgent, unexpected appointment elsewhere. Moreover, the leader in the preceding summary example frames the conflict as a chance to learn, simultaneously demonstrating an ability to manage and contain the conflict so it can be conflict. If time is running short, a summary may also simply entail a quick check-in on emotions in which the leader asks for one word from each member to describe their emotions.

INTERVENTION SELECTION USING THE GROUP GOAL LAP SHEET

Selecting interventions can be one of the most challenging aspects in group therapy. Many threads can be pulled on, and at any one moment, the group leader can choose to focus on the individual, interpersonal relationship, or group as a whole (Gelso & Williams, 2022). FBGT has a method for helping leaders decide which thread to follow based on goal achievement.

The group leader takes a blank sheet of paper that is filled with members' names in order of seating, which is organized in a circle. This sheet is similar to the one used in Session 1 (see Chapter 7). This time, though, the leader makes abbreviated notes under each member's name to indicate their goals. For example, these are the shorthand/abbreviated listed goals for group member Brian:

Brian
1. Ask follow-up questions
2. Feedback: Obtain
3. Initiate conversation at least ×1 [at least once]

As a group member achieves their goals, the leader places a check mark next to each goal. This allows them to track who has accomplished their goals; therefore, at key moments, they can direct traffic toward members who may need time or attention. It is particularly important that leaders track carefully and ensure members get feedback from the group as they accomplish goals because those members will be highly anxious that their new behaviors may have left them rejected or ostracized by the group. Once a group member has received feedback on a specific goal, the leader should place an asterisk next to the check mark for that goal. The leader needs to keep the sheet and use it every session to promote continuity between sessions. While leaders should not spend the session staring down at their sheet, robotically checking off goals, it is vital that they keep track because this is the proposed mechanism of change.

Figure 8.1, which depicts goals accomplished in Session 3, shows that several members (introduced in Chapter 7) have received considerable attention from the group and have achieved their goals already as well as received feedback. Marco and Joe appear to have been focusing well on their goals, and Joe, in particular, has completed his goals and also received feedback. Pi, Ann, and Shannah have achieved partial success, but Ann has not yet received feedback on goal completion, so this should be a main target of the group leaders as soon as possible. Ash has not yet attempted either of their listed goals because they have indicated they find it difficult to wait for others or to ask follow-up questions. Ash may need a process intervention to uncover what worries are making this goal difficult to accomplish. Pi is still someone of concern in this group because they were already identified as someone who had not become cohered to the group. If the leaders had still not managed to facilitate connection and cohesion to Pi, and Pi had accomplished a goal but had not yet received feedback, then their anxiety about the group's perception of them might be extremely high. Without the anchor of cohesion, there is a possibility that this added anxiety of trying a new behavior might lead to a desire to seek interpersonal safety by missing the next session. The role of feedback in this case not only reinforces the behavior and removes the anxiety, but also begins to build cohesion. At this point, the leader might also invite further feedback from other members to reinforce the cohesion.

THE FINAL SESSION

Similar to Session 1, the last session—Session 8—is highly structured, requiring the use of both activities and careful management of time. It can be an intense session for the therapist because it involves juggling many tasks simultaneously while managing time. And it is a session in which there is considerable pent-up energy. Some group members are working hard to distance themselves to obviate the pain of ending, whereas others are negotiating the stages of grief as they end by bargaining for more time, being in denial, or expressing sadness or anger. This makes ending the session challenging on emotional and cognitive levels for the group leader, so doing so requires considerable skill.

FIGURE 8.1. Goal Accomplishment Check Sheet

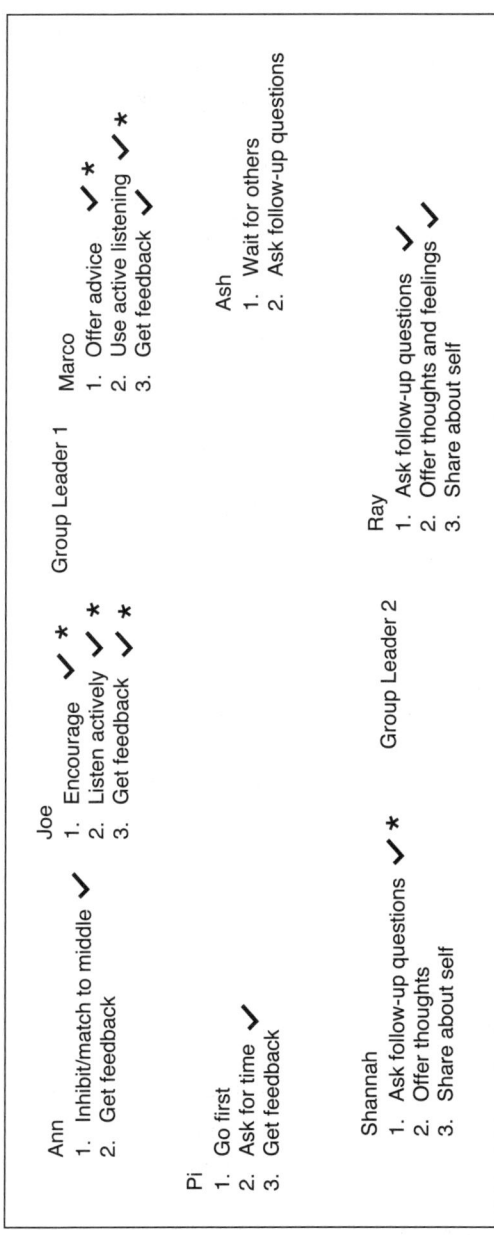

Two Primary Tasks

The group leader carries out two main tasks in Session 8: (a) reflecting on work accomplished and (b) saying goodbye. Of the two tasks, saying goodbye can be the most challenging. Clients are often highly ambivalent about leaving a cohesive group that they have found to be helpful and where they have felt safe and connected. No one wants to leave a place where they feel they belong.

Normal feelings of sadness emerge, and groups often bargain with the group leader to keep the group running beyond its boundaries. To have a healthy and boundaried ending, it is vital that the leader close the group and ensure that members have the opportunity to acknowledge what the group and its members have done for them.

Leadership Functions

Leadership functions related to structuring and the executive role in group management become particularly important during the ending of groups. Ensuring that groups end well is a complex process, and time boundaries can easily be violated by the group as they resist closure (Kobos, 1993). Therefore, strong but empathic leadership is necessary during the adjournment of the group. Activities can also greatly assist in this process (Shapiro & Ginzberg, 2002).

Time Management

The leadership function central to Session 8 is time management. There is a lot to accomplish in the final session, and the group leader must ensure that the executive functions of leadership predominate. The leader must begin by explaining the purpose of the session and prepare clients for the reimposition of structure. The leader needs to warn members that they may be interrupted for the sake of time management and that this interruption may feel jarring. Acknowledging how this may feel and apologizing in advance for it helps mitigate the potential of the interruption to be an alliance rupture.

The leadership stance that is most helpful in this final session is to acknowledge the imperfection of endings and to work to hold, contain, and sometimes express—using self-involving self-disclosure and reflection of feelings—the mixed emotions that come from leaving. For example, the group leader might say,

> I am experiencing a lot of emotion in the room. There is a lot of happiness and sense of connection, along with a sense of sadness and a desire to keep the warm connection that has been built. I wonder who else is experiencing this?

The connections established in FBGT, although limited in duration, can be highly impactful for clients. It is quite typical for clients to express considerable sadness at ending and also to ask the group leader if the group can continue in some other form after the group has ended. This fantasy reflects important feelings. For many in the group, the wish to connect in a rich way has been an elusive goal, and the fantasy that continuing the group will continue that feeling is one that is powerful. However, leaders must enforce the boundary while acknowledging the wish. The group leader should consider reframing this desire as representing an ongoing wish to connect to others. However, the leader should emphasize that this group is a place to practice how to attain more meaningful connections in life—that is, the group should be a spur to do so and not an end in itself. The final session, then, is a helpful time for group members to explore how they have been successful in connecting and to get further praise for the goals they have accomplished.

Time management is extremely challenging during the last session because members often have unfinished business of their own and with each other. It is not unusual for members to use *doorknob* comments (Arnd-Caddigan, 2013), which are often dramatic admissions or revelations delivered just as a group is closing. These last-minute admissions or self-disclosures are sometimes highly activating for both the group and the individual who makes them. For example, someone may suddenly disclose a past trauma or a shocking secret, such as feelings of attraction for another group member. Doorknob comments happen for numerous reasons. In some cases, they reflect the person's ambivalence about revealing themselves and represent a lower risk way of speaking a truth while avoiding judgment. They can also reflect a desire to continue the group—a last gasp effort to engage the group with material so dramatic, it makes an ending seem impossible. Regardless of the reason, they place the group in an emotional quandary.

Because doorknob comments are delivered at the last possible moment, that makes it impossible for the group to fully process them, which can take away from feelings that the group is finished and leave group members feeling upset and wishing for more time to work them through together. In some cases, groups are flexible enough to be extended. However, the therapist should resist this temptation. The group is ending, and despite many different reasons why the group may wish to continue, endings, separations, and loss are also a part of life that cannot be avoided. The therapist can acknowledge the wish for the group to continue but with the caveat that the skills learned and used created this feeling of belonging. It is these skills that allowed for this depth, and the purpose of the group is to be thankful for the help others gave while recognizing and being recognized for what was accomplished.

The job of the group leader is also to acknowledge what can be a larger truth: that endings are often complex and can involve conflicting feelings of both closure and sometimes unfinished business. Embracing this kind of complexity can give permission to clients to also begin to reset expectations of other endings from their past or that may lie in their future.

Final Session Structure

The first part of the group typically involves having members reflect on goals. Again, note cards are used, and members can comment on how they have accomplished their goals and felt helped by other members. The group leader needs to carefully set up this part of the group, alerting members that they have limited time and that the leader may need to interrupt to ensure that the group has enough time to get to the final activity. Therefore, the group leader should become comfortable with interrupting in an appropriate way, as needed. Apologizing for the need to interrupt in the moment can offset group members' hurt feelings, providing the group has been forewarned.

The Ending Activity

The final part of the group is devoted to an ending activity. Many such activities are available, and which one to choose is according to the group leader's preference. Any activity that promotes appreciation and honors accomplishments can serve as an effective ritual and provide closure. One simple example of such an activity is to hand out a piece of paper and a pen to every member. The member puts their name at the top. They then make a fold in the paper and hand it to the person next to them who then writes a brief appreciation on it. This continues around the group with each member writing a comment and then making a fold so the prior person cannot see it. The end result looks like a concertina or folder fan and has comments from every group member. Members have reported enjoying this activity because it gives a chance for everyone to be appreciated and to have a say without needing to open up a larger discussion. Members have also reported treasuring the paper and using it—after the group has ended—as a device to empower themselves when they are having a difficult day.

Members typically report wishing to continue the group elsewhere. They may ask for each other's contact details. Encourage members to see this as a self-contained experience and to process the goodbye with all the finality it implies. Allow people to express feelings but process feelings around an ending.

At the end of the group, the therapist gives members the IIP-32 and quality of life measure (e.g., the 30-item Outcome Questionnaire; Ellsworth et al., 2006) to fill out. Members also need to schedule an individual debriefing session with the therapist. These last two administrative tasks are extremely important. Debriefings are an essential part of FBGT, and the posttests are a vital part of assessing outcomes. Chapter 9 explores how to interpret the data.

SUMMARY

The group process involves several key concerns. The working alliance and group cohesion remain an important thread that must be kept as the drumbeat underlying the group. This does not mean that certain aspects of group like conflict must be avoided but, rather, that the therapist should titrate them and ensure that the process is well managed based on engaging in therapeutic tact and giving meaning to events. The two main processes that then drive change are the activation of goals and use of feedback, processes that are key to group member progress. Group leaders should note the number of times members accomplish these two processes, using the notes as a guide to select interventions that allow each member time to work on their goals. Techniques such as engaging feedback loops, working through ruptures and making repairs, working the axes, and holding feet to the fire all form important parts of the middle and later group processes.

The final group involves establishing that group has ended and saying goodbye. Members often resist termination and sometimes bargain, wishing for group to continue or suggesting that the group all meet socially. The need to enforce that the group is ending and that saying goodbye is a part of that ending is essential. It is also important for the therapist to note that the work of the group is designed to help people with their lives outside of the group. Therefore, the ending should be processed as an experience that allows its members to take learnings into their real-world settings. The therapist should readminister assessment tools in preparation for the triangulation of data and debriefing session.

9 MAKING SENSE OF CLIENT CHANGE

Triangulation of Data

Triangulation of data is an important part of focused brief group therapy (FBGT) because it allows the therapist to detect changes that might otherwise be obscured to them (Whittingham, 2015). It is easy to see success if a client has accomplished their goals and seems happy with treatment and sad for the group to end. However, while those measures of success have some merit as ways to evaluate progress, they seldom tell the whole story.

Triangulation of data allows that information to be blended with data about changes in overall quality of life or symptoms, risk factors, measures of interpersonal functioning, and changes in scores that were the focus of treatment. It also allows for the integration of data about the distress that comes from change—subjects that need to be broached in the debriefing session (discussed in Chapter 10). Triangulation of data also sometimes provides surprising results in which data points seem discrepant, contradictory, or hard to reconcile. These then often lead to new clinical directions that can further facilitate client change and progress. Therefore, it is essential to remember that this process is for clinical reasons—to help better understand and facilitate the change process—and therefore should not be skipped.

https://doi.org/10.1037/0000389-010
Focused Brief Group Therapy: An Integrative Approach to Reducing Interpersonal Distress, by M. Whittingham

ORIGINS OF TRIANGULATION

One of the most fascinating and revealing aspects of conducting FBGT when it was first being implemented were the processes of data triangulation (Whittingham, 2015) and debriefing. Although on many occasions, the data lined up in ways that intuitively made sense, at other times, data emerged that were seemingly at odds with the total picture or were initially confusing. Using multiple data points during therapy and integrating them with clinical judgment were processes that required a balance between trust in the theory and responsiveness to each individual as a person. The deep structure of the premises of the theory never failed to illuminate, and it became clear at an early stage that the mechanisms of change, when performed with skill, were active ingredients in change. It also became clear that clients approach change processes idiosyncratically and that failing to appreciate that could lead clinicians into misunderstandings and mistaken conclusions.

As a result, when analyzing the data, the approach has shifted to viewing the data with humility and with an open mind—to consider one's hypotheses about what happened as possibilities that need verifying and may be missing important information. However, it is important to avoid "throwing out the baby with the bathwater"—to use an expression that suggests people should not reject the whole premise because some part of it does not work as anticipated—in the face of information that is seemingly contradictory.

HOW TO TRIANGULATE

When triangulating data, the therapist collects all data points and uses them to develop a tentative hypothesis regarding each group members' progress in group. Triangulation involves comparing and contrasting several data points:

- Did the client complete their goals during the group (e.g., What did the therapist observe, and did the client realize and acknowledge it?)?

- What did the therapist observe in terms of client behavior (e.g., a change in body language, an improvement in overall interpersonal functioning) during the group that indicated the client had been successful?

- What change was observed from prepost on the 32-item Inventory of Interpersonal Problems (IIP-32; Horowitz et al., 2000) change score that was the agreed on focus of treatment (e.g., Did the score on the social inhibition scale [Scale 4: Socially Inhibited; see Figure 1.2 in Chapter 1] change from the start of group to the end of group?)?

- What change was observed on the IIP-32 total distress score (e.g., Did overall distress change from the start to the end of group?)?

- What change was noted on the quality of life prepost change score (e.g., Did the 30-item Outcome Questionnaire [OQ-30; Ellsworth et al., 2006] score decrease reliably, as indicated by the analytics?)?

- When comparing and contrasting the results, what tentative hypothesis can be developed using clinical judgment?

- Are there discrepancies between instruments (e.g., Did one measure show the client improved, but another showed no improvement or worsening?)? If so, then explore with the client during the debriefing session and also consult with other data sources, if available (e.g., confer with the client's individual therapist).

Comparing and Contrasting

The therapist should carefully and thoughtfully compare and contrast each of these observations—whether assessment data, behavior, or goal completion—with the other data points. In many cases, these comparisons prove consistent with each other and trend in the same direction. For example, in triangulating the data for a member who was working on focusing on the needs of others, multiple observations are made. First, the group leader notes that the member completed their goals, successfully asking for help twice and going first in the group twice. The leader also notes that the member received positive feedback, and as the group progressed, the member seemed to appear more confident and self-assured in looking after their own needs.

Next, in looking at the scale data, the group leader notes that the member's score on Scale 6: Focused on the Needs of Others went down significantly. They also note that, as expected, the opposite scale, Scale 2: Focused on the Needs of the Self, went up slightly but not by as much as the scores that were the focus of treatment (which is a typical pattern for people experiencing the discomfort of change). The therapist also notes that the client's total interpersonal distress score went down. The therapist compares this information to the client's OQ-30 (Ellsworth et al., 2006) score, which went down by a statistically significant amount. The OQ-30 analytic printout describes this as "reliable change." In this case, all data points align. The therapist develops the tentative hypothesis that the client had a successful group experience and prepares to discuss this hypothesis with the client in the debriefing session.

The therapist also observes that this particular scale score change, although well received in the group, may receive negative feedback from people in real life. They note that it is important for this client to understand that some people in their life outside of group therapy may not respond well to a change in the terms of relationship. People in the client's life who are used to a one-way, service-based relationship with no boundaries may become angry when limits are set or when the client asks for their needs to be met as well. The therapist notes the need to discuss with the client attempts to make these changes with people who may be more receptive and also prepare themself for the end of some one-way relationships if they choose to confront them.

Making Sense of Discrepancies

Not every set of scores is consistent with each other. There can be confounds and complications with respect to these scores, and these need investigating during the debriefing session. They may either be related to external issues that are unrelated to treatment (e.g., a death in the family, which leads to sadness that is unrelated to the work of the group), issues related to implementing treatment (e.g., ending an unhealthy relationship as a result of working on assertiveness but now grieving it while also believing it was the right thing to do), or issues related to difficulties in implementing the learning in the real world (e.g., only using the new behavior online and not in person). Therefore, investigating discrepancies can be an important part of helping the client understand the impact of treatment and to find ways to effectively implement the changes once treatment has ended.

Consider this example, which illustrates the method of exploring discrepancies. A group member has been working on their goals related to being socially inhibited. The therapist notes that the member has succeeded in completing all their goals: They worked on asking follow-up questions and initiating conversations. The therapist also observes that the member has managed to form connections with others in the group and is looking less at the floor and is giving eye contact and nonverbal indications that they are listening. They also seem to be enjoying the group and finding its members helpful. The scale scores showed improvement on social inhibition and total distress on the IIP-32 (Horowitz et al., 2000) as well as an expected increase on the opposite scale as a result of anxiety around growth and the awkwardness that comes with new behaviors. However, the client's OQ-30 (Ellsworth et al., 2006) score has not changed: It has remained high. Equally, the cotherapist (who is high in warmth) remarks that they did not really feel the client had grown at all and that the changes seem too small and insignificant. Thus, the information seems contradictory. The hypothesis then becomes a more tentative one. It appears that the client has been successful in achieving their goals—the main mechanism of change—and their IIP-32 scores have moved in the right direction. However, the OQ-30 score suggests that either something has not translated well into real life, or external circumstances have impacted this member's feelings about their life in general. The therapist agrees to ask the client more about the scores to try to understand what the discrepancy means.

So, the therapist discusses with the cotherapist how they each perceive the changes. They state that they cannot see how small changes such as asking follow-up questions can achieve so much change. They note the lack of crying that has accompanied the change and that the client did not then become more extraverted. The therapist explains that what seems like a small change to someone who is more extraverted is actually a profound one for someone who is more inhibited. They remind the group leader of how terrified the client was to join the group and that the client had rated those goals a 9 out of 10 for difficulty. The coleader engages in some introspection and notes that their own style—of being at ease with warmth—may have led them to minimize the difficulty of the goals. The coleader realizes the seemingly small changes in fact required tremendous courage on the part of the client.

The OQ-30 discrepancy in this example could have been explained by many things. The therapy certainly seemed successful, given the change in scores on the IIP-32, but the therapists needed to explore how these changes were playing out in real life. For example, if the client was not yet implementing the changes in their work, leisure, or friendships, that could explain the lack of movement on the OQ-30. Equally, if the client had a successful experience and had also transferred these changes to the real world but had a negative life event, such as failing an exam or experiencing financial problems, then this could also explain the discrepancy. It is also possible that the change in OQ-30 scores is the result of a good thing. For example, perhaps the client is beginning to believe in their ability to find new relationships, so they have ended an unhappy romantic relationship. They feel good about the decision but then also experience feelings of sadness and loneliness that lead to a higher score on the OQ-30. Remember that positive changes in one's life are not always accompanied by pleasant feelings. That is where informed consent becomes important in debriefings as therapists discuss the possibility of pain that can arise from new choices.

Using Clinical Judgment

Several processes within data triangulation are important. First, remember that assessment augments but does not replace clinical judgment (Whittingham et al., 2023). The data are always illuminating and typically are vital. However, the therapist should always retain their clinical judgment. In many instances, clinical judgment becomes highly important at the end of the therapy during the triangulation of data.

In some cases, assessments may be filled out incorrectly, leading to odd or incongruent or seemingly impossible results. When in distress, clients may become flustered or emotional, which can impact the way they complete instruments. Clients are also sometimes tempted to hide the true extent of their feelings or may increase or decrease their true scores for a multitude of reasons. For example, they may believe that they need to appear worse to obtain treatment, or, in some cases, they may fake being good to please a therapist or to ensure that they can leave treatment (Grieve & de Groot, 2011).

Catching these incorrect scores requires a combination of technical and clinical judgment. For example, a client completes their IIP-32 (Horowitz et al., 2000) at the end of treatment. The therapist notes that they have changed from someone high on Scale 8: Unassertive to someone high on Scale 2: Focused on the Needs of the Self and with no distress on unassertiveness whatsoever. The therapist finds this odd because the client had reported being unassertive, and every other clinical indicator shows that the initial report is accurate. The therapist notes that it is highly unlikely that someone would suddenly have a very high score on Scale 2: Focused on the Needs of the Self and no distress on Scale 5: Unassertive, their previous highest score. This pattern seems highly unlikely. So, the therapist calls the client and asks, "How was it filling out the form on the last day?" The client reports being tired that day and in a hurry to leave. They explain that they may have scored them "backward" by mistake because they did not recheck what the high scores meant and had misremembered a high score as meaning low distress. They apologize and offer to come in to rescore the instrument.

The completion of goals is the main mechanism of change in FBGT. Within this is also the assumption that the group leader has ensured that clients have received feedback on their goals. Because goal completion is observable, and the group leader has been tracking and recording incidences of success, these data should be clear. Partial completion of goals (e.g., having a goal of completing twice and only completing once) should be acknowledged as a success while working to understand the context around not completing twice.

Further, in some instances, a group member may complete a goal outside of the group but not inside the group. Consider this example: A member arrives flustered and upset, and recounts an incident in which they had been involved in an altercation on the way to work in the subway. They state that someone harassed them but that they had stood up to that person and asserted strongly that they should be left alone. The group supports them and also mentions that this is a goal completion. The group and the member explore what it was like for this member to stand up for themself, and the group provides feedback. The member also explores what has been holding them back from being assertive in the group. At the end of the group, the member acknowledges that this external incident has been important and is a significant accomplishment.

Determining the Types of Change

The central mechanism of change is the client goal that was developed based on their highest scale score. The key *process variable* is whether the group member completed their scale group goals (e.g., asking follow-up questions twice as a goal for social inhibition). The key *outcome variable* is whether this resulted in reductions in distress on the targeted scale (this then led to a reduction of 10 points on the Scale 4: Socially Inhibited distress score). It would be expected that these scores should also then correlate with other outcome measures. For example, did the changes made have an impact on the client's quality of life measure score (e.g., their OQ-30 [Ellsworth et al., 2006] score went down by an amount rated as clinically reliable)? In other words, did changes made in group have a concrete impact on the person's life?

The overall IIP-32 (Horowitz et al., 2000) total score change is also assessed. Typically, the total distress scale shows a reduction in distress, but this may be small because of the increases in distress on other scales that often come with changes in the targeted scale. Growth is painful. Typically, as FBGT clinical observations and research have found, these increases remit over time as the client habituates to the change. They are important to discuss with the client (as discussed in Chapter 10). However, they represent the normal process of change and are not a failure of the therapy.

Starting the Two-Step Process

The therapist must then combine all data points. Note that clinical judgment should be the ultimate arbiter, but only after all data have been reviewed, including client comments and feedback. Thus, the process consists of two steps. First, the therapist evaluates change by integrating multiple data points to form a tentative hypothesis.

Second, the therapist asks the client for their perceptions of treatment and then presents the hypothesis for discussion during debriefing. The therapist should carry out this second step carefully and thoughtfully, making sure they are integrating new information the client presents and are listening carefully. A hypothesis is typically only confirmed with client agreement. However, hypothesis formation is the first crucial step.

Exploring Indicators of Progress

This is completed as follows: A hypothesis is generated by combining indicators of progress and then using clinical judgment to form an initial impression of change. Each indicator is now addressed.

IIP-32 Change Scores

The first question to establish is whether the targeted scale of change shows any prepost difference. Given that the accomplishment of goals based on their highest scale score is the intended mechanism of change, it is important to understand if and how the score altered from prepost. Any positive change is worthy of discussion and comment. However, what qualifies as significant change relies somewhat on local norms and benchmarking. Use of reliable change indices (Jacobson & Truax, 1992) can be helpful in determining whether a local change score is statistically significant.

Next, the therapist evaluates the client's total interpersonal distress score. It is typical for the client's score to lower when their distress scores improve on the targeted scale. However, the total interpersonal distress score typically reduces at a lower rate than the targeted score because change scores on the targeted scale are almost always mirrored by some increase in distress on the opposite scales as clients habituate to change. The therapist then reviews other scale scores to determine whether they increased or decreased. They note and integrate this information into the discussion about habituation.

The therapist observes the amount of change that happened between the pre- and postscores and makes an initial, tentative hypothesis about whether there change occurred on the targeted scale and if it impacted overall interpersonal distress. The therapist then considers whether this lines up with their clinical judgment and the behavioral change they had observed the client make during group.

Quality of Life Measure

The therapist then notes changes from prepost in the quality of life measure. The nature of these changes depends on the quality of life measure used. In some cases, there is a global distress score, whereas for other instruments, there is a more fine-grained analysis. The therapist looks for reductions in distress. If any of these scores increased, then the therapist considers further intervention as appropriate and notes to discuss this matter nonjudgmentally with the client. Edbrooke-Childs et al. (2015) pointed out that goals of treatment typically achieve higher gains on outcome measures than quality of life measures. This is consistent with what was clinically found in FBGT: Quality of life improvement is a function of goal improvement but is also confounded by multiple other factors. FBGT, like any other brief treatment, is not a panacea; rather, it is a stepping stone that leads a client on the road toward self-improvement in a specific area. Brief therapies are designed to achieve an improvement in symptoms and to set clients on a course for improved functioning.

Goal Attainment

Goal attainment typically refers to goals accomplished within the life of the group. The most important indicator of a process goal achieved is whether the client has successfully enacted their focused goals during group therapy. How many goals they have accomplished and how often they have accomplished them speak to whether the client has been successful in completion. This is a key element of success in the group. Achievement of goals is typically, but not always, predictive of treatment success. As group therapy has gone on, the therapist should be noting goals on the group goal lap sheet (see Chapter 8) and also entering them in group therapy notes for each individual client.

In some cases, clients accomplish goals outside of the group and report them back. Consider this example: A group member reports that although they did not yet work on their goal of being assertive, they were highly assertive on the way to the group with a store owner who had been verbally abusive toward them. The group recognizes the work and processes it with that group member during the group session. When the client asks if this means that they have accomplished their goal, the group is clear and effusive that they have. It is essential to recognize what is important to each member with respect to change. Because there were no other opportunities during the time the group had left for the client to accomplish this goal (and because doing so would have felt to the client that they were "forcing" a conflict), the group leader concurred with the group's recognition of the goal. Therefore, notation of goal accomplishment should respect behavioral change that takes part outside of the group.

Behavioral Observations

The next data point is whether the client has noticeably changed their behavior in the direction of their goals. This should be evident from the notes the therapist has made following each session. For example, did the therapist observe someone who is socially inhibited giving good eye contact and asking follow-up questions in a way that was not previously part of their typical behavior? Overall, did they seem to be benefiting from group therapy as evidenced by changes in behavior related directly or indirectly to goals? For example, did the therapist see them smiling more as group progressed and giving more non-verbal indications that they were connecting well to other members? Verbal and nonverbal changes are worthy of note and should form another data point to support or disconfirm hypotheses.

Interpreting the Data

Combining data points then leads to a variety of different possibilities. Sometimes data points agree, and there is a clear pattern of progress. However, there also may be discrepancies between data points or, in rarer cases, clinical worsening. Each data point is now explored in turn.

Agreement of Information Points

The therapist must then use their clinical judgment to determine whether the information points agree. When all data points align, this decision-making process can be very straightforward. The client's targeted scale score improved, their quality of life score improved, the therapist noted that the client achieved all goals during group (along with positive feedback from the group), and the client showed nonverbal behaviors consistent with this set of other changes. The therapist then has an initial hypothesis that the client has changed and can now plan for debriefing with this hypothesis in mind. However, the therapist should be aware of the possibility that even in cases that are seemingly straightforward, clients can sometimes differ in their appraisals of how group went. This is an issue for the debriefing session (see Chapter 10).

Mixed Data

Many other data combinations are possible, making results less clear. And, in some cases, instruments disagree. For example, say the IIP-32 (Horowitz et al., 2000) shows improvement in distress but the quality of life measure worsens. The therapist must note this finding, and they may begin to wonder what might be causing discrepancy. Remember that if the client has completed all their goals and their IIP-32 scores have improved, the quality of life scores may reflect something else going on outside of group that is either related or unrelated to the work of the group. For example, the death of a relative might explain a lowered quality of life score that is unrelated to treatment. In other cases, reductions on a quality of life score can be related to treatment and should be explored. For example, a client who has been working on assertiveness decides to end a relationship, leading to mixed feelings of experiencing pride in being assertive enough to end a bad relationship but experiencing sadness and loneliness from the ending. Reductions on a quality of life score also be related to problems in translating gains into the real world in a way that is consistent with embracing strengths of existing styles. For example, someone may have overgeneralized a new skill and tried it out in a setting where it was not well received. The resulting negative feedback may have caused them distress. This is an important issue to debrief. If the IIP-32 scores did not decrease, then the therapist should make checks against other data points, such as whether behavioral goals have been met.

Worsening Indicated by All Scales

The first thing the therapist needs to check is whether the client may actually have worsened and find out why. Clinical worsening, although carefully controlled for in FBGT, is a feature of every treatment (Lambert, 2013), and it is the height of hubris to imagine that no client ever worsens under treatment, no matter how expert the clinician or how well researched the techniques. For instance, the client may be experiencing a crisis that is related or unrelated to the work of the group. For example, the person misapplied a new technique or attempted it on a person who received it poorly and received negative reactions outside of group. Alternatively, they had a trauma in their outside life, and it led to an overall perception of distress in all areas. Equally, a client may be moving toward a better interpersonal place but experiencing distress as they go. For example, by becoming more assertive about getting their own needs met, friendships may have been lost, and the transition to new relationships is proving challenging. This issue requires significant debriefing.

Further, external factors, such as bereavement or failing an exam, might contribute to overall worsening. The skill of the clinician in exploring reasons for worsening scores is essential. The therapist should explore these possibilities and more in the debriefing session with a view to helping the client reduce their distress, whether by another round of treatment or other types of continuity of care.

Considering Hypothesis Formation Versus Idiographic Validity

It is vital to remember that standardized measures are only one data point of many. They should be used to augment and not replace clinical judgment. However, clinical judgment should be carefully balanced against idiographic validity. No set of standardized data points should ever replace clinical judgment based on careful appraisal of the client's assessment of the change process.

Behavioral Observation

Consider the following case example in which the therapist forms a tentative hypothesis and integrates data about the distress that comes from change. Here, the therapist reviews their behavioral observations of the client:

> Joe [discussed in Chapter 8] appeared to try and be more focused on asking for help, and as they progressed and got feedback, they visibly appeared to become more confident and happier. They seemed anxious initially as they asked for time, but as the group progressed, they seemed to visibly become more confident and assured. At times, they reverted to being helpful to other group members and also received acknowledgment that their comments and support were helpful. They seemed emotionally ambivalent when receiving this feedback, appearing to be both happy and slightly wistful.

Goal Achievement and Feedback

Continuing with the preceding case example, the therapist then reviews the following notes about data on the client's accomplishment of goals and feedback from the group:

> Leaders assess [Joe's] data. In their opinion, Joe met their goals well, as evidenced by performing Goal 1 twice and Goal 2 once. Joe identified during group that they felt they had accomplished their goals and were pleased with their progress. Joe also received feedback from group members as to how their goal achievement impacted them. Joe reported being nervous about the feedback but feeling relieved that they did not react badly and were supportive of the changes.
>
> As can be seen from the prepost scores, the targeted highest scale, Scale 6: Focused on the Needs of Others, was dropped by a significant amount. This change is noteworthy and suggestive of change in the desired direction on the targeted scale. This is also the highest change of any other scale. There is also a smaller change on Scale 7: Warm/Self-Sacrificing, suggestive of a diffuse effect. That is, the client is also now slightly less worried about being too warm and too self-sacrificing.

Notably, there is an expected increase in Scale 2: Focused on the Needs of the Self (see Figures 9.1 and 9.2). This is typical for FBGT in which a reduction in distress on the targeted scale is accompanied by a slight increase on the opposite scale. The client is now worried that the successful scale change will be met with displeasure and rejection from others on the other scale. In other words, their becoming less focused on their own needs and asking more from friends may well be met with rejection and the ending of relationships.

This idea is reality based and could well be an outcome for some relationships. Recall that relationships are based on homeostasis. Friendships and other relationships are based on the idea of predictable interactions, whether those interactions are mutually satisfying or not. The client will likely receive negative feedback from some relationships as they ask for help from others or will, at times, refuse to meet unreasonable demands from others. In some cases, the relationship may end, and it is unrealistic to pretend to the client that this will not be the case. The client needs coaching during the debriefing that some relationships may recalibrate but others may not survive the change.

Clients should be prepared for this eventuality and must make decisions as to where and when to attempt new behaviors. In some cases, they may choose not to at all, such as in rigidly hierarchical family systems during the holidays during which the consequences for not being the family glue could be problematic for more than just the client. The client may still choose to play with options but should carefully and realistically appraise the consequences for changes in behavior and determine the cost–benefit ratio carefully. They may

FIGURE 9.1. Pretreatment Score for Joe

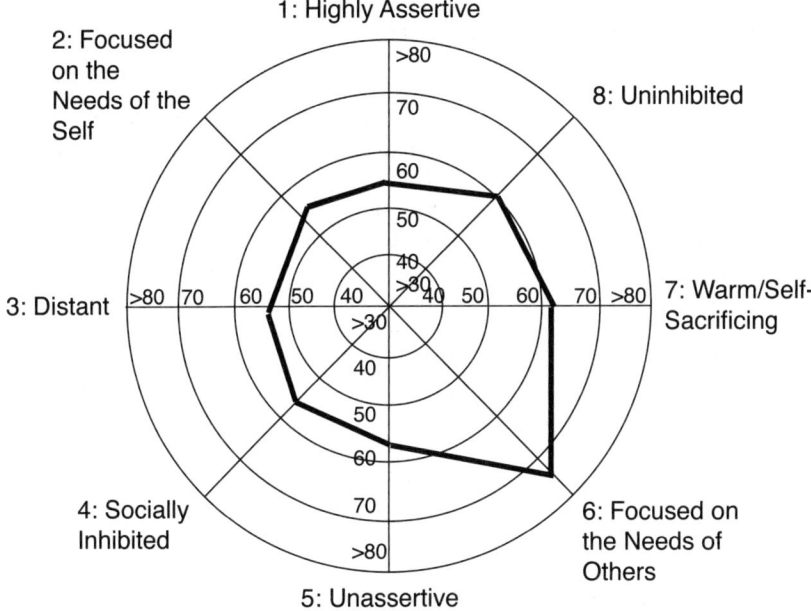

Note. Adapted from the manual for the Inventory of Interpersonal Problems by special permission of the Publisher, Mind Garden, Inc. Further reproduction requires the Publisher's written consent. Copyright © 2000 by Leonard M. Horowitz, Lynn E. Alden, Jerry S. Wiggins, & Aaron L. Pincus. All rights reserved in all media. Published by Mind Garden, Inc., www.mindgarden.com

choose to strongly assert themselves in a very different way, and this is also a viable choice; however, they need to be realistic about the potential outcomes and be prepared to deal with the repercussions. While people hope that positive changes in our behavior will be met with universally positive reception from all, debriefings should always encompass radical acceptance of reality and being prepared to accept consequences of decisions. In some cases, booster sessions, support groups, or further therapy might be considered as ways to consolidate and process changes.

Quality of Life Scores

Next, the therapist reviews the quality of life scores and sees that the client's score has improved by a clinically significant level: The OQ-30 (Ellsworth et al., 2006) shows a reduction in overall distress. This indicates a reduction in overall quality of life distress and improvement in functioning. The therapist notes that this is the hoped-for direction.

FIGURE 9.2. Posttreatment Score for Joe

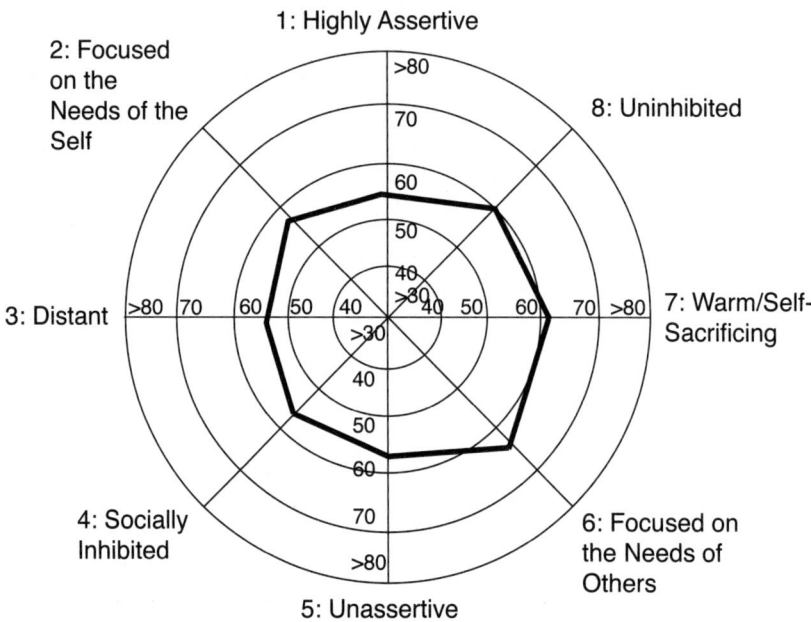

Note. Adapted from the manual for the Inventory of Interpersonal Problems by special permission of the Publisher, Mind Garden, Inc. Further reproduction requires the Publisher's written consent. Copyright © 2000 by Leonard M. Horowitz, Lynn E. Alden, Jerry S. Wiggins, & Aaron L. Pincus. All rights reserved in all media. Published by Mind Garden, Inc., www.mindgarden.com

Reasons for Score Changes Per Clinical Judgment

Both group leaders feel that Joe has achieved their goals and has had a successful group experience. In their clinical judgment, the scores changed in expected directions, and the client has appeared to benefit from group. They anticipate being able to congratulate Joe on their progress and to talk to them about generalization and transfer. In particular, the group leaders plan to focus on Joe's choices and to prepare Joe for the fact that not every relationship will survive changes in behavior.

They also plan to discuss how Joe wants to make decisions about what is worth keeping as it is, what they want to change, and how they will prepare themselves for when some things go badly. They will encourage Joe to see things as a work in progress and that they must make sure that in new relationships, they set the stage for mutuality early on. The group leaders also plan to discuss how Joe can make choices early on that consolidate and support change rather than choose situations that are likely to end poorly. The leaders also realize it is important to discuss with Joe the idea of building on change without entirely letting go of the existing skills of warmth and self-sacrifice so the client can appreciate the strengths of what they did before while now considering how and when to achieve more balance in getting their own needs met at times. The group leaders decide to approach the debriefing session with this hypothesis in mind. However, they are ready for the possibility that this could be wrong or other processes may be involved about which they are unaware. Therefore, the hypothesis is held lightly.

SUMMARY

Triangulation of data involves combining multiple formal and informal data points and then using clinical judgment to form a hypothesis. The first check should be an initial read on whether the therapists believed the client has improved, stayed the same, or worsened. At this stage, the therapists should make a very tentative hypothesis. They should evaluate whether the client has completed their goals. It is then important for them to determine whether the IIP-32 (Horowitz et al., 2000) scale score that was the target of change has been impacted. Then they can check the IIP-32 total distress score to determine if change has occurred overall. They then note any increases in IIP-32 scales (indicative of increased distress on that scale) so they can discuss them with the client. If the increase is on the opposite (or next to opposite) scale of the decrease in distress, they make notes to discuss these findings in terms of habituation. For example, if the focus for treatment is Scale 4: Socially Inhibited, and it has reduced as expected, an increase in distress on Scale 8: Uninhibited (or sometimes on Scale 1: Highly Assertive or Scale 7: Warm/Self-Sacrificing) would be an expected part of schema change and habituation.

If the data are all consistent, then the therapist can make a hypothesis with a greater degree of certainty. However, they should await meeting with the client before validating the finding. In some cases of positive change, the client may have misattributed change or may have been exposed to contextual variables (e.g., pushback from the person's family or friends) that means they need longer time to process. Negative change requires processing nonjudgmentally and plans made for continuity of care as appropriate. When data are in disagreement, differences are then noted, and the therapist considers hypotheses as to what may have happened.

10 DEBRIEFING AS AN ESSENTIAL BOOKEND

Debriefing is one of the most illuminating processes in focused brief group therapy (FBGT). It allows tentative hypotheses formed during triangulation of data to be confirmed, amended, or discarded and for further therapeutic work to commence. The process can sometimes be simple, involving cheerleading successes and planning ways to implement changes in real-world settings. Even in more straightforward cases, an essential need in the debriefing process is to understand and discuss habituation to change, homeostatic pushback from the environment, and the selection of environments and people on which to attempt new behaviors. For more complex cases, the debriefing session becomes a layered exercise in listening, assimilating new information, and sometimes engaging in detective work in collaboration with the client around constructs, events, contexts, and processes that may be involved in having an uneven change process.

https://doi.org/10.1037/0000389-011
Focused Brief Group Therapy: An Integrative Approach to Reducing Interpersonal Distress, by M. Whittingham

UNDERSTANDING THE CLIENT'S VIEW OF CHANGE

As Edbrooke-Childs et al. (2015) described, *idiographic validity*—the elucidation and agreement of the client with assessment interpretation—is essential to the validity of any findings. They pointed out that the goals of treatment typically achieve higher gains on outcome measures than on quality of life measures. This finding is consistent with what I have found in FBGT: Quality of life improvement is a function of goal improvement but is also confounded by multiple other factors. FBGT, like any other brief treatment, is a stepping-stone that leads a client on the road toward self-improvement in a specific area.

In my clinical experience, learnings from hundreds of debriefings have shown that the debriefing session frequently illuminates issues that might provide barriers to change and might impact the learning the client obtains from the group. Remember that during the termination session, the client faces significant pressure to conform to the group's belief that the group went well. Members reflect on successes, express sadness, and often convey strong wishes to carry on with the group beyond its boundaries, thus leaving little room for dissent. Members also express gratitude and thankfulness but seldom discuss what went wrong or did not work for them in the group. The purpose of the debriefing almost always is to bring to light a more nuanced picture than the simple dichotomy of the notion of an unadulterated success or complete failure.

Intervening Variables

Intervening variables (e.g., attribution style, levels of perfectionism, ego strength) and frequent struggles as clients attempt to integrate new skills and behaviors into their lives may have escaped the group leader's notice. Moreover, data are also best understood through the client's eyes, often shedding light on seemingly incongruent data.

Consider, for example, a client who broke up with their romantic partner after realizing in group therapy that they only were with that partner because they had not considered their own needs is making a positive life choice. However, this choice may have repercussions, such as feelings of loneliness, sadness, and longing as well as potential pushback from friends or family if they perceived the relationship as successful. Therefore, in this case, the client's scores on the 32-item Inventory of Interpersonal Problems (IIP-32; Horowitz et al., 2000) may go down in the expected direction, but their quality of life score, reflecting overall life happiness, may temporarily go down as they answer questions about feeling more sad or lonely. These changes in scores need to be part of the debriefing discussion so clients can make sense of change and the emotional repercussions that accompany it.

Scores, Results, and Necessary Discussions

Debriefing involves showing the client their scores and discussing the results of the group. This process is intended to promote understanding of what happened (for both client and therapist). It is also designed to increase agency, promote generalization and transfer to the outside world, and manage continuity of care as necessary. Debriefing should be performed by one of the group leaders who was present for the work of the group because they can sometimes share examples from group that the client may not have remembered or had discounted, or they can use techniques (e.g., reframing, recalling instances that counter the client's narrative, asking the client for examples that counter that narrative) born from their observations of the client or the group. For example, a client may state that they doubt the group really likes them and that they still have reservations that their attempts to befriend others were successful. Because the group leader has concrete evidence—witnessing that members nodded and agreed with or smiled at the client as they spoke—they can counter the client's effort to return to their prior maladaptive schemas.

The debriefing process follows six steps requiring several discussions to take place around each step: (a) Invite comments from the client on how the group went, (b) share prepost results and show the assessments, (c) discuss and invite the client's response, (d) discuss habituation and feelings of anxiety that accompany change, (e) discuss homeostasis, and (f) discuss generalization and transfer to the real world as well as consider continuity of care. Debriefing should always be conducted as a set of tentative hypotheses that require client confirmation. The session should be encouraging and positive with a focus on strengths and accomplishments.

Client Agency and Locus of Control

The client, in most cases, should also be the "star" of debriefing. While some clients wish to endow the therapist with the credit for success, the therapist should acknowledge thankfulness but avoid accepting credit unless that is culturally contraindicated. Thanks can be given for appreciations, but goals of debriefing are for the client to understand their own autonomy, choices, and ability to change and for them to see how their actions have led to remission of symptoms or to growth, or both.

The notion of client-enhanced internal locus of control (i.e., to what degree a client believes they have control over their lives as opposed to being controlled by external forces) is helpful to many clients in their movement forward after treatment. This concept has received increased attention in the past few years and has shown considerable promise as a key mechanism of change and action because it has been linked to personal empowerment, improved self-esteem, task motivation, and coping strategies (Galvin et al., 2018). However, the group leader should take care to ensure that this notion is culturally consistent with the client's worldview. In some cultures, attribution for success may be mediated through other processes (e.g., belief that their success was aided by their connection to their spiritual beliefs or helped by ancestors' guidance), and so the leader should approach locus of control with a degree of cultural humility and a desire to continue learning about and understanding those cultural beliefs.

Return to Strengths

Equally, client strengths should be a main focus of debriefing. The therapist must take time to remind the client that their preexisting skills and strategies have always been useful and that their personality is not something that needs "fixing" because it was never broken. Rather, treatment just offered the client a chance to add new skills to their repertoire so they have more choices moving forward.

This is an important distinction. It is not uncommon for clients to see changes they have made as a negative reflection on past failures, and the specter of shame and guilt for past mistakes looms large in the mind. The therapist must take time to reinforce the validity of past strategies and that many of those past strategies still have their place in the future. However, the group merely provided opportunities to integrate new possibilities into the client's possible choices in future interactions. Remember: The client is always doing their best with what they knew. The message is one of self-forgiveness, self-acceptance, and being at play with new options.

Celebration of Success

With respect to change, the debriefing should also include some therapeutic cheerleading or celebrating of accomplishments when they have taken place. Examples include reviewing outcomes, focusing on the courage needed to risk activating behavior, and acknowledging the impact of their behavior on the group. Whenever possible, the therapist should use examples of the group's reaction to new behaviors to reinforce learning.

Notably, clients frequently recall with uncertainty events that happened in the group. Risking new behaviors was challenging for them, so integrating new schemas will take time. In many cases, the old schemas are still working to reactivate, so cognitions will return, suggesting to the client that perhaps the group did not receive the new behaviors well. Anxiety about changes can often lead clients to reimagine the group as having been hostile or rejecting, when the reverse was true. The therapist needs to challenge and reframe this perception using concrete evidence from the group process. It is important for them to cite examples of the group or of specific members' responding positively.

Habituation and the Discomfort of Change

In my clinical work with FBGT, case studies have repeatedly shown that when a client has achieved change on their highest score, that change is typically accompanied by a smaller increase on the score at the opposite axis. So, consider, for example, that a client achieves a 10-point reduction in distress on Scale 8: Uninhibited (see Figure 1.2 in Chapter 1). This change is usually accompanied by an increase in distress on Scale 4: Socially Inhibited—the opposite end of that axis. However, this increase in distress is seldom, if ever, an equal change. Ordinarily, it would be a lesser change in magnitude on the IIP-32 (Horowitz et al., 2000) than the magnitude of change on the scale that they were working on. After looking at the results on aggregate as well as discussing those results with the client, this change was eventually conceptualized as being a result of a disruption to internal homeostasis. The client who made changes was experiencing discomfort resulting from growth.

It is easy to forget that any change in interpersonal behavior feels uncomfortable and awkward. A person's interpersonal schemas have kept behavioral options restricted for many years by predicting that changes in behaviors will likely result in disaster, ranging from negative evaluation by others to outright rejection. Therefore, when growth takes place, the feelings around this change are often relief and excitement but also apprehension and discomfort. Without immediate feedback from group members in a session that the new behavior is not going to result in rejection, the discomfort is far greater and more immediate. As a result, clients sometimes do not return or report that they did not sleep that night because they were worrying that they had offended and upset the group with their behaviors. Thus, ensuring immediate feedback for new behaviors became an essential part of the FBGT approach. The provision of immediate feedback has improved attendance and also allowed schemas to be challenged in real time while also reinforcing behaviors. However, even with feedback, new behaviors are still a source of anxiety for clients that needs addressing in debriefing. The need to normalize the feelings of discomfort as representing growth is a central task of the debriefing session and represents the need to address threats to internal homeostasis.

Managing Homeostatic Responses

Homeostasis, however, is not purely internal. When the client returns to their contexts, they are returning to homeostatic contexts that prefer interactions to be stable and predictable. If the client introduces new interactional strategies, people and systems often react by attempting to return the interactions to stability. In some cases, changes are welcome, but in others, they may not be. For example, clients with scores on Scale 6: Focused on the Needs of Others likely, as a result of a series of invitations resulting in complementarity, have developed a series of one-way relationships. They may have friends, romantic relationships, and work relationships that are entirely predicated on their providing emotional and task-related support to others without any expectation of their own needs being met.

Once a client attempts to make their own needs known, not everyone in their social circle will welcome the change. People prefer social interactions to be stable and predictable because they prefer homeostasis (Matthews & Tye, 2019). While some group members may express feeling closer and more attuned and having a greater sense of intimacy, others may ignore attempts by the client to set boundaries or dismiss the client's self-expression. For example, a friend who is used to getting complete support at any time of day and night—and finds the client setting better boundaries—might become angry and upset. Some of these relationships may come to an end. The client needs to be prepared for this eventuality. Not every change, no matter how healthy for the client, will result in outcomes that are without pain or consequences. To pretend otherwise, or to fail to address this possibility in debriefing, is sending the client out into the real world unprepared.

Discussion of systems responses should entail the client's seeking to achieve small challenges with a higher level of success before moving onto bigger challenges. The client should also consider whether they are prepared for any consequences and be ready to develop a support system to help them deal with consequences that may accrue. The therapist should encourage the client to start small and build up skills in the desired area before attempting to move onto bigger challenges with more uncertain outcomes. For example, refusing to go out late at night with an acquaintance before an exam or important work event has a lower but still significant potential consequence (i.e., loss of an acquaintance) than setting a firm boundary with an assertive and volatile boss at work (i.e., potential loss of employment). While setting a firm boundary with a volatile boss might be a worthy goal, the client should be ready to embark on that challenge thoughtfully and strategically and be prepared with a contingency plan in case it does not go well.

Every scale has its challenges in terms of adjusting styles to be more flexible. The therapist should remind clients that if their main interpersonal style works in some contexts, do not try and "fix" it. For example, a client who is the boss of a company works on becoming more sensitive to their children's and marital partner's needs. They decide to improve their listening skills and to be less domineering—a goal of Scale 1: Highly Assertive. They achieve that goal, but in doing so, overcompensate and apply that style at work too— a place dominated by brutal internal politics and a hierarchical structure that is unlikely to change quickly. Their employees, who are used to having a decisive boss, now experience them as fallible and unsure. A whispering campaign ensues, suggesting that this person is not the leader they once thought. Challenges to the client's authority surface, and the client is forced to act in increasingly hostile ways to fend off attacks.

The consequences of not reinforcing preexisting strategies for coping and behaving are quite real. When discussing change, it is also important that the client evaluates the arenas not only where change is needed, but also where it is completely unnecessary. The therapist should ensure that they reinforce the client's prior strengths, support changes, and help the client develop a thoughtful way of moving changes into their different contexts that are helpful.

Having the Habituation Discussion

Explaining habituation and homeostasis is therefore crucial. Any new behavior initially feels uncomfortable because it lacks fluency and easy integration. Therapists in training often experience that their new skill set initially feels awkward and does not come naturally. However, after an adjustment period, new therapists often find they have to restrain themselves from using their now fluent and congruent skills across situations in which those skills would not be appropriate. This is the same with clients attempting new skills: The lack of fluency, awkwardness, and adjustments to find out where new skills do and do not fit are key to growth. Therefore, the therapist should discuss with the client how the process of change necessarily entails some discomfort and that this should be seen as a positive sign of change. Two important discussions need to happen with each client: (a) the habituation discussion and (b) the homeostasis discussion. Both can help the client prepare for internal and external reactions to change.

These discussions about change can also illuminate a range of other issues facing clients. These may range from attributional issues (i.e., seeing positive change as the result of luck and not the client's own efforts), contextual overgeneralization (i.e., implementing change made in group into contexts where no change was necessary), and issues with incorporating changes into identity (i.e., the client's worrying that they cannot reintegrate changes into a coherent self-image). Each of these issues can be worthy of discussion, depending on the client. For example, helping a client reintegrate new skills into an existing identity typically involves highlighting that new skills are just behavioral choices and that the client does not need to give anything up that was previously successful.

In cases in which clients may present with more complex issues or are in settings where the approach is part of a larger treatment package for more complex cases, the need to manage continuity of care also becomes important. In rarer cases, this can also be the result of clients' not doing well in the group.

MANAGING CONTINUITY OF CARE

Group therapy may not go well for a client for many reasons: They experienced a life crisis in the middle of group, the group leader did not calibrate the goals well, a rupture in the group or with the leader occurred and was not repaired sufficiently, cultural issues were not dealt with adequately, or the client was not ready to change or actively resisted change. In response, the therapist must avoid shaming or blaming and help the client avoid self-castigation. The therapist should always seek to align with the client empathically around lack of success and seek to understand what happened and collaboratively determine a path forward. Typically, this involves understanding why the group did not go well.

The therapist must use their clinical judgment carefully in managing this discussion. The key is to be accurate in appraising the reasons why the group did not go well and help the client make sense of the set of circumstances. For example, some clients may realize they need a longer treatment duration to find efficacy, and the therapist may realize they had underestimated the severity of a problem. In such a case, the therapist should nonjudgmentally and supportively explore options for continuity of care. One purpose of the individualized debriefing is to understand and collaborate with the client around what the next steps are for them, so if this outcome sharpens the focus around what the client may need next, then the client is still progressing forward on their treatment journey.

Examination of Different Perceptions

Inviting comments on how group went requires the therapist be open to any possible response. In many cases, the therapist's perception of how group went matches the data and the client's interpretation. However, in some cases, it does not. The therapist must be open to hearing the client's perspective and be willing to then explore where differences in the data have occurred.

At times, the therapist must be prepared to ask questions that go beyond the life of the group. For example, if a quality of life score has worsened but all other evidence points to the group's going well, is there an incident or are there factors in the client's life that may account for the worsening? Bear in mind that some clients may tell the group that the group went well for them even though it did not. The therapist must be open to all possibilities.

Exploration of Assessments and Results

Results are presented as a tentative hypothesis, never as a certainty. The therapist should begin by asking for a general response from the client regarding how the group went for them, such as: "How did group go for you?" This can be a good beginning step to confirm or disconfirm the results of triangulation of data. For example, when all data points are in agreement that the client did well and achieved strong results, and the client says, "Group went really well" as a first statement, then the discussion can then move on to reinforcing positives and discussing habituation, homeostasis, and next steps.

However, in some cases, the data are confusing, or the client reports that group therapy is not going well, or both. This issue requires collaborative exploration with the client. Consider this example in which the therapist explores changes in scores with their client, Nick:

> The therapist observes that Nick has achieved all of their group goals. They have asked group members follow-up questions three times. And they received positive feedback on their goals. Nick also initiated conversations at least once and has received feedback.
>
> In the therapist's clinical judgment, Nick has done well in group therapy: They have been successful and have achieved their goals. The therapist, though, is somewhat puzzled that Nick's overall score on the 30-item Outcome Questionnaire (OQ-30; Ellsworth et al., 2006) is worsening. The therapist is not surprised by Nick's increases in Scale 7: Warm/Self-Sacrificing and Scale 8: Uninhibited because this is typical worsening of the opposite scale after change. So, the therapist makes a note to discuss this matter as part of the habituation discussion.
>
> The therapist also notes that a major national holiday is approaching and that the client is going home to be with family. There, the likelihood of any new interpersonal behaviors might be met with either surprise or pushback from family members who will seek to maintain the family homeostasis. The therapist

makes a note to discuss with Nick their need to pick and choose their moments to experiment with new behaviors and to discuss that families can be resistant to change. The therapist also reminds themself to follow the same rules as the group when delivering feedback: to begin with positives and then explore negatives.

The following is a strengths-based approach the therapist uses to engage in a collaborative exploration with their client, Nick. The therapist always leads with client strengths and reinforces those strengths whenever appropriate:

THERAPIST: So, Nick, how did group go?

NICK: It went well.

THERAPIST: So, what went well and how are things overall with you?

NICK: I really felt I accomplished a lot with my goals. I was worried people would be really upset with me, but it seemed to go well when I asked questions.

THERAPIST: Yes, I saw you do really well. You really were making such great efforts to activate your goals, and I saw you getting good feedback too. Good for you. Was it hard?

NICK: Yes. It was a struggle at times, but I pushed through it.

THERAPIST: Let's have a quick look at your results. Bear in mind these are only as truthful as makes sense to you, so I want to explore with you whether they ring true. Some of it really made sense to me, but some of the results weren't clear, so I wanted to ask you about them.

NICK: Hmm. Okay.

THERAPIST: First, your IIP-32 [Horowitz et al., 2000] score on Scale 4 [Socially Inhibited] went down. That was what you wanted to change. You accomplished all your goals, and this was the result: an overall reduction in your distress on that scale. What do you think?

NICK: I think that sums it up well. I feel really good about what I did, and I am glad to see it made a difference.

THERAPIST: Now one thing to prepare you for: Your score on Scales 7 and 8 [Warm/Self-Sacrificing and Uninhibited, respectively] went up, meaning you are now worried that the changes you made could be upsetting others, and this is leaving you feeling anxious. Is that right?

NICK: Yes. I am still worried about this.

THERAPIST: That is normal. Whenever people make changes, it always feels uncomfortable and slightly scary. Over time, this dissipates as we get used to the new behaviors. The process is called habituation. It is getting comfortable with newness.

NICK: Okay. So, as I do it more, then it will feel more comfortable?

THERAPIST: Yes. (*A brief discussion ensues.*)

THERAPIST: I am wondering about this score, though? (*Shows client that the OQ-30 [Ellsworth et al., 2006] score has increased.*) This score went up, and I was wondering what might explain it. Was it to do with the group or something else?

NICK: Yes, when I took that instrument, we had just finished group, and I was about to head off to an organic chemistry exam, so I was pretty stressed about it. I thought I was going to fail. I was really catastrophizing all week, so I hadn't been sleeping well and was really in a bad place.

THERAPIST: Okay. That makes sense. So, overall, apart from that day, would you say the overall impact of the group has been positive?

NICK: Yes. I really feel my relationships are improving slowly but surely.

In this case, the therapist was lacking important information that made sense of the data. Although the group was going well, the client had experienced a distressing day. The client's awareness of catastrophizing and lack of sleep as issues demonstrated good insight, allowing the therapist to consider whether to recommend cognitive behavior therapy to further work on catastrophizing. However, it is also possible that the explanations or configurations of data could have resulted in a very different debriefing.

Clients not accomplishing their goals is always possible. FBGT is not Pollyannaish in its philosophy. It is not a cure-all that always works with any client at any time. No therapy does. Even the most evidence-based therapies with large effect sizes have many, often unreported, treatment failures (Jonsson et al., 2014).

FBGT is designed to accommodate the possibility of a need for continuity of care when clients have not completed their goals or because of other reasons that become clear during the debriefing session. The therapist should deal with any lack of change or progress in treatment in a person-centered, nonshaming, nonblaming way that allows for continuity of care. If more treatment is needed, then the decision should revolve around what is good for the client. This may be adding another sequence of FBGT, but referral to another type of treatment altogether may prove a helpful option if it fits with what the client needs.

Referral to another type of treatment depends on an accurate appraisal of what happened and where treatment was successful and unsuccessful. In some cases, the initial assessment was incorrect, or goals were set up poorly. For example, if goals were set up that were unrealistic (e.g., asking a person high on Scale 6: Focused on the Needs of Others to strongly disagree with another group member), then the leader and client must determine whether to try again with better goals or to shift to other treatment. In other cases, a client may be better suited to a different type of therapy, and the therapist should also consider this possibility.

The general principle behind FBGT is care for the client. The debriefing session should always focus on what is best for the client. It should use as many data points as possible to ensure the therapist is aware of a possibility of client worsening so that they can then take steps to respond compassionately and with continuity of care uppermost in mind.

If It Isn't Broken . . . But Now You Have Choices

However, when FBGT is run as intended, the focus on a strong working, including clear goals, provides the building blocks for success. However, as mentioned previously, this success needs to be applied in very specific ways to the situations that were identified as problematic during the TPS session. It is vital to remind clients that many of their behaviors worked previously and should not be adjusted if they were successful in a specific context. For example, a client who was a successful politician and whose interpersonal strategies in that world provided them with considerable respect and success should likely not change those core strategies. However, if during the therapy, pregroup preparation, and screening session they preidentified that they wished to be more successful in being a good parent, and the skills they learned in group—asking follow-up questions and offering support and encouragement—were successful in that arena, then they should be practiced there.

It is not uncommon for clients, particularly ones who are highly driven and motivated to succeed, to want to overgeneralize their changes into environments where it is not necessary (and, in some cases, might be harmful to them) to do so. A boss who runs their business successfully by making decisions quickly, decisively, and without consultation in a fast-paced industry might find themselves paralyzed by indecision and find their team confused if they suddenly switch to a caring, empathic mode that is not well suited to the demands of the context. Thoughtful discussion needs to take place about being careful to experiment with new behaviors in contexts and situations in which they are likely to be successful. Clients need to remember that if their strategies were effective in certain contexts, they should keep those strategies and use them whenever necessary. Matching the interpersonal skill set to the environment where it is most adaptive is key to understanding where and when to implement skills.

The key to change in FBGT is to remain flexible and at play with options. Selection of interpersonal skills depends on evaluation of their likely success in each context, and this process takes time, practice, and trial and error. Continuing with strengths is an essential part of this change.

Group: A Good Beginning

It is incumbent on the therapist to explain that the progress made during group should be a beginning and not an end point. A client can sometimes see therapy as the only place in which changes can be made. Encouraging the client to build on success and proceed with sharpening their skill set are vital to progress. The therapist should encourage the client to continue the process of observing others and practicing new interpersonal techniques in low-risk situations. They should also help the client to see their progress in group as an exemplar of their ability to make changes in their life by being at play with interpersonal skills and strategies. Further, the therapist should urge the client to watch others around them and look for examples of effective social skills that they might eventually integrate into their own repertoire.

SUMMARY

Debriefing is an essential part of FBGT. Failure to debrief frequently results in poor generalization and transfer or in missing important information necessary for ethical continuity of care. The debriefing session, which involves multiple steps, starts asking for the client's perception of how group went. Subsequent steps include showing results and discussing agreement over change or discrepancies (if any) in data points, or both, in a nonjudgmental way; aligning on an assessment of the degree to which group therapy resulted in change; reminding the client that group is a beginning, not an end, to change; helping the client understand habituation and homeostasis (from both an internal sense of discomfort as well as anticipating pushback from contexts); and working on continuity of care.

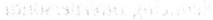

11

RESEARCH AND FUTURE DIRECTIONS

From the beginning at a counseling center at Wright State University (WSU), focused brief group therapy (FBGT) was designed with the idea that it needed to measurably work in a real-world setting; therefore, the approach developed with those real-world applications and a problem-solving mentality in mind. Assessment was also intentionally woven into the therapy to enhance collaboration with the client. All assessments used in FBGT are shared with the client and used to refine treatment in real time, a method of using instruments that is now becoming more accepted under the label of "measurement-based care" (Lewis et al., 2019).

RESEARCH IN NATURALISTIC SETTINGS

Because of the limitations of the WSU quarter system, FBGT needed to start, run, and finish in 10 weeks. The model was set up with the lofty goal of no dropouts and to show measurable outcomes in eight or fewer sessions.

Research took place at multiple levels. The outcome data built into the model allowed for tracking of prepost change across a range of variables,

https://doi.org/10.1037/0000389-012
Focused Brief Group Therapy: An Integrative Approach to Reducing Interpersonal Distress, by M. Whittingham

including depression, social anxiety, interpersonal distress, and hostility, using the 62-item Counseling Center Assessment of Psychological Symptoms (CCAPS-62; B. D. Locke et al., 2011; Youn et al., 2015) rather than the 30-item Outcome Questionnaire (OQ-30; Ellsworth et al., 2006) because CCAPS was required at the counseling center and was normed against the university student population. Interpersonal distress as a total score and scale scores were also collected for each student. During regular analyses outcomes, the research team looked for patterns within individual cases, group dynamics, and across scales that would suggest ways to improve treatment. This was a particularly important part of FBGT's process because it involved diligent work to catch any treatment failures and to learn from them.

Several techniques evolved from this process, ranging from inoculation to noticing patterns that were predictive of poor outcomes, such as poor attendance and its antecedents: low initial motivation with poor goal selection and lower working alliance. Patterns also emerged in the data that led to the primacy of the quarter turn as a means to select goals.

RESEARCH FINDINGS

Research findings have so far been quasi-experimental, and these findings have proven remarkably consistent in effectiveness studies and clinical reports from practitioners. Depression, social anxiety, hostility, and interpersonal distress have all been studied in the United States in a university counseling center and found to show statistically significant change, demonstrating equivalence to individual therapy and superiority to wait-list (Rotsinger-Stemen & Whittingham, 2013). In Singapore, research found statistically significant change in depression and quality of life in a hospital setting (Whittingham & Liew, 2020) with effect sizes for depression and overall quality of life being in the large range ($d = 0.93$ and $d = 1.15$, respectively). Research also found low dropout rates: 6.7% in Singapore (Whittingham & Liew, 2020) and 17% in the United States (Rotsinger-Stemen & Whittingham, 2013). The 17% figure reflects early adjustments in the model, and the modal dropout from groups was zero. Dropout reduction for FBGT is a main goal, and the model is designed to reduce premature termination at every stage.

With models of therapy, it is important to recognize and acknowledge their limitations. In the United States, measures of generalized anxiety did not show significant change or only showed small changes after longer treatment durations (Rotsinger-Stemen & Whittingham, 2013). This makes sense when one considers that the mechanisms of change for generalized anxiety do not seem to relate as much to relationships than to the ability to self-regulate internal states. These mechanisms of change for generalized anxiety also tend to be better treated with cognitive- or exposure-based treatments.

Changes in interpersonal subtype scores have also proven highly encouraging, showing predominately large to very large effect sizes for the scales targeted by FBGT (Allison & Whittingham, 2017; Whittingham & Liew, 2020). When looking at the impact of treatment on the scales that were the highest peaks—and therefore the target of treatment—the change scores were almost all in the large to very large effect size (ES = 0.83–1.58; Allison & Whittingham, 2017). This is a highly encouraging finding because it provides initial support for the central mechanism of change: that reducing distress on a specific subtypes scale is both possible and meaningful. This same study (Allison & Whittingham, 2017) also found a diffuse effect for those scores; the research suggested that not only were the highest scores impacted, but also the next highest scores. That is, the specific effect of targeting and improving the highest scores had a knock-on effect to the next highest scores as well (Allison & Whittingham, 2017). Overall, the research has proven highly promising.

Other research has taken place on the specific scales used in FBGT. Yutrzenka (2012) studied socially inhibited subtypes and found that, overall, people at university counseling centers had very high social anxiety as a baseline. Results from the study showed large effects of the treatment ($d = 1.156$). Sobon and Whittingham (2013) studied FBGT participants with high scores on Scale 6: Focused on the Needs of Others and also found statistically significant change.

PROGRAM EVALUATION

Therapists can use FBGT as a tool to evaluate their own groups and programs. Measurement-based care is designed to enhance care in real time but can also be used to review therapist performance either for the purposes of self-reflection and learning or for supervision or consultation. FBGT also should be used for periodic program evaluation to either make the case to administrators for the continuation of groups or to prove effectiveness to third-party payers or other stakeholders. Research is most useful when it evaluates outcomes at the local level and provides a means for therapists to understand and improve their work with the clients and groups under their care.

FBGT was developed within a real-world, naturalistic setting from a scientist–practitioner perspective, which means treating each client in a naturalistic setting and giving them the optimal combination of therapies that they need. Unlike approaches devised in a laboratory in which internal validity is tightly controlled, FBGT was designed with a close eye on external validity and applicability and integration within a wider treatment paradigm. Therefore, research conducted was quasi-experimental and had confounds that render the approach promising. The next step needed is a randomized clinical trial with longitudinal follow-up.

PROCESS RESEARCH

Process research has proven promising with notably large effect sizes for targeted scales (Allison & Whittingham, 2017; Whittingham & Liew, 2020), which were higher than the effect sizes for other outcomes, such as depression, social anxiety, and hostility (Rotsinger-Stemen & Whittingham, 2013). These preliminary data suggest that the central mechanism of change—looking to change a person's highest level of interpersonal distress—is an active component of treatment. More research is needed using path analysis on larger samples to determine this mechanism of change.

Rotsinger-Stemen and Whittingham (2013) completed some dose–effect analyses and found that FBGT showed no difference in change at four sessions than at seven and nine sessions. This is not to suggest that no further sessions are needed after the fourth session but, rather, that the impact of the therapy, pregroup preparation, and screening (TPS) session and early group sessions propel clients into change quickly. As Thomas and Persons (2013) suggested, these sudden gains only indicate that things started well, so this does not mean FBGT is necessarily improved with shorter treatment. Indeed, treatment length and whether FBGT would be better as an 8-session, 15-session, or longer treatment needs further study.

RESEARCH DIRECTIONS

The research so far has taken place in naturalistic, real-world settings using a quasi-experimental design. This approach has made FBGT very responsive to real-world concerns, such as reducing dropout and fine-tuning techniques to work for clients with different presenting problems and diagnoses. Premature dropout rates suggest that the approach is promising with respect to client retention. This is a particularly important outcome, given the need for brief group therapies to keep dropout to a minimum.

The Local Clinical Scientist

It is the intent of FBGT that those using this model become local clinical scientists. Because the measures are an element of routine clinical practice, they are part of not only ensuring real-time success in therapy but also have the option of aggregating data to develop a bird's-eye view of how a practice is performing. These data can then be used for reporting purposes or research purposes, assuming that the clinician has carefully considered informed consent and institutional review board protocols.

To conduct local clinical science on this model requires an understanding of what constitutes client change. It is important that quality of life measures are valid; reliable; sensitive to change; and, whenever possible, normed against the population of interest. Ideally, they should also contain analytics and provide the ability to benchmark against other treatment and setting types. For example, the OQ-30 (Ellsworth et al., 2006) provides scoring as reliable change indices (Jacobson & Traux, 1992) so that it is possible to understand individual change scores. This is an important metric in clinical work that allows the clinician to understand individual change.

These changes can also be transposed into charts and summaries outlining the number of clients who achieved significant change, those who did not change at clinically significant levels, and those who worsened. In cases of client worsening, further analysis is warranted to understand why and to determine any need for continuity of care. This analysis then forms the basis of good practice in which therapists are clear about treatments gains and are no longer hampered by the blind spot to client worsening and premature dropout that typically exists among therapists in group and individual therapy (Chapman et al., 2012; Lambert & Harmon, 2018). Given that routine therapy in many settings provides equivalent outcomes to evidence-based models in tightly controlled labs, this kind of analysis provides extra guarantees the practitioners are providing therapy that is evidence based at the local level and is responsive to local clinical variation.

The local clinical scientist should determine what their goals are in collecting data. They can use data purely to account for individual change within the group as a clinical aid. However, they may also use data for quality improvement initiatives—for example, by looking at how groups are performing overall, whether individual clinicians are equally successful, and if there are any blind spots in how treatment is delivered (e.g., consistently poorer results than might be expected for a particular interpersonal style; Whittingham et al., 2023).

Cultural Differences and Adopt Versus Adapt

Cultural adaptations of FBGT are an extremely important consideration. Liew (Hewitt & Liew, 2023), who implemented FBGT in a longer term inpatient–outpatient setting in Singapore, noted that clinicians should assess several variables: the validity of the assessments in terms of cultural difference, any cultural adaptations, and the role of within-region diversity issues. Liew conducted item analysis on each instrument, sought feedback from clients on both the instruments and the therapy, and implemented minor changes in protocols to account for client feedback. Liew (Hewitt & Liew, 2023) also observed that clients found the 32-item Inventory of Interpersonal Problems (Horowitz et al., 2000) extremely helpful in focusing goals, and despite what these researchers anticipated might be cultural differences in the working alliance around task, they also found that clients were highly amenable to the therapy approach in general. Because interpersonal process was a new concept for Singapore, Liew expressed surprise that clients enjoyed it and also found it intuitive (Hewitt & Liew, 2023).

Liew also noticed within-country differences (Hewitt & Liew, 2023). Singapore is a diverse country with several distinct ethnic groups (e.g., Chinese, Indian, Singaporean) living in culturally different neighborhoods that are quite varied in their cultural atmosphere. She suggested that not only would the therapy need some slight adaptation to Singapore in general, but also, at times, to differences within the culture, such as when noticing interpersonal cultural differences in norms between Muslim women and other group members who identify as Christian or Buddhist.

Liew (Hewitt & Liew, 2023) observed that her identity as ethnically Chinese also meant that some members from that same background may have identified with her more strongly than those from a different ethnic or cultural background. She noted the implications for the working alliance. These adaptations are important. However, she also noted, as did several clinicians from China, that their individual and group outcomes were surprisingly strong. The low dropout and overall improvement in functioning replicated well from studies performed in the United States (Rotsinger-Stemen & Whittingham, 2013), and specific scale score changes were also statistically significant, suggesting the approach is highly promising across cultures. However, this process of considering when to adapt and when to adopt should not be short circuited. Liew's success was in carefully considering each aspect of the therapy on an ongoing basis, carefully monitoring outcomes, and making adjustments as the therapy progressed.

Cultural variations also take place in sometimes unexpected ways in terms of techniques that may be essential in some cultures but being less so in others. For example, something as mundane as selecting activity questions in icebreakers can have different cultural meanings and may need adjusting. As previously mentioned in this book, a popular icebreaker moment in the United States is when, in Session 1, clients are asked to share their favorite dessert. That activity allows clients to share an often "guilty pleasure" that enables them to connect to each other and enjoy memories of pleasurable events. In China, dessert is not a part of meals; therefore, the intent of the icebreaker is lost. So, the therapist needs to consider the original intent of the activity (to build cohesion and a positive climate) and modify it to a different format.

Cultural variations are also important to consider in data collection and analysis. Most measures are normed on a predominately White, Western norm group, although there are now studies exploring their generalizability to other groups (e.g., A. O. Lopez et al., 2021) that are finding acceptable applicability, depending on their use for some instruments. Therefore, data should be assessed carefully in terms of selection of instruments, benchmarking, and inference. Ideally, the selection of instruments should be able to draw on norm groups that are culturally relevant to the setting being studied. When this is not the case, results from instruments should be treated with considerable caution.

Data-Informed Self-Reflection and Growth

The FBGT approach asks the therapist to make a big leap, and this leap takes some courage. It invites the therapist to really reflect on their outcomes at the local level and to accurately measure how they are doing. This process can feel worrisome to some therapists. On the plus side, therapists get to see and receive feedback on successes. Rather than just relying on client self-report, symptom remission, and feedback, they have another set of data points that let them know how they are doing. This can be positive and can really help with feelings of self-competence, which can alleviate burnout.

However, the more challenging invitation of the work is to evaluate what happened when things go wrong. FBGT is designed to promote accuracy in answers when clients are not successful. The model invites the clinician to evaluate multiple data points and to consider what actually happened rather than rely on self-serving biases that place fault in circumstances or random factors that are outside of the therapist's control. Using the FBGT approach, the therapist is reality based and fully investigates what went right and what went wrong. The goal is to continually improve and grow. If things go poorly, the therapist considers all the possible factors involved in continuous quality improvement. Factors may include understanding how to formulate goals more effectively; learning how to remain mindfully centered as a participant–observer; managing one's own hooked responses; learning to become more proficient with certain types of group members (based on interpersonal style or cultural difference, or both); understanding group dynamics and predicting into problems; becoming more skilled at managing critical incidents; becoming more skilled at managing process versus goal attainment; interpreting instruments; developing skills in the TPS session; and maintaining clear and realistic expectations of client change.

This list of major areas in which therapists can continue to grow is not intended as an exercise in self-blame or self-castigation. Instead, the list reflects a way to improve while exercising self-compassion. Learning to work with groups is an exciting challenge but is not easy. True expertise comes from a continual process of learning, feedback, consultation, and improvement. Being open to learning in the form of practice, plus supervisory feedback, is essential to this process (Harwell & Southwick, 2021). Each therapist is a work in progress, and those who become the most expert are the most aware of this idea. Similar to the FBGT approach itself, that means focusing on strengths by valuing and owning successes, which should always precede understanding and learning from failures. With increased skill in the techniques and greater exposure to typical and atypical cases, therapists gain a more nuanced understanding of what success in therapy actually looks like from the client's perspective.

CURRENT DEVELOPMENTS IN FBGT

Since launching at WSU, FBGT has become widely used across the United States, primarily in counseling and outpatient settings, and internationally, where the model is being used across various settings and populations (Denduluri & Kasper, 2022; Jia, 2021; Whittingham & Liew, 2020). Equally, cross-cultural, adoption–adaptation continues, particularly in China and Singapore, with ongoing research on the impact of the method in both cultures (e.g., Whittingham & Liew, 2020). In Singapore, research has taken place on outcomes and process to ensure the theory fits the culture and also that it is responsive to cultural differences. It is my hope that regardless of setting and geography, therapists take time to not only evaluate outcomes member by member, but also ensure no client is left behind and conduct periodic evaluation of the results for the whole program of therapy. This local clinical scientist model—in which therapists become responsible for and accountable to their own outcomes at the local level by reviewing their own data—has the potential to truly narrow the gap between science and practice in ways that can benefit both clients and the therapists conducting the therapy.

FUTURE DIRECTIONS

Research on FBGT is going in some exciting directions. Currently, the approach is being used in university counseling centers in the United States as well as being piloted across the world in a variety of other treatment settings (e.g., Denduluri & Kasper, 2022; Jia, 2021). The potential for applications to longer term hospital and agency-based care is an exciting one. The model also has potential applications for trauma-related care. Recent work with the Institute for Disaster Mental Health at the State University of New York (Whittingham et al., 2023) has focused on considering what different growth pathways after trauma would look like depending on individual interpersonal style. Given the role of social support in recovery and thriving after trauma, a finer-grain analysis of which styles find it most difficult to attract social support has important implications for long-term recovery.

Equally, the literature on loneliness has been accelerating recently with an increasing focus on the mental and physical health correlates of this condition (Hickin et al., 2021; Steptoe, 2023). FBGT has implications for treatment of loneliness because it directly addresses the interpersonal difficulties that make absence or dissatisfaction with relationships (both of which are connected to poor mental and physical health) so problematic. More studies are needed to determine the longer term effects of FBGT on loneliness and mental and physical health.

On my travels, I also have received considerable interest from people in the field of pediatrics and work with children and adolescents. Although the FBGT model would need adapting (e.g., to ensure correct instruments are chosen that are valid, reliable, and sensitive to change for children), it has gained enough strong interest from those working with children to suggest an adaptation in the future would be worth exploring. Equally, several clinicians have personally reached out to me to report strong results with special populations, such as men's groups or lesbian, gay, bisexual, transgender, questioning, or queer groups. However, while these clinical anecdotes are promising, more research is needed on these and other populations.

SUMMARY

Research on FBGT is promising and shows significant change in depression, social anxiety, hostility, total interpersonal distress, stress, and anxiety in quasi-experimental, naturalistic studies. More research is needed that focuses on experimental design and generalizability to other populations.

Therapists should carefully consider when to adopt versus adapt the model. Data in all forms should inform their decision on how to tailor to the approach to fit different populations and cultures. To allow the FBGT approach to inform learning, therapist courage is needed to help clinicians confront the realities of therapeutic success and failure. Periodic review of outcomes at the aggregate level may be helpful for program evaluation.

Visit https://www.focusedbriefgrouptherapy.com for updates on FBGT training, materials, and model developments.

References

Abouguendia, M., Joyce, A. S., Piper, W. E., & Ogrodniczuk, J. S. (2004). Alliance as a mediator of expectancy effects in short-term group psychotherapy. *Group Dynamics: Theory, Research, and Practice, 8*(1), 3–12. https://doi.org/10.1037/1089-2699.8.1.3

Abraham, P. P., Lepisto, B. L., & Schultz, L. (1995). Adolescents' perceptions of process and specialty group therapy. *Psychotherapy, 32*(1), 70–76. https://doi.org/10.1037/0033-3204.32.1.70

Agazarian, Y. M. (2011). *Systems-centered therapy: Clinical practice with individuals, families and groups*. Routledge. https://doi.org/10.4324/9780429480737

Agazarian, Y. M. (2018). *Systems-centered therapy for groups*. Routledge. https://doi.org/10.4324/9780429480744

Aggarwal, N. K. (2011). Intersubjectivity, transference, and the cultural third. *Contemporary Psychoanalysis, 47*(2), 204–223. https://doi.org/10.1080/00107530.2011.10746451

Alden, L. E., Wiggins, J. S., & Pincus, A. L. (1990). Construction of circumplex scales for the Inventory of Interpersonal Problems. *Journal of Personality Assessment, 55*(3–4), 521–536. https://doi.org/10.1080/00223891.1990.9674088

Allison, J., & Whittingham, M. (2017, March 6–11). *Focused brief group therapy change scores for interpersonal subtypes: The impact of an eight session model on targeted interpersonal distress* [Paper presentation]. 74th Annual American Group Psychotherapy Association Conference, New York, NY, United States.

American Psychiatric Association. (2013). *Diagnostic and statistical manual of mental disorders* (5th ed.). https://doi.org/10.1176/appi.books.9780890425596

American Psychological Association. (2017). *Ethical principles of psychologists and code of conduct* (2002, amended effective June 1, 2010, and January 1, 2017). https://www.apa.org/ethics/code/

Anders, C., Kivlighan, D. M., III, Porter, E., Lee, D., & Owen, J. (2021). Attending to the intersectionality and saliency of clients' identities: A further investigation of therapists' multicultural orientation. *Journal of Counseling Psychology*, *68*(2), 139–148. https://doi.org/10.1037/cou0000447

Arnd-Caddigan, M. (2013). Don't let the doorknob hit you: A relational-intersubjective exploration of leaving and remaining within the therapeutic frame. *Psychoanalytic Social Work*, *20*(2), 134–149. https://doi.org/10.1080/15228878.2013.791868

Arnold, R. A. (2021). *The relationship of alliance, cohesion, and group climate with outcome* [Master's thesis, Brigham Young University]. BYU ScholarsArchive. https://scholarsarchive.byu.edu/cgi/viewcontent.cgi?article=10571&context=etd

Aronson, E. (with Aronson, J.). (2018). *The social animal* (12th ed.). Worth Publishers.

Awad, M. N., & Connors, E. H. (2023). Active bystandership by youth in the digital era: Microintervention strategies for responding to social media-based microaggressions and cyberbullying. *Psychological Services*. Advance online publication. https://doi.org/10.1037/ser0000749

Bailey, C., Abate, A., Sharp, C., & Venta, A. (2018). Psychometric evaluation of the Inventory of Interpersonal Problems 32. *Bulletin of the Menninger Clinic*, *82*(2), 93–113. https://doi.org/10.1521/bumc.2018.82.2.93

Bakan, D. (1966). *The duality of human existence: An essay on psychology and religion*. Rand McNally.

Baker, E., Burlingame, G. M., Cox, J. C., Beecher, M. E., & Gleave, R. L. (2013). The Group Readiness Questionnaire: A convergent validity analysis. *Group Dynamics*, *17*(4), 299–314. https://doi.org/10.1037/a0034477

Barry, K. G. (2011). *Predicting conflict in group psychotherapy: A model integrating interpersonal and group-as-a-whole theories* [Doctoral dissertation, Wright State University]. CORE Scholar. https://corescholar.libraries.wright.edu/etd_all/1120/

Baumeister, R. F., DeWall, C. N., Ciarocco, N. J., & Twenge, J. M. (2005). Social exclusion impairs self-regulation. *Journal of Personality and Social Psychology*, *88*(4), 589–604. https://doi.org/10.1037/0022-3514.88.4.589

Baumeister, R. F., Twenge, J. M., & Nuss, C. K. (2002). Effects of social exclusion on cognitive processes: Anticipated aloneness reduces intelligent thought. *Journal of Personality and Social Psychology*, *83*(4), 817–827. https://doi.org/10.1037/0022-3514.83.4.817

Beck, L. (2007). Social status, social support, and stress: A comparative review of the health consequences of social control factors. *Health Psychology Review*, *1*(2), 186–207. https://doi.org/10.1080/17437190802217246

Beutel, M. E., Klein, E. M., Brähler, E., Reiner, I., Jünger, C., Michal, M., Wiltink, J., Wild, P. S., Münzel, T., Lackner, K. J., & Tibubos, A. N. (2017). Loneliness in the general population: Prevalence, determinants and relations to mental health. *BMC Psychiatry, 17*(1), Article 97. https://doi.org/10.1186/s12888-017-1262-x

Boswell, J. F., Iles, B. R., Gallagher, M. W., & Farchione, T. J. (2017). Behavioral activation strategies in cognitive-behavioral therapy for anxiety disorders. *Psychotherapy, 54*(3), 231–236. https://doi.org/10.1037/pst0000119

Bronfenbrenner, U. (1979). *The ecology of human development: Experiments by nature and design.* Harvard University Press.

Bronfenbrenner, U. (1992). Ecological systems theory. In R. Vasta (Ed.), *Six theories of child development: Revised formulations and current issues* (pp. 187–249). Jessica Kingsley Publishers.

Brossart, D. F. (1996). *An investigation of the adequacy of two counseling group development theories using Tuckerized growth curves* (Publication No. 9712794) [Doctoral dissertation, University of Missouri-Columbia]. ProQuest Dissertations and Theses Global.

Burlingame, G. M., & Jensen, J. L. (2017). Small group process and outcome research highlights: A 25-year perspective. *International Journal of Group Psychotherapy, 67*(Suppl. 1), S194–S218. https://doi.org/10.1080/00207284.2016.1218287

Burlingame, G. M., McClendon, D. T., & Yang, C. (2018). Cohesion in group therapy: A meta-analysis. *Psychotherapy, 55*(4), 384–398. https://doi.org/10.1037/pst0000173

Burlingame, G. M., & Strauss, B. (2021). Efficacy of small group treatments: Foundation for evidence-based practice. In M. Barkham, W. Lutz, & L. G. Castonguay (Eds.), *Bergin and Garfield's handbook of psychotherapy and behavior change: 50th anniversary edition* (pp. 583–624). John Wiley & Sons.

Burlingame, G. M., Strauss, B., Joyce, A., MacNair-Semands, R., MacKenzie, K. R., Ogrodniczuk, J., & Taylor, S. (2006). *CORE Battery–Revised: An assessment tool kit for promoting optimal group selection, process, and outcome.* American Group Psychotherapy Association.

Buss, D. M. (1991). Evolutionary personality psychology. *Annual Review of Psychology, 42*, 459–491. https://doi.org/10.1146/annurev.ps.42.020191.002331

Campbell, J. C. (2004). Helping women understand their risk in situations of intimate partner violence. *Journal of Interpersonal Violence, 19*(12), 1464–1477. https://doi.org/10.1177/0886260504269698

CAPSBoulder. (2012, February 1). *Introduction to group therapy* [Video]. YouTube. https://www.youtube.com/watch?v=qrUy6nWJrqg&t=2s&ab_channel=CAPSBoulder

Carson, R. C. (1969). *Interaction concepts of personality.* Aldine Publishing Company.

Carter, E. F., Mitchell, S. L., & Krautheim, M. D. (2001). Understanding and addressing clients' resistance to group counseling. *The Journal for Specialists in Group Work, 26*(1), 66–80. https://doi.org/10.1080/01933920108413778

Chao, R. C.-L., Mallinckrodt, B., & Wei, M. (2012). Co-occurring presenting problems in African American college clients reporting racial discrimination distress. *Professional Psychology: Research and Practice, 43*(3), 199–207. https://doi.org/10.1037/a0027861

Chapman, C. L., Burlingame, G. M., Gleave, R., Rees, F., Beecher, M., & Porter, G. S. (2012). Clinical prediction in group psychotherapy. *Psychotherapy Research, 22*(6), 673–681. https://doi.org/10.1080/10503307.2012.702512

Chelmardi, A. K., Naeeni, Y. J., & Mazaheri, Z. (2018). Validation of Interpersonal Circumplex questionnaire in Iranian couples. *Journal of Family Research, 14*(1), 57–73.

Chen, E. C., Kkad, D., & Balzano, J. (2008). Multicultural competence and evidence-based practice in group therapy. *Journal of Clinical Psychology, 64*(11), 1261–1278. https://doi.org/10.1002/jclp.20533

Chen, Z., Poon, K.-T., DeWall, C. N., & Jiang, T. (2020). Life lacks meaning without acceptance: Ostracism triggers suicidal thoughts. *Journal of Personality and Social Psychology, 119*(6), 1423–1443. https://doi.org/10.1037/pspi0000238

Clements-Hickman, A. L., & Reese, R. J. (2020). Improving therapists' effectiveness: Can deliberate practice help? *Professional Psychology: Research and Practice, 51*(6), 606–612. https://doi.org/10.1037/pro0000318

Clifton, S. (2018). *Operationalising the interpersonal circumplex in South Africa* (Publication No. 2528080174) [Doctoral dissertation, University of Johannesburg]. ProQuest Dissertations and Theses Global.

Clough, B., Spriggens, L., Stainer, M., & Casey, L. (2022). Working together: An investigation of the impact of working alliance and cohesion on group psychotherapy attendance. *Psychology and Psychotherapy: Theory, Research and Practice, 95*(1), 79–97. https://doi.org/10.1111/papt.12364

Cole, S. W., Capitanio, J. P., Chun, K., Arevalo, J. M. G., Ma, J., & Cacioppo, J. T. (2015). Myeloid differentiation architecture of leukocyte transcriptome dynamics in perceived social isolation. *Proceedings of the National Academy of Sciences of the United States of America, 112*(49), 15142–15147. https://doi.org/10.1073/pnas.1514249112

Collins, N. L. (1996). Working models of attachment: Implications for explanation, emotion and behavior. *Journal of Personality and Social Psychology, 71*(4), 810–832. https://doi.org/10.1037/0022-3514.71.4.810

Collins, N. L., & Feeney, B. C. (2004). Working models of attachment shape perceptions of social support: Evidence from experimental and observational studies. *Journal of Personality and Social Psychology, 87*(3), 363–383. https://doi.org/10.1037/0022-3514.87.3.363

Collins, N. L., & Read, S. J. (1990). Adult attachment, working models, and relationship quality in dating couples. *Journal of Personality and Social Psychology, 58*(4), 644–663. https://doi.org/10.1037/0022-3514.58.4.644

Connors, E. H., Arora, P. G., Resnick, S. G., & McKay, M. (2023). A modified measurement-based care approach to improve mental health treatment engagement among racial and ethnic minoritized youth. *Psychological Services, 20*(Suppl. 1), 170–184. https://doi.org/10.1037/ser0000617

Connors, M. E. (1997). The renunciation of love: Dismissive attachment and its treatment. *Psychoanalytic Psychology, 14*(4), 475–493. https://doi.org/10.1037/h0079736

Corpas, J., Moriana, J. A., Venceslá, J. F., & Gálvez-Lara, M. (2021). Brief psychological therapies for emotional disorders in primary care: A systematic review and meta-analysis. *Clinical Psychology: Science and Practice, 28*(4), 363–376. https://doi.org/10.1037/cps0000009

Costa, P. T., Jr., & McCrae, R. R. (2011). The five-factor model, five-factor theory, and interpersonal psychology. In L. M. Horowitz & S. Strack (Eds.), *Handbook of interpersonal psychology* (pp. 91–104). John Wiley & Sons. https://doi.org/10.1002/9781118001868.ch6

Cox, J. C. (2008). Selecting members for group therapy: A validation study of the Group Selection Questionnaire. *Dissertation Abstracts International: B. The Sciences and Engineering, 69*(3-B), 1947.

Crocker, L. D., Heller, W., Warren, S. L., O'Hare, A. J., Infantolino, Z. P., & Miller, G. A. (2013). Relationships among cognition, emotion, and motivation: Implications for intervention and neuroplasticity in psychopathology. *Frontiers in Human Neuroscience, 7*, Article 261. https://doi.org/10.3389/fnhum.2013.00261

Csikszentmihalyi, M., Montijo, M. N., & Mouton, A. R. (2018). Flow theory: Optimizing elite performance in the creative realm. In S. I. Pfeiffer, E. Shaunessy-Dedrick, & M. Foley-Nicpon (Eds.), *APA handbook of giftedness and talent* (pp. 215–229). American Psychological Association. https://doi.org/10.1037/0000038-014

Dandachi-FitzGerald, B., Meijs, L., Moonen, I. M. A. J., & Merckelbach, H. (2021). No self-serving bias in therapists' evaluations of clients' premature treatment termination: An approximate replication of Murdock et al. (2010). *Clinical Psychology & Psychotherapy*. Advance online publication. https://doi.org/10.1002/cpp.2677

Delgadillo, J., Deisenhofer, A.-K., Probst, T., Shimokawa, K., Lambert, M. J., & Kleinstäuber, M. (2022). Progress feedback narrows the gap between more and less effective therapists: A therapist effects meta-analysis of clinical trials. *Journal of Consulting and Clinical Psychology, 90*(7), 559–567. https://doi.org/10.1037/ccp0000747

Denduluri, M., & Kasper, L. (2022, December 18). *Time-limited interpersonal group therapy* [Distance learning event]. American Group Therapy Association.

D'Ippolito, S., Shams, M., Ambrosini, E., Calì, G., & Pastorelli, D. (2017). The effect of loneliness on cancer mortality. *Annals of Oncology: Abstracts Session R—Psychological and Psychosocial Aspects, 28*(Suppl. 6), Article V18. https://doi.org/10.1093/annonc/mdx434

Donegan, E., & Dugas, M. J. (2012). Generalized anxiety disorder: A comparison of symptom change in adults receiving cognitive-behavioral therapy or applied relaxation. *Journal of Consulting and Clinical Psychology, 80*(3), 490–496. https://doi.org/10.1037/a0028132

Dozier, M., Stovall, K. C., & Albus, K. E. (1999). Attachment and psychopathology in adulthood. In J. Cassidy & P. R. Shaver (Eds.), *Handbook of attachment: Theory, research, and clinical applications* (pp. 497–519). Guilford Press.

Edbrooke-Childs, J., Jacob, J., Law, D., Deighton, J., & Wolpert, M. (2015). Interpreting standardized and idiographic outcome measures in CAMHS: What does change mean and how does it relate to functioning and experience? *Child and Adolescent Mental Health, 20*(3), 142–148. https://doi.org/10.1111/camh.12107

Eisenberger, N. I., Lieberman, M. D., & Williams, K. D. (2003). Does rejection hurt? An fMRI study of social exclusion. *Science, 302*(5643), 290–292. https://doi.org/10.1126/science.1089134

Ellsworth, J. R., Lambert, M. J., & Johnson, J. (2006). A comparison of the Outcome Questionnaire-45 and Outcome Questionnaire-30 in classification and prediction of treatment outcome. *Clinical Psychology & Psychotherapy, 13*(6), 380–391. https://doi.org/10.1002/cpp.503

Elsaadawy, N., & Carlson, E. N. (2022). Do you make a better or worse impression than you think? *Journal of Personality and Social Psychology, 123*(6), 1407–1420. https://doi.org/10.1037/pspp0000434

Erkic, M., Bailer, J., Fenske, S. C., Schmidt, S. N. L., Trojan, J., Schröder, A., Kirsch, P., & Mier, D. (2018). Impaired emotion processing and a reduction in trust in patients with somatic symptom disorder. *Clinical Psychology & Psychotherapy, 25*(1), 163–172. https://doi.org/10.1002/cpp.2151

Ernst, M., Niederer, D., Werner, A. M., Czaja, S. J., Mikton, C., Ong, A. D., Rosen, T., Brähler, E., & Beutel, M. E. (2022). Loneliness before and during the COVID-19 pandemic: A systematic review with meta-analysis. *American Psychologist, 77*(5), 660–677. https://doi.org/10.1037/amp0001005

Falender, C. A., Shafranske, E. P., & Falicov, C. J. (Eds.). (2014). *Multiculturalism and diversity in clinical supervision: A competency-based approach.* American Psychological Association. https://doi.org/10.1037/14370-000

Feldman, R. (2017). The neurobiology of human attachments. *Trends in Cognitive Sciences, 21*(2), 80–99. https://doi.org/10.1016/j.tics.2016.11.007

Fisher, A. J., & Boswell, J. F. (2016). Enhancing the personalization of psychotherapy with dynamic assessment and modeling. *Assessment, 23*(4), 496–506. https://doi.org/10.1177/1073191116638735

Flores, P. J. (2004). *Addiction as an attachment disorder.* Jason Aronson.

Flores, P. J. (2006). Conflict and repair in addiction treatment: An attachment disorder perspective. *Journal of Groups in Addiction & Recovery, 1*(1), 5–26. https://doi.org/10.1300/J384v01n01_02

Flores, P. J., & Porges, S. W. (2017). Group psychotherapy as a neural exercise: Bridging polyvagal theory and attachment theory. *International Journal of Group Psychotherapy, 67*(2), 202–222. https://doi.org/10.1080/00207284.2016.1263544

Fonagy, P. (1999). Psychoanalytic theory from the viewpoint of attachment theory and research. In J. Cassidy & P. R. Shaver (Eds.), *Handbook of attachment: Theory, research, and clinical applications* (pp. 595–624). Guilford Press.

Fonagy, P., & Bateman, A. W. (2006). Mechanisms of change in mentalization-based treatment of BPD. *Journal of Clinical Psychology, 62*(4), 411–430. https://doi.org/10.1002/jclp.20241

Fonagy, P., Gergely, G., Jurist, E. L., & Target, M. (2002). *Affect regulation, mentalization, and the development of the self*. Other Press.

Fonagy, P., & Target, M. (1997). Attachment and reflective function: Their role in self-organization. *Development and Psychopathology, 9*(4), 679–700. https://doi.org/10.1017/S0954579497001399

Forsyth, D. R. (2021). Recent advances in the study of group cohesion. *Group Dynamics, 25*(3), 213–228. https://doi.org/10.1037/gdn0000163

Fortney, J. C., Unützer, J., Wrenn, G., Pyne, J. M., Smith, G. R., Schoenbaum, M., & Harbin, H. T. (2017). A tipping point for measurement-based care. *Psychiatric Services, 68*(2), 179–188. https://doi.org/10.1176/appi.ps.201500439

Fournier, M. A., Moskowitz, D. S., & Zuroff, D. C. (2011). Origins and applications of the interpersonal circumplex. In L. M. Horowitz & S. Strack (Eds.), *Handbook of interpersonal psychology: Theory, research, assessment, and therapeutic interventions* (pp. 57–73). John Wiley & Sons.

Freud, S. (1989). The ego and the id (1923). *TACD Journal, 17*(1), 5–22. https://doi.org/10.1080/1046171X.1989.12034344 (Original work published 1923)

Galvin, B. M., Randel, A. E., Collins, B. J., & Johnson, R. E. (2018). Changing the focus of locus (of control): A targeted review of the locus of control literature and agenda for future research. *Journal of Organizational Behavior, 39*(7), 820–833. https://doi.org/10.1002/job.2275

García-Mieres, H., Usall, J., Feixas, G., & Ochoa, S. (2020). Placing cognitive rigidity in interpersonal context in psychosis: Relationship with low cognitive reserve and high self-certainty. *Frontiers in Psychiatry, 11*, Article 594840. https://doi.org/10.3389/fpsyt.2020.594840

Garris, C. P., Ohbuchi, K., Oikawa, H., & Harris, M. J. (2011). Consequences of interpersonal rejection: A cross-cultural experimental study. *Journal of Cross-Cultural Psychology, 42*(6), 1066–1083. https://doi.org/10.1177/0022022110381428

Gelso, C. J., & Williams, E. N. (2022). *Counseling psychology*. American Psychological Association. https://doi.org/10.1037/0000249-016

Girard, J. M., Wright, A. G. C., Beeney, J. E., Lazarus, S. A., Scott, L. N., Stepp, S. D., & Pilkonis, P. A. (2017). Interpersonal problems across levels of the psychopathology hierarchy. *Comprehensive Psychiatry, 79*, 53–69. https://doi.org/10.1016/j.comppsych.2017.06.014

Gold, P. B., & Kivlighan, D. M. (2011, August 4–7). *Pattern of endorsement of therapeutic factors over time and change in group member interpersonal problems*

[Conference session]. American Psychological Association 119th Annual Convention, Washington, DC, United States.

Grieve, R., & de Groot, H. T. (2011). Does online psychological test administration facilitate faking? *Computers in Human Behavior, 27*(6), 2386–2391. https://doi.org/10.1016/j.chb.2011.08.001

Grimes, J. L., & Kivlighan, D. M., III. (2022). Whose multicultural orientation matters most? Examining additive and compensatory effects of the group's and leader's multicultural orientation in group therapy. *Group Dynamics, 26*(1), 58–70. https://doi.org/10.1037/gdn0000153

Gurtman, M. B. (2009). Exploring personality with the interpersonal circumplex. *Social and Personality Psychology Compass, 3*(4), 601–619. https://doi.org/10.1111/j.1751-9004.2009.00172.x

Halberstadt, A. L., Pincus, A. L., Mogle, J., & Ansell, E. B. (2023). Interpersonal complementarity and affect in daily life. *Motivation and Emotion.* Advance online publication. https://doi.org/10.1007/s11031-022-10003-0

Hardy, A. O., Tracey, T. J., Glidden-Tracey, C., Hess, T. R., & Rohlfing, J. E. (2011). Interpersonal contribution to outcome: The relation of interpersonal distress and symptomatic improvement as a result of psychotherapy. *Clinical Psychology & Psychotherapy, 18*(3), 225–233. https://doi.org/10.1002/cpp.709

Harwell, K., & Southwick, D. (2021). Beyond 10,000 hours: Addressing misconceptions of the expert performance approach. *Journal of Expertise, 4*(2), 220–233.

Hayes, J. A., McAleavey, A. A., Castonguay, L. G., & Locke, B. D. (2016). Psychotherapists' outcomes with White and racial/ethnic minority clients: First, the good news. *Journal of Counseling Psychology, 63*(3), 261–268. https://doi.org/10.1037/cou0000098

Hayes, J. A., Owen, J., & Bieschke, K. J. (2015). Therapist differences in symptom change with racial/ethnic minority clients. *Psychotherapy, 52*(3), 308–314. https://doi.org/10.1037/a0037957

Hayes, S., Carlyle, M., Haslam, S. A., Haslam, C., & Dingle, G. (2022). Exploring links between social identity, emotion regulation, and loneliness in those with and without a history of mental illness. *British Journal of Clinical Psychology, 61*(3), 701–734. https://doi.org/10.1111/bjc.12358

Hayes, S. C., Hofmann, S. G., Stanton, C. E., Carpenter, J. K., Sanford, B. T., Curtiss, J. E., & Ciarrochi, J. (2019). The role of the individual in the coming era of process-based therapy. *Behaviour Research and Therapy, 117,* 40–53. https://doi.org/10.1016/j.brat.2018.10.005

Heu, L. C., van Zomeren, M., & Hansen, N. (2019). Lonely alone or lonely together? A cultural-psychological examination of individualism–collectivism and loneliness in five European countries. *Personality and Social Psychology Bulletin, 45*(5), 780–793. https://doi.org/10.1177/0146167218796793

Hewitt, P. L., & Liew, S. M. (2023). Enhancing group therapy outcomes with measurement-based care: Two case examples. In R. MacNair-Semands &

M. Whittingham (Eds.), *Group psychotherapy assessment and practice: A measurement-based care approach* (pp. 162–187). Routledge.

Hickin, N., Käll, A., Shafran, R., Sutcliffe, S., Manzotti, G., & Langan, D. (2021). The effectiveness of psychological interventions for loneliness: A systematic review and meta-analysis. *Clinical Psychology Review, 88*, Article 102066. https://doi.org/10.1016/j.cpr.2021.102066

Hofmann, S. G., & Hayes, S. C. (2019). The future of intervention science: Process-based therapy. *Clinical Psychological Science, 7*(1), 37–50. https://doi.org/10.1177/2167702618772296

Horevitz, E., Organista, K. C., & Areán, P. A. (2015). Depression treatment uptake in integrated primary care: How a "warm handoff" and other factors affect decision making by Latinos. *Psychiatric Services, 66*(8), 824–830. https://doi.org/10.1176/appi.ps.201400085

Horowitz, L. M. (2004). *Interpersonal foundations of psychopathology*. American Psychological Association. https://doi.org/10.1037/10727-000

Horowitz, L. M., Alden, L. E., Wiggins, J. S., & Pincus, A. L. (2000). *Inventory of Interpersonal Problems*. The Psychological Corporation.

Horowitz, L. M., & Strack, S. (Eds.). (2011). *Handbook of interpersonal psychology: Theory, research, assessment, and therapeutic interventions*. John Wiley & Sons. https://doi.org/10.1002/9781118001868

Horowitz, L. M., Wilson, K. R., Turan, B., Zolotsev, P., Constantino, M. J., & Henderson, L. (2006). How interpersonal motives clarify the meaning of interpersonal behavior: A revised circumplex model. *Personality and Social Psychology Review, 10*(1), 67–86. https://doi.org/10.1207/s15327957pspr1001_4

Horvath, A. O., & Greenberg, L. S. (1989). Development and validation of the Working Alliance Inventory. *Journal of Counseling Psychology, 36*(2), 223–233. https://doi.org/10.1037/0022-0167.36.2.223

Hurt, A. C. (2012). The Punctuated-Tuckman: A conceptual model for the integration of Tuckman, PEM, and systems group development theories. *Leadership & Organizational Management Journal, 2012*(1), 143–152.

Imel, Z. E., & Wampold, B. E. (2008). The importance of treatment and the science of common factors in psychotherapy. In S. D. Brown & R. W. Lent (Eds.), *Handbook of counseling psychology* (pp. 249–266). John Wiley & Sons.

Jackson, D. D. (1981). The question of family homeostasis. *International Journal of Family Therapy, 3*, 5–15. https://doi.org/10.1007/BF00936266

Jacobson, N. S., & Truax, P. (1992). Clinical significance: A statistical approach to defining meaningful change in psychotherapy research. In A. E. Kazdin (Ed.), *Methodological issues and strategies in clinical research* (pp. 631–648). American Psychological Association. https://doi.org/10.1037/10109-042

Jia, Y. (2021). The historical development and related research exploration of focus brief group therapy. *The Frontiers of Society, 3*(3), Article 030301. https://doi.org/10.25236/FSST.2021.030301

The Joint Commission. (n.d.). *Performance measurement*. https://www.jointcommission.org/measurement/

Jonsson, U., Alaie, I., Parling, T., & Arnberg, F. K. (2014). Reporting of harms in randomized controlled trials of psychological interventions for mental and behavioral disorders: A review of current practice. *Contemporary Clinical Trials, 38*(1), 1–8. https://doi.org/10.1016/j.cct.2014.02.005

Jung, C. G. (1968). *The collected works of C. G. Jung: Vol. 9. The archetypes and the collective unconscious* (H. Read, M. Fordham, & G. Adler, Eds., & R. F. C. Hull, Trans.; 2nd ed.). Princeton University Press. (Original work published 1959)

Karatzias, T., Shevlin, M., Hyland, P., Brewin, C. R., Cloitre, M., Bradley, A., Kitchiner, N. J., Jumbe, S., Bisson, J. I., & Roberts, N. P. (2018). The role of negative cognitions, emotion regulation strategies, and attachment style in complex post-traumatic stress disorder: Implications for new and existing therapies. *British Journal of Clinical Psychology, 57*(2), 177–185. https://doi.org/10.1111/bjc.12172

Kassel, J. D., Stroud, L. R., & Paronis, C. A. (2003). Smoking, stress, and negative affect: Correlation, causation, and context across stages of smoking. *Psychological Bulletin, 129*(2), 270–304. https://doi.org/10.1037/0033-2909.129.2.270

Kellermann, P. F. (1996). Interpersonal conflict management in group psychotherapy: An integrative perspective. *Group Analysis, 29*(2), 257–275. https://doi.org/10.1177/0533316496292012

Kiesler, D. J. (1996). *Contemporary interpersonal theory and research: Personality, psychopathology, and psychotherapy.* John Wiley & Sons.

Killgore, W. D. S., Cloonan, S. A., Taylor, E. C., & Dailey, N. S. (2020). Loneliness: A signature mental health concern in the era of COVID-19. *Psychiatry Research, 290*, Article 113117. https://doi.org/10.1016/j.psychres.2020.113117

Kim, H., & Rose, K. M. (2014). Concept analysis of family homeostasis. *Journal of Advanced Nursing, 70*(11), 2450–2468. https://doi.org/10.1111/jan.12496

King, D. D., Fattoracci, E. S. M., Hollingsworth, D. W., Stahr, E., & Nelson, M. (2023). When thriving requires effortful surviving: Delineating manifestations and resource expenditure outcomes of microaggressions for Black employees. *Journal of Applied Psychology, 108*(2), 183–207. https://doi.org/10.1037/apl0001016

Kinner, V. L., Kuchinke, L., Dierolf, A. M., Merz, C. J., Otto, T., & Wolf, O. T. (2017). What our eyes tell us about feelings: Tracking pupillary responses during emotion regulation processes. *Psychophysiology, 54*(4), 508–518. https://doi.org/10.1111/psyp.12816

Kiss, I., Levy-Gigi, E., & Kéri, S. (2011). CD 38 expression, attachment style and habituation of arousal in relation to trust-related oxytocin release. *Biological Psychology, 88*(2–3), 223–226. https://doi.org/10.1016/j.biopsycho.2011.08.005

Kitayama, S., Salvador, C. E., Nanakdewa, K., Rossmaier, A., San Martin, A., & Savani, K. (2022). Varieties of interdependence and the emergence of the Modern West: Toward the globalizing of psychology. *American Psychologist, 77*(9), 991–1006. https://doi.org/10.1037/amp0001073

Kivlighan, D., Whittingham, M., & Tasca, G. (2017, August 3–6). Innovations in group psychotherapy—Integrating theories and targeted treatment. In C. L. Marmarosh (Chair), *The power of us* [Symposium]. American Psychological Association 125th Annual Convention, Washington, DC, United States.

Kivlighan, D. M., III, Ali, R. W., & Garrison, Y. L. (2020). Is there an optimal level of positive and negative feedback in group therapy? A response surface analysis. *Psychotherapy, 57*(2), 174–183. https://doi.org/10.1037/pst0000244

Kivlighan, D. M., III, Aloe, A. M., Adams, M. C., Garrison, Y. L., Obrecht, A., Ho, Y. C. S., Kim, J. Y. C., Hooley, I. W., Chan, L., & Deng, K. (2020). Does the group in group psychotherapy matter? A meta-analysis of the intraclass correlation coefficient in group treatment research. *Journal of Consulting and Clinical Psychology, 88*(4), 322–337. https://doi.org/10.1037/ccp0000474

Kivlighan, D. M., & Angelone, E. O. (1992). Interpersonal problems: Variables influencing participants' perception of group climate. *Journal of Counseling Psychology, 39*(4), 468–472. https://doi.org/10.1037/0022-0167.39.4.468

Kivlighan, D. M., Jr., Gullo, S., Giordano, C., Di Blasi, M., Giannone, F., & Lo Coco, G. (2021). Group as a social microcosm: The reciprocal relationship between intersession intimate behaviors and in-session intimate behaviors. *Journal of Counseling Psychology, 68*(2), 208–218. https://doi.org/10.1037/cou0000495

Kivlighan, D. M., III, Swancy, A. G., Smith, E., & Brennaman, C. (2021). Examining racial microaggressions in group therapy and the buffering role of members' perceptions of their group's multicultural orientation. *Journal of Counseling Psychology, 68*(5), 621–628. https://doi.org/10.1037/cou0000531

Kliman, J. (2010). Intersections of social privilege and marginalization: A visual teaching tool. *Expanding our social justice practices: Advances in theory and training*. American Family Therapy Academy.

Klonsky, E. D., Pachkowski, M. C., Shahnaz, A., & May, A. M. (2021). The three-step theory of suicide: Description, evidence, and some useful points of clarification. *Preventive Medicine, 152*(Pt. 1), Article 106549. https://doi.org/10.1016/j.ypmed.2021.106549

Kobos, J. C. (1993, Summer). Aspects of termination in group psychotherapy. *The Psychotherapy Bulletin, 28*(2), 31–32.

Krogel, J., Burlingame, G., Chapman, C., Renshaw, T., Gleave, R., Beecher, M., & MacNair-Semands, R. (2013). The Group Questionnaire: A clinical and empirically derived measure of group relationship. *Psychotherapy Research, 23*(3), 344–354. https://doi.org/10.1080/10503307.2012.729868

Kross, E., Berman, M. G., Mischel, W., Smith, E. E., & Wager, T. D. (2011). Social rejection shares somatosensory representations with physical pain. *Proceedings of the National Academy of Sciences of the United States of America, 108*(15), 6270–6275. https://doi.org/10.1073/pnas.1102693108

Lambert, M. J. (2013). Outcome in psychotherapy: The past and important advances. *Psychotherapy, 50*(1), 42–51. https://doi.org/10.1037/a0030682

Lambert, M. J., & Harmon, K. L. (2018). The merits of implementing routine outcome monitoring in clinical practice. *Clinical Psychology: Science and Practice, 25*(4), Article e12268. https://doi.org/10.1111/cpsp.12268

Lambert, M. J., Whipple, J. L., & Kleinstäuber, M. (2018). Collecting and delivering progress feedback: A meta-analysis of routine outcome monitoring. *Psychotherapy, 55*(4), 520–537. https://doi.org/10.1037/pst0000167

Leary, T. (1957). *Interpersonal diagnosis of personality*. The Ronald Press Company.

Leavitt, C. E. (2022, November 11). How to combat loneliness with relationships. *Psychology Today*. https://www.psychologytoday.com/us/blog/sexual-mindfulness/202211/how-combat-loneliness-within-relationships

Leising, D., Rehbein, D., & Sporberg, D. (2006). Does a fish see the water in which it swims? A study of the ability to correctly judge one's own interpersonal behavior. *Journal of Social and Clinical Psychology, 25*(9), 963–974. https://doi.org/10.1521/jscp.2006.25.9.963

Levenson, H. (2010). Time-limited dynamic psychotherapy. In L. M. Horowitz & S. Strack (Eds.), *Handbook of interpersonal psychology: Theory, research, assessment, and therapeutic interventions* (pp. 545–563). John Wiley & Sons. https://doi.org/10.1002/9781118001868.ch32

Lewis, C. C., Boyd, M., Puspitasari, A., Navarro, E., Howard, J., Kassab, H., Hoffman, M., Scott, K., Lyon, A., Douglas, S., Simon, G., & Kroenke, K. (2019). Implementing measurement-based care in behavioral health: A review. *JAMA Psychiatry, 76*(3), 324–335. https://doi.org/10.1001/jamapsychiatry.2018.3329

Linehan, M. M., & Wilks, C. R. (2015). The course and evolution of dialectical behavior therapy. *American Journal of Psychotherapy, 69*(2), 97–110. https://doi.org/10.1176/appi.psychotherapy.2015.69.2.97

Livingston, E. M., Siegel, L. S., & Ribary, U. (2018). Developmental dyslexia: Emotional impact and consequences. *Australian Journal of Learning Difficulties, 23*(2), 107–135. https://doi.org/10.1080/19404158.2018.1479975

Locke, B. D., Buzolitz, J. S., Lei, P.-W., Boswell, J. F., McAleavey, A. A., Sevig, T. D., Dowis, J. D., & Hayes, J. A. (2011). Development of the Counseling Center Assessment of Psychological Symptoms-62 (CCAPS-62). *Journal of Counseling Psychology, 58*(1), 97–109. https://doi.org/10.1037/a0021282

Locke, K. D. (2015). Agentic and communal social motives. *Social and Personality Psychology Compass, 9*, 525–538. https://doi.org/10.1111/spc3.12201

Lo Coco, G., Gullo, S., Prestano, C., & Burlingame, G. M. (2015). Current issues on group psychotherapy research: An overview. In O. C. G. Gelo, A. Pritz, & B. Rieken (Eds.), *Psychotherapy research: Foundations, process, and outcome* (pp. 279–292). Springer-Verlag Publishing. https://doi.org/10.1007/978-3-7091-1382-0_14

Lo Coco, G., Gullo, S., Profita, G., Pazzagli, C., Mazzeschi, C., & Kivlighan, D. M., Jr. (2019). The codevelopment of group relationships: The role of individual group member's and other group members' mutual influence and shared group environment. *Journal of Counseling Psychology*, *66*(5), 640–649. https://doi.org/10.1037/cou0000349

Lopez, A. O., Martinez, M. N., Garcia, J. M., Kunik, M. E., & Medina, L. D. (2021). Self-report depression screening measures for older Hispanic/Latin American adults: A PRISMA systematic review. *Journal of Affective Disorders*, *294*, 1–9. https://doi.org/10.1016/j.jad.2021.06.049

Lopez, F. G., & Brennan, K. A. (2000). Dynamic processes underlying adult attachment organization: Toward an attachment theoretical perspective on the healthy and effective self. *Journal of Counseling Psychology*, *47*(3), 283–300. https://doi.org/10.1037/0022-0167.47.3.283

Lorentzen, S., Strauss, B., & Altmann, U. (2018). Process-outcome relationships in short- and long-term psychodynamic group psychotherapy: Results from a randomized clinical trial. *Group Dynamics*, *22*(2), 93–107. https://doi.org/10.1037/gdn0000084

Lutz, P.-E., Courtet, P., & Calati, R. (2020). The opioid system and the social brain: Implications for depression and suicide. *Journal of Neuroscience Research*, *98*(4), 588–600. https://doi.org/10.1002/jnr.24269

MacKenzie, K. R. (1983). The clinical application of group measure. In R. R. Dies & K. R. MacKenzie (Eds.), *Advances in group psychotherapy: Integrating research and practice* (pp. 159–170). International Universities Press.

MacNair-Semands, R., & Whittingham, M. (Eds.). (2023). *Group psychotherapy assessment and practice: A measurement-based care approach*. Routledge.

MacNair-Semands, R. R., & Corazzini, J. (1998). *Manual for the Group Therapy Questionnaire (GTQ)*. Virginia Commonwealth University, Counseling Services, and University of North Carolina at Charlotte, Counseling Center.

MacNair-Semands, R. R., Ogrodniczuk, J. S., & Joyce, A. S. (2010). Structure and initial validation of a short form of the Therapeutic Factors Inventory. *International Journal of Group Psychotherapy*, *60*(2), 245–281. https://doi.org/10.1521/ijgp.2010.60.2.245

Markin, R. D., & Marmarosh, C. (2010). Application of adult attachment theory to group member transference and the group therapy process. *Psychotherapy*, *47*(1), 111–121. https://doi.org/10.1037/a0018840

Marmarosh, C. L. (2015). Emphasizing the complexity of the relationship: The next decade of attachment-based psychotherapy research. *Psychotherapy*, *52*(1), 12–18. https://doi.org/10.1037/a0036504

Marmarosh, C. L. (2017). Attachment in group psychotherapy: Bridging theories, research, and clinical techniques. *International Journal of Group Psychotherapy*, *67*(2), 157–160. https://doi.org/10.1080/00207284.2016.1267573

Marmarosh, C. L. (2021). Ruptures and repairs in group psychotherapy: Introduction to the special issue. *Group Dynamics: Theory, Research, and Practice*, *25*(1), 1–12. https://doi.org/10.1037/gdn0000150

Marmarosh, C. L., Franz, V. A., Koloi, M., Majors, R. C., Rahimi, A. M., Ronquillo, J. G., Somberg, R. J., Swope, J. S., & Zimmer, K. (2006). Therapists' group attachments and their expectations of patients' attitudes about group therapy.

International Journal of Group Psychotherapy, 56(3), 325–338. https://doi.org/10.1521/ijgp.2006.56.3.325

Marmarosh, C. L., Markin, R. D., & Spiegel, E. B. (2013). *Attachment in group psychotherapy*. American Psychological Association. https://doi.org/10.1037/14186-000

Marmarosh, C. L., Whipple, R., Schettler, M., Pinhas, S., Wolf, J., & Sayit, S. (2009). Adult attachment styles and group psychotherapy attitudes. *Group Dynamics, 13*(4), 255–264. https://doi.org/10.1037/a0015957

Martínez-Arias, R., Silva, F., Díaz-Hidalgo, M. T., Ortet, G., & Moro, M. (1999). The structure of Wiggins' interpersonal circumplex: Cross-cultural studies. *European Journal of Psychological Assessment, 15*(3), 196–205. https://doi.org/10.1027/1015-5759.15.3.196

Maslow, A. H. (1971). *Farther reaches of human nature*. Viking.

Matthews, G. A., & Tye, K. M. (2019). Neural mechanisms of social homeostasis. *Annals of the New York Academy of Sciences, 1457*(1), 5–25. https://doi.org/10.1111/nyas.14016

McDiarmid, T. A., Yu, A. J., & Rankin, C. H. (2019). Habituation is more than learning to ignore: Multiple mechanisms serve to facilitate shifts in behavioral strategy. *BioEssays, 41*(9), Article e1900077. https://doi.org/10.1002/bies.201900077

McIvor, O., Napoleon, A., & Dickie, K. M. (2009). Language and culture as protective factors for at-risk communities. *International Journal of Indigenous Health, 5*(1), 6–25. https://doi.org/10.18357/ijih51200912327

Meehan, K. B., Cain, N. M., Roche, M. J., Clarkin, J. F., & De Panfilis, C. (2019). Rejection sensitivity and self-regulation of daily interpersonal events. *Journal of Contemporary Psychotherapy, 49*(4), 223–233. https://doi.org/10.1007/s10879-019-09424-9

Meyer, M. L., Williams, K. D., & Eisenberger, N. I. (2015). Why social pain can live on: Different neural mechanisms are associated with reliving social and physical pain. *PLOS ONE, 10*(6), Article e0128294. https://doi.org/10.1371/journal.pone.0128294

Mikulincer, M. (1995). Attachment style and the mental representation of the self. *Journal of Personality and Social Psychology, 69*(6), 1203–1215. https://doi.org/10.1037/0022-3514.69.6.1203

Mikulincer, M. (1998). Attachment working models and the sense of trust: An exploration of interaction goals and affect regulation. *Journal of Personality and Social Psychology, 74*(5), 1209–1224. https://doi.org/10.1037/0022-3514.74.5.1209

Miles, J. R., Anders, C., Kivlighan, D. M., III, & Belcher Platt, A. A. (2021). Cultural ruptures: Addressing microaggressions in group therapy. *Group Dynamics, 25*(1), 74–88. https://doi.org/10.1037/gdn0000149

Miller, S. D., Duncan, B. L., Brown, J., Sparks, J., & Claud, D. (2003). The Outcome Rating Scale: A preliminary study of the reliability, validity, and feasibility of a brief visual analog measure. *Journal of Brief Therapy, 2*(2), 91–100.

Miller, W. R., & Rollnick, S. (2002). *Motivational interviewing: Preparing people for change* (2nd ed.). Guilford Press.

Moeller, S. K., Lee, E. A., & Robinson, M. D. (2011). You never think about my feelings: Interpersonal dominance as a predictor of emotion decoding accuracy. *Emotion, 11*(4), 816–824. https://doi.org/10.1037/a0022761

Morran, D. K., Stockton, R., Cline, R. J., & Teed, C. (1998). Facilitating feedback exchange in groups: Leader interventions. *Journal for Specialists in Group Work, 23*(3), 257–268. https://doi.org/10.1080/01933929808411399

Morran, D. K., Stockton, R., & Whittingham, M. H. (2004). Effective leader interventions for counseling and psychotherapy groups. In J. L. DeLucia-Waack, D. A. Gerrity, C. R. Kalodner, & M. T. Riva (Eds.), *Handbook of group counseling and psychotherapy* (pp. 91–103). SAGE Publications. https://doi.org/10.4135/9781452229683.n7

Moss, E. (2008). The holding/containment function in supervision groups for group therapists. *International Journal of Group Psychotherapy, 58*(2), 185–201. https://doi.org/10.1521/ijgp.2008.58.2.185

Mushtaq, R., Shoib, S., Shah, T., & Mushtaq, S. (2014). Relationship between loneliness, psychiatric disorders and physical health: A review on the psychological aspects of loneliness. *Journal of Clinical & Diagnostic Research, 8*(9), WE01-WE4. https://doi.org/10.7860/JCDR/2014/10077.4828

Nadal, K. L. Y. (2023). *Dismantling everyday discrimination: Microaggressions toward LGBTQ people* (2nd ed.). American Psychological Association. https://doi.org/10.1037/0000335-000

Nepon, T., Flett, G. L., Hewitt, P. L., & Molnar, D. S. (2011). Perfectionism, negative social feedback, and interpersonal rumination in depression and social anxiety. *Canadian Journal of Behavioural Science, 43*(4), 297–308. https://doi.org/10.1037/a0025032

Nissen-Lie, H. A., Rønnestad, M. H., Høglend, P. A., Havik, O. E., Solbakken, O. A., Stiles, T. C., & Monsen, J. T. (2017). Love yourself as a person, doubt yourself as a therapist? *Clinical Psychology & Psychotherapy, 24*(1), 48–60. https://doi.org/10.1002/cpp.1977

Norcross, J. C., & Wampold, B. E. (2011). What works for whom: Tailoring psychotherapy to the person. *Journal of Clinical Psychology, 67*(2), 127–132. https://doi.org/10.1002/jclp.20764

O'Connor, B. P., & Dyce, J. (1997). Interpersonal rigidity, hostility, and complementarity in musical bands. *Journal of Personality and Social Psychology, 72*(2), 362–372. https://doi.org/10.1037/0022-3514.72.2.362

Ogrodniczuk, J. S., Sivagurunathan, M., Kealy, D., Rice, S. M., Seidler, Z. E., & Oliffe, J. L. (2023). Suicidal ideation among men during COVID-19: Examining the roles of loneliness, thwarted belongingness, and personality impairment. *Scandinavian Journal of Psychology.* Advance online publication. https://doi.org/10.1111/sjop.12904

Owen, J. J., Tao, K., Leach, M. M., & Rodolfa, E. (2011). Clients' perceptions of their psychotherapists' multicultural orientation. *Psychotherapy, 48*(3), 274–282. https://doi.org/10.1037/a0022065

Parcover, J. A., Dunton, E. C., Gehlert, K. M., & Mitchell, S. L. (2006). Getting the most from group counseling in college counseling centers. *Journal for Specialists in Group Work, 31*(1), 37–49. https://doi.org/10.1080/01933920500341671

Pietromonaco, P. R., & Collins, N. L. (2017). Interpersonal mechanisms linking close relationships to health. *American Psychologist, 72*(6), 531–542. https://doi.org/10.1037/amp0000129

Pincus, A. L., & Hopwood, C. J. (2012). A contemporary interpersonal model of personality pathology and personality disorder. In T. A. Widiger (Ed.), *Oxford handbook of personality disorders* (pp. 372–398). Oxford University Press.

Pinner, D. H., & Kivlighan, D. M., III. (2018). The ethical implications and utility of routine outcome monitoring in determining boundaries of competence in practice. *Professional Psychology: Research and Practice, 49*(4), 247–254. https://doi.org/10.1037/pro0000203

Piper, W. E., & Ogrodniczuk, J. S. (2004). Brief group therapy. In J. L. DeLucia-Waack, D. A. Gerrity, C. R. Kalodner, & M. T. Riva (Eds.), *Handbook of group counseling and psychotherapy* (pp. 641–650). SAGE Publications. https://doi.org/10.4135/9781452229683.n46

Porges, S. W. (2007). The polyvagal perspective. *Biological Psychology, 74*(2), 116–143. https://doi.org/10.1016/j.biopsycho.2006.06.009

Porges, S. W., & Dana, D. (2018). *Clinical applications of the polyvagal theory: The emergence of polyvagal-informed therapies.* W. W. Norton & Company.

Quadt, L., Esposito, G., Critchley, H. D., & Garfinkel, S. N. (2020). Brain–body interactions underlying the association of loneliness with mental and physical health. *Neuroscience and Biobehavioral Reviews, 116,* 283–300. https://doi.org/10.1016/j.neubiorev.2020.06.015

Rahmawati, Y., & Taylor, P.C. (2018). "The fish becomes aware of the water in which it swims": Revealing the power of culture in shaping teaching identity. *Culture Studies of Science Education, 13,* 525–537. https://doi.org/10.1007/s11422-016-9801-1

Rholes, W. S., Simpson, J. A., Campbell, L., & Grich, J. (2001). Adult attachment and the transition to parenthood. *Journal of Personality and Social Psychology, 81*(3), 421–435. https://doi.org/10.1037/0022-3514.81.3.421

Ridley, C. R. (2005). *Overcoming unintentional racism in counseling and therapy: A practitioner's guide to intentional intervention* (2nd ed.). SAGE Publications. https://doi.org/10.4135/9781452204468

Robert, G., & Zadra, A. (2014). Thematic and content analysis of idiopathic nightmares and bad dreams. *Sleep, 37*(2), 409–417. https://doi.org/10.5665/sleep.3426

Rodrigo, A. H., Di Domenico, S. I., Wright, L., Page-Gould, E., Fournier, M. A., Ayaz, H., & Ruocco, A. C. (2022). Interpersonal traits and the neural representations of cognitive control in the prefrontal cortex. *Cognitive, Affective, & Behavioral Neuroscience, 22*(5), 1001–1020. https://doi.org/10.3758/s13415-022-00986-1

Rogers, C. R. (1957). The necessary and sufficient conditions of therapeutic personality change. *Journal of Consulting Psychology, 21*(2), 95–103. https://doi.org/10.1037/h0045357

Rotsinger-Stemen, S., & Whittingham, M. (2013, July 31–August 4). *Focused brief group therapy: An effectiveness study* [Poster presentation]. American Psychological Association 121st Annual Convention, Honolulu, HI, United States.

Ruiz, M. A., Pincus, A. L., Borkovec, T. D., Echemendia, R. J., Castonguay, L. G., & Ragusea, S. A. (2004). Validity of the Inventory of Interpersonal Problems for predicting treatment outcome: An investigation with the Pennsylvania Practice Research Network. *Journal of Personality Assessment, 83*(3), 213–222. https://doi.org/10.1207/s15327752jpa8303_05

Rutan, J. S., Stone, W. N., & Shay, J. J. (2014). *Psychodynamic group psychotherapy* (5th ed.). Guilford Press.

Sadler, P., Ethier, N., & Woody, E. (2011). Interpersonal complementarity. In L. M. Horowitz & S. Strack (Eds.), *Handbook of interpersonal psychology: Theory, research, assessment, and therapeutic interventions* (pp. 123–143). John Wiley & Sons.

Safran, J. D., & Muran, J. C. (2006). Has the concept of the therapeutic alliance outlived its usefulness? *Psychotherapy, 43*(3), 286–291. https://doi.org/10.1037/0033-3204.43.3.286

Santos, M. M., Puspitasari, A. J., Nagy, G. A., & Kanter, J. W. (2021). Behavioral activation. In A. Wenzel (Ed.), *Handbook of cognitive behavioral therapy: Overview and approaches* (pp. 235–273). American Psychological Association. https://doi.org/10.1037/0000218-009

Schore, A. N. (2000). Attachment and the regulation of the right brain. *Attachment & Human Development, 2*(1), 23–47. https://doi.org/10.1080/146167300361309

Scott, K., & Lewis, C. C. (2015). Using measurement-based care to enhance any treatment. *Cognitive and Behavioral Practice, 22*(1), 49–59. https://doi.org/10.1016/j.cbpra.2014.01.010

Sedikides, C., & Skowronski, J. J. (2020). In human memory, good can be stronger than bad. *Current Directions in Psychological Science, 29*(1), 86–91. https://doi.org/10.1177/0963721419896363

Seshadri, G. (2019). Homeostasis in family systems theory. In J. L. Lebow, A. L. Chambers, & D. C. Breunlin (Eds.), *Encyclopedia of couple and family therapy* (pp. 1395–1399). Springer. https://doi.org/10.1007/978-3-319-49425-8_267

Set, Z. (2019). Potential regulatory elements between attachment styles and psychopathology: Rejection sensitivity and self-esteem. *Archives of Neuropsychiatry/Nöropsikiatri Arşivi, 56*(3), 205–212.

Sexton, T. L. (2012, August 2–5). *Creativity and structure in functional family therapy* [Conference session abstract]. American Psychological Association 120th Annual Convention, Orlando, FL, United States.

Shafranske, E. P., & Falender, C. A. (2008). Supervision addressing personal factors and countertransference. In C. A. Falender & E. P. Shafranske (Eds.),

Casebook for clinical supervision: A competency-based approach (pp. 97–120). American Psychological Association. https://doi.org/10.1037/11792-005

Shapiro, E. L., & Ginzberg, R. (2002). Parting gifts: Termination rituals in group therapy. *International Journal of Group Psychotherapy, 52*(3), 319–336. https://doi.org/10.1521/ijgp.52.3.319.45507

Shaver, P. R., & Mikulincer, M. (2011). An attachment-theory framework for conceptualizing interpersonal behavior. In L. M. Horowitz & S. Strack (Eds.), *Handbook of interpersonal psychology: Theory, research, assessment, and therapeutic interventions* (pp. 17–35). John Wiley & Sons.

Sheffield, M., Carey, J., Patenaude, W., & Lambert, M. J. (1995). An exploration of the relationship between interpersonal problems and psychological health. *Psychological Reports, 76*(3), 947–956. https://doi.org/10.2466/pr0.1995.76.3.947

Simpson, J. A., Rholes, W. S., & Phillips, D. (1996). Conflict in close relationships: An attachment perspective. *Journal of Personality and Social Psychology, 71*(5), 899–914. https://doi.org/10.1037/0022-3514.71.5.899

Slade, A., & Holmes, J. (2019). Attachment and psychotherapy. *Current Opinion in Psychology, 25*, 152–156. https://doi.org/10.1016/j.copsyc.2018.06.008

Sobon, M., & Whittingham, M. (2013, July 31–August 4). *Assessing change patterns of the overly accommodating subtype within focused brief group therapy* [Poster presentation]. American Psychological Association 121st Annual Convention, Honolulu, HI, United States.

Stein, A. T., Carl, E., Cuijpers, P., Karyotaki, E., & Smits, J. A. J. (2021). Looking beyond depression: A meta-analysis of the effect of behavioral activation on depression, anxiety, and activation. *Psychological Medicine, 51*(9), 1491–1504. https://doi.org/10.1017/S0033291720000239 (Addendum published 2021, *Psychological Medicine, 51*(9), 1505–1506. https://doi.org/10.1017/S0033291720003050)

Steptoe, A. (2023). Loneliness, health and applied psychology. *Applied Psychology. Health and Well-Being, 15*(1), 259–266. https://doi.org/10.1111/aphw.12417

Strupp, H. H. (1993). The Vanderbilt psychotherapy studies: Synopsis. *Journal of Consulting and Clinical Psychology, 61*(3), 431–433. https://doi.org/10.1037/0022-006X.61.3.431

Sullivan, H. S. (1947). *Conceptions of modern psychiatry*. William Alanson White Psychiatric Foundation.

Tasca, G. A., & Maxwell, H. (2021). Attachment and group psychotherapy: Applications to work groups and teams. In C. D. Parks & G. A. Tasca (Eds.), *The psychology of groups: The intersection of social psychology and psychotherapy research* (pp. 149–167). American Psychological Association. https://doi.org/10.1037/0000201-009

Thomas, C., & Persons, J. B. (2013). Sudden gains can occur in psychotherapy even when the pattern of change is gradual. *Clinical Psychology: Science and Practice, 20*(2), 127–142. https://doi.org/10.1111/cpsp.12029

Tuckman, B. W., & Jensen, M. A. C. (2010). Stages of small-group development Revisited1. *Group Facilitation, 10*, 43–48.

Van Denburg, T. F., & Kiesler, D. J. (1993). Transactional escalation in rigidity and intensity of interpersonal behaviour under stress. *British Journal of Medical Psychology, 66*(1), 15–31. https://doi.org/10.1111/j.2044-8341.1993.tb01723.x

Van der Kolk, B. (2014). *The body keeps the score: Brain, mind, and body in the healing of trauma*. Penguin Publishing Group.

Van Houdenhove, E., Gijs, L., T'Sjoen, G., & Enzlin, P. (2014). Asexuality: Few facts, many questions. *Journal of Sex & Marital Therapy, 40*(3), 175–192. https://doi.org/10.1080/0092623X.2012.751073

Vargas, S. M., Huey, S. J., Jr., & Miranda, J. (2020). A critical review of current evidence on multiple types of discrimination and mental health. *American Journal of Orthopsychiatry, 90*(3), 374–390. https://doi.org/10.1037/ort0000441

von der Lippe, A. L., Monsen, J. T., Rønnestad, M. H., & Eilertsen, D. E. (2008). Treatment failure in psychotherapy: The pull of hostility. *Psychotherapy Research, 18*(4), 420–432. https://doi.org/10.1080/10503300701810793

Waldinger, R., & Schulz, M. (2023). *The good life: Lessons from the world's longest scientific study of happiness*. Simon & Schuster.

Wampold, B. E., Baldwin, S. A., Holtforth, M. g., & Imel, Z. E. (2017). What characterizes effective therapists? In L. G. Castonguay & C. E. Hill (Eds.), *How and why are some therapists better than others? Understanding therapist effects* (pp. 37–53). American Psychological Association. https://doi.org/10.1037/0000034-003

Wampold, B. E., & Imel, Z. E. (2015). *The great psychotherapy debate: The evidence for what makes psychotherapy work* (2nd ed.). Routledge. https://doi.org/10.4324/9780203582015

Watanabe, N., & Yamamoto, M. (2015). Neural mechanisms of social dominance. *Frontiers in Neuroscience, 9*, Article 154. https://doi.org/10.3389/fnins.2015.00154

Wei, M., Mallinckrodt, B., Arterberry, B. J., Liu, S., & Wang, K. T. (2021). Latent profile analysis of interpersonal problems: Attachment, basic psychological need frustration, and psychological outcomes. *Journal of Counseling Psychology, 68*(4), 467–488. https://doi.org/10.1037/cou0000551

Weissbourd, R., Batanova, M., Lovison, V., & Torres, E. (n.d.). *Loneliness in America: How the pandemic has deepened an epidemic of loneliness and what we can do about it* [Press release]. Harvard University. https://static1.squarespace.com/static/5b7c56e255b02c683659fe43/t/6021776bdd04957c4557c212/1612805995893/Loneliness+in+America+2021_02_08_FINAL.pdf

Whittingham, M. (2007). *How do power, affiliation and status satisfaction impact the dynamics of conflict within small groups? An analysis of the perceptions of group members* (Publication No. 3252770) [Doctoral dissertation, Indiana University]. ProQuest Dissertations and Theses Global.

Whittingham, M. (2015). Focused brief group therapy: A practice-based evidence approach. In E. S. Neukrug (Ed.), *The SAGE encyclopedia of theory in counseling and psychotherapy* (pp. 419–423). SAGE Publications.

Whittingham, M. (2017). Attachment and interpersonal theory and group therapy: Two sides of the same coin. *International Journal of Group Psychotherapy*, *67*(2), 276–279. https://doi.org/10.1080/00207284.2016.1260463

Whittingham, M. (2021). Change processes of interpersonal functioning in group therapy: Implications for team functioning. In C. D. Parks & G. A. Tasca (Eds.), *The psychology of groups: The intersection of social psychology and psychotherapy research* (pp. 249–265). American Psychological Association. https://doi.org/10.1037/0000201-014

Whittingham, M. (2022, October 20–21). *How interpersonal style predicts trauma pathways* [Workshop presentation]. 18th Annual IDMH [Institute for Disaster Mental Health] Conference, New Paltz, NY, United States.

Whittingham, M., Burlingame, G., & Arnold, R. (2023). Assessment in group therapy: An introduction and overview. In R. MacNair-Semands & M. Whittingham (Eds.), *Group psychotherapy assessment and practice: A measurement-based care approach* (pp. 1–30). Routledge.

Whittingham, M., Lefforge, N. L., & Marmarosh, C. (2021). Group psychotherapy as a specialty: An inconvenient truth. *Psychotherapy*, *74*(2), 60–66. https://doi.org/10.1176/appi.psychotherapy.20200037

Whittingham, M., & Liew, S. M. (2020, March 5–7). *Time-limited process groups based on focused brief group therapy in Singapore: A pilot and feasibility study* [Paper presentation]. 77th Annual American Group Psychotherapy Association Conference [Virtual meeting].

Wike, T., Tomlinson, C. A., Wagaman, A., Matijczak, A., Murphy, J., Watts, K., O'Connor, K., & McDonald, S. (2023). The role of thwarted belongingness on the relationship between microaggressions and mental health for LGBTQ+ emerging adults. *Journal of Youth Studies*, *26*(2), 286–303. https://doi.org/10.1080/13676261.2021.2010687

Wilcox, M. M., Franks, D. N., Taylor, T. O., Monceaux, C. P., & Harris, K. (2020). Who's multiculturally competent? Everybody and nobody: A multimethod examination. *The Counseling Psychologist*, *48*(4), 466–497. https://doi.org/10.1177/0011000020904709

Wright, A. G. C., Pincus, A. L., & Hopwood, C. J. (2023). Contemporary integrative interpersonal theory: Integrating structure, dynamics, temporal scale, and levels of analysis. *Journal of Psychopathology and Clinical Science*, *132*(3), 263–276. https://doi.org/10.1037/abn0000741

Wright, A. G. C., Ringwald, W. R., Hopwood, C. J., & Pincus, A. L. (2022). It's time to replace the personality disorders with the interpersonal disorders. *American Psychologist*, *77*(9), 1085–1099. https://doi.org/10.1037/amp0001087

Wright, A. G. C., & Zimmermann, J. (2019). Applied ambulatory assessment: Integrating idiographic and nomothetic principles of measurement. *Psychological Assessment*, *31*(12), 1467–1480. https://doi.org/10.1037/pas0000685

Wu, L. Z., Roche, M. J., Dowgwillo, E. A., Wang, S., & Pincus, A. L. (2015). A Chinese translation of the Inventory of Interpersonal Problems–Short Circumplex. *Journal of Personality Assessment, 97*(2), 153–162. https://doi.org/10.1080/00223891.2014.971461

Wu, T., Jia, X., Shi, H., Niu, J., Yin, X., Xie, J., & Wang, X. (2021). Prevalence of mental health problems during the COVID-19 pandemic: A systematic review and meta-analysis. *Journal of Affective Disorders, 281*, 91–98. https://doi.org/10.1016/j.jad.2020.11.117

Yalom, I. D. (1966). A study of group therapy dropouts. *Archives of General Psychiatry, 14*(4), 393–414. https://doi.org/10.1001/archpsyc.1966.01730100057008

Yalom, I. D., & Leszcz, M. (2020). *The theory and practice of group psychotherapy* (6th ed.). Basic Books.

Youn, S. J., Castonguay, L. G., Xiao, H., Janis, R., McAleavey, A. A., Lockard, A. J., Locke, B. D., & Hayes, J. A. (2015). The Counseling Center Assessment of Psychological Symptoms (CCAPS): Merging clinical practice, training, and research. *Psychotherapy, 52*(4), 432–441. https://doi.org/10.1037/pst0000029

Yutrzenka, D. A. (2012). *Assessing change in socially inhibited interpersonal subtype through focused brief group therapy* [Doctoral dissertation, Wright State University]. COREScholar. https://corescholar.libraries.wright.edu/etd_all/660

Index

About the Author

Martyn Whittingham, PhD, CGP, FAPA, FAGPA, is a licensed psychologist in Ohio and a consultant with a private practice. He has received national awards for practice and teaching, including the Group Practice Award (with Erin Frick) in 2010 from the Association for Specialists in Group Work and the Excellence in Teaching Group Dynamics Award from the American Psychological Association (APA) in 2021. Dr. Whittingham is a former president of APA Division 49 (Society of Group Psychology and Group Psychotherapy), and formerly chaired the Service Task Force of the American Group Psychotherapy Association (AGPA). He has authored numerous book chapters and journal articles, and he regularly presents on focused brief group therapy throughout the United States, China, United Kingdom, and Singapore. Dr. Whittingham is a Fellow of both the APA and the AGPA. He lives in Cincinnati, where he derives the greatest joy from moments spent with his wife, Felisa, and daughter, Felisa Iris, and their cat, Envelope.